Dash Diet

Easy Recipes and 21 Days Meal Plan to Burn Fat and Jumpstart Your Weight Loss, Lowering Blood Pressure and Improve Your Health

MARTHA MOORE BONICA

Contents

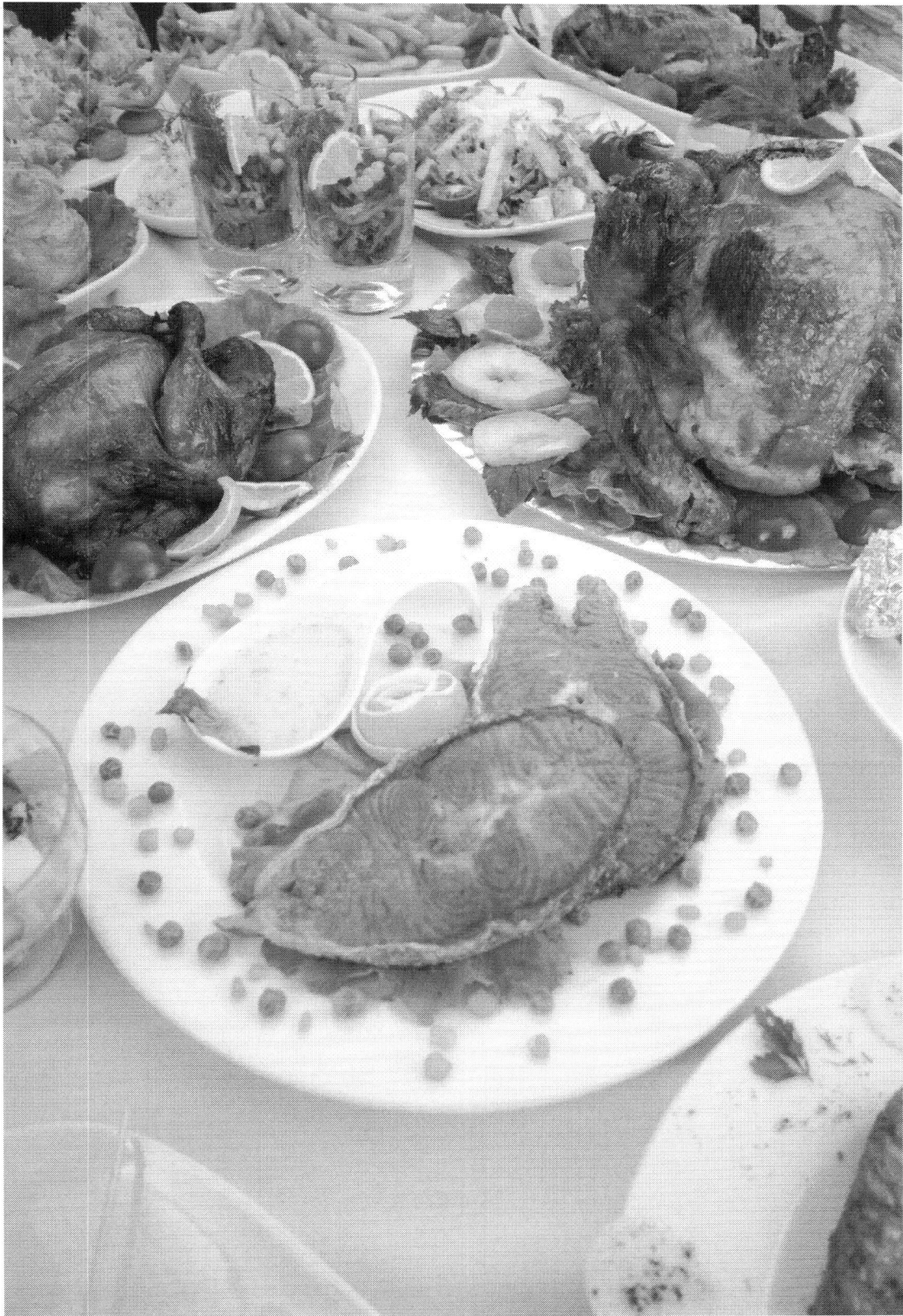

Introduction

The Dash Diet has proven to be one of the healthiest, most effective diets out there that have benefits in a lot of different health-related areas. From cancer to type 2 diabetes, from coronary heart disease to overall immunity enhancement and many more, diet-related problems. Dash diet has the power to prevent and even reverse some of the just mentioned diseases.

The Dash Diet has proven to be one of the healthiest, most effective diets out there that works not only to lower the body's blood pressure but to ensure weight loss, as well. When taking the first steps on a new diet program, however, it can be overwhelming to try and come up with meal ideas and recipes that will keep you in shape and in line with the diet. However, this does not have to be as daunting an experience as you think, which is why this e-book featuring "Dash Diet & 21 Days Dash Diet Meal Plan" is perfect for you. You now have a comprehensive list of delicious, healthy, Dash Diet-friendly meals you can prepare every day for an entire year! This book will allow you to discover all of the benefits of Dash Diet cooking and will even help you to discover some new meals that will quickly become your favorites.

DASH is an acronym for Dietary Approaches to Stop Hypertension, which was the name of the original study. The study organizers wanted to take the best elements of vegetarian diets, which were known to be associated with lower blood pressure, and design a plan that would be flexible enough to appeal to the vast majority of Americans, who are dedicated meat eaters. They developed what they believed was the healthiest omnivore diet plan. And the research has borne out this hope. The DASH diet helps lower blood pressure as well as the first-line medication for hypertension. It also lowers cholesterol. When evaluated over very long periods of time, the DASH eating pattern has been shown to help lower the risk for many diseases and life-threatening medical conditions or events, including stroke, heart attack, heart failure, type 2 diabetes, kidney disease, kidney stones, and some types of cancer. Not only is DASH recommended for people who have these conditions or are at risk for them, but it is recommended for everyone in the Dietary Guidelines for Americans. And the DASH diet is fabulous for weight loss, since it is loaded with bulky, filling fruits and vegetables and has plenty of protein to provide satiety.

Unfortunately, most people who are reading this book haven't noticed any major health problems as of yet, and their main concern is their current shape and how to make it better in a specific period of time. Fortunately for you, you will lose weight fast and naturally while following the Dash diet approach we represent in this book.

While still speaking about a perfect shape, it is also worth mentioning you will also be able to build lean mass and achieve any other fitness-oriented goal you want.

Along with meal plan, you will discover a huge variety of over 100 delicious Dash Diet recipes that will make you excited every time you cook or make your meal prep for the next days. Breakfast, lunch, dinner, various healthy snacks, and side-dishes will definitely satisfy your taste. And even if you have no previous cooking experience, this book also has recipes with less than 5 ingredients to start.

So don't wait, start your new healthy lifestyle right now!

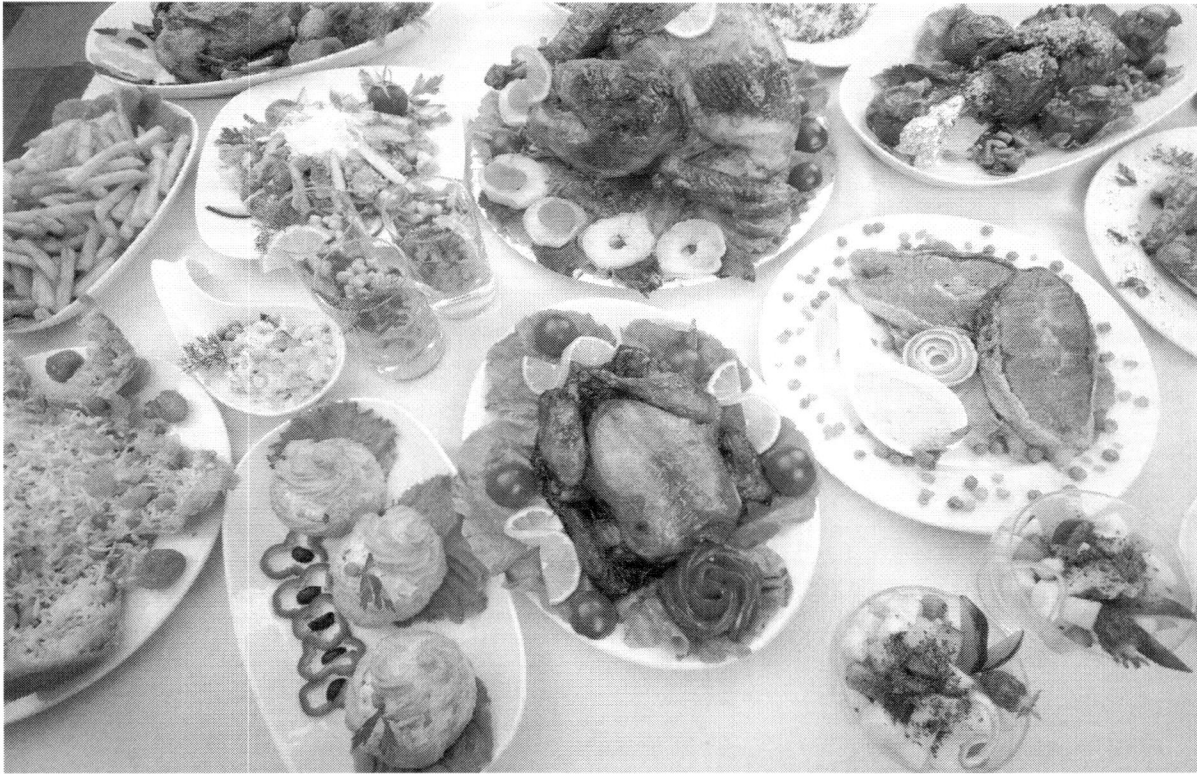

The Dash Diet

CHAPTER ONE

The Psychology of Diet Preparation

Since we have numerous reasons, we resolve to lose weight: we don't like how we look, our clothes don't match, our wellbeing is in danger, the others are wandering, and our work is in danger, or our children are humiliated. We generally think about weight loss as something that only includes our body; definitely, no one has ever wanted to lose weight due to a fat brain or a bloated intellect.

But "we decide" is a function of the mind. It depends on our minds and not on our bodies when and why we take such a decision. We will decide whether we are five pounds heavier than we want, or after two hundred pounds and real medical obesity has passed. The actual body size does not cause the option of losing weight, as this is achieved in the brain.

Since the start (and follow-up) of a dietary program is a mental operation, it seems worth exploring what factors such decisions might cause.

1. Self-Image.

- one of us has a dual picture: our face to the world and our inner idea of how we look. Although we dress and groom to be seen by others as desirable, we are far less affected by others than by our satisfaction or disappointment with us.

Explore this idea by looking at yourself and others over the next week. You will find you are always complimented on the clothes you wear that you don't feel right. Wear a favorite costume perfectly suited, that you think looks amazing and that makes you particularly feel stirring - and nobody notices! The same thing happens with a hairstyle. One morning, you can't get your hair to do something, hurried for time, so you can pull it back with clips with frustration, and hope no one important is looking so bad. That's it! Three people say they like what you did with your hair.

When it comes to our weight, there is the same disconnect. When we look good in our eyes, we don't feel overweight, even though friends and colleagues gossip about our steady increase in weight. However, if we feel overweight, no reassurance from those around us will make us feel less fat. This mental image of our body size, taken to the extreme, can lead to anorexia Nervosa in eating disorders where excessively thin individuals keep their caloric intake dangerously reduced because they constantly feel too large.

We then decide to take a diet in response to our internal self-image. Some of the advantages that we expect are lean and fit take into account others: I'll be more attractive to the opposite sex; I will be noted when it comes to promotion at work; my family and friends will be jealous and have to reassess me as a stronger person than they thought. But what it does for us individually is the true incentive for getting in shape. It is the need to feel better about ourselves, which leads us to diet and exercise through pain and Monotony. It is the vision of us in the future that leads us to our target. Losing this hope or concluding, we won't feel that much better about ourselves are the reasons we give up and slip into the relative convenience of "okay." settling.

2. Body versus Mind dominance.

We all fight for a lifelong inner struggle between our mind and body. Each stage of development is dominant. As kids, we are just a series of sensations. We discover the exciting new world around us by touching everything within reach, sampling everything we can put in our mouths, looking around at the gestures and all the sounds we hear, until finally, we learn to mimic them.

When we step into our early years of education, we begin to reflect on our minds. We eat vast quantities of knowledge voraciously. We learn to read, and our planet extends its borders by 1000 percent. We learn to use the internet, and we have an infinite world at hand.

Then we pass into puberty, and our beauty becomes the primary factor of daily life overnight. We sail through the pitfalls and joys of adolescence, where success and coolness are much more important than learning or mental growth. We spend a very long time on our bodies. We're trying new clothing, new hairstyles, and new maquillage. We have pierced body parts and are exposed to tattoo discomfort because it would make us stand out. We primp, groom, and push ourselves into the models that have been judged by our peers as in."

When we mature, we aspire to reconcile our physical and mental selves. While our corps is supreme in the world of attracting one, we need to practice our minds to advance our careers and establish deep relationships that go far beyond physical attraction.

When we settle down and start creating the good life we want, our energies and efforts turn to things outside of us: children, significant others, friends, family, and jobs. We have so much going on around us that we lose contact with our bodies and minds. We fall into our own comfort zone where food meets so much of our needs. It eases our tension, alleviates our daily tensions, and makes constant blues endurable. It eats away our social connections. It becomes a crucial part of how we express love for those we love. We always see ourselves as we once were and ignore the love handles and pockets of fat that we strongly overlook parts of our body. Our bodies and our inner image of our bodies are becoming increasingly discordant.

3. Our sense of self-efficacy.

Self-efficacy is a psychological concept to describe the perception of a person that any action they take influences the outcome. It is neither self-confidence nor the assumption that you are capable of doing something, although it can include both. It represents our inner hope that what we do will bring about our desired results.

If we begin a diet, want to shape, or begin to take better care of ourselves is essentially a personal choice that may or may not is made as we have expected. The difference lies in the assumption of success, and it's always easier to go on a path that we expect to be successful than to travel to a target where disappointment is the most likely result.

How do we incorporate these principles to make us lean, healthy, and attractive?

We start by looking at our self-image and how we appear to others. Only telling someone Do you think I'm getting too heavy?" does not work unless you have a brutally frank friend or ask somebody who you don't like. Most of us are culturally trained to save the feelings of others so that the answers to such a question are more respectful than real.

Specific focusing can provide better feedback. Tell others that you have a survey for a class you take. Offer a short one-page questionnaire that allows any friend or colleague to list three adjectives that identify various aspects of your physical appearance. Complete yourself one of the sheets. Make sure the responses are confidential by demanding that no names be used and that someone else gathers the sheets completed.

Once the answers are available, compare them to your own answers and see where the descriptions are different. You might find yourself a little defensive. It's not an exercise to make you feel bad about yourself or to gloat about the unexpected compliments. It is an orchestrated endeavor to help you assess the distance between your self-image and your image in the world. Those areas of divergence are a starting point to overlap the two photos.

After defining areas of work, it is time to draw on the unmistakable power of our wonderful mind to start imposing the structure and organization, which we will have to introduce the desired changes. Our mind can only take us where we want to go if it is supported by confidence in our ability to achieve success. Now is the time to reject any failure expectations. Many failed diet and exercise attempts have been made in the past. Leave the past. Leave the past. We are not destined to continue unproductive behavior. We have the gem of a creation, the human mind, able to do almost everything. If we concentrate on any mission, it will succeed if our concerns and doubts do not interfere.

By exploring our memories, we draw on our optimistic aspirations to build up a long list of past achievements. There can be big benchmarks such as endorsing a campaign we liked, planning a great event, or establishing an intense relationship with ourselves. The smallest personal victories are, however, the most important but are generally easily overlooked or dismissed.

Studies and a strong degree in a challenging class show clearly the ability to produce the results you want. Go for quantity: the day you grinned over someone in a smoky room and finished with a short but beautiful affair; the timing study that no-one expected; the night you spin on ice skates. Continue: make the drill squad, shoot a stolen basket, make your own promotional outfit, dying in a wonderful color in your own bathroom, catch a ball, find new apps on your machine and burn your first CD. The list can be infinite and will linger while you recall snippets of the past that you have been burying for a long time.

Hold this list close and read it on a regular basis. It's your self-effective pep band.

You now know the fields in which you can operate and trust the success of your efforts. You must now identify the internal benefits that good weight loss brings. Feel strong, enjoy step-by-step, and quickly zipping your clothes are quick starters. Unconsciously heading to the pool in a short suit is a fantasy enhancing. Making a sales success with the belief that you look best is a picture you will appreciate as you fall asleep. Having someone you like admires or seeing your rivals, jealously emphasizes your determination and maintains the inconvenience of dieting and the demands of repetitive workout routines.

You know where you are going, you know what it will take, and you know that you will succeed. Your mind is set, just waiting for your decision day. Whenever you choose, you will make a choice because you are now under power.

What is Dash Diet Eating Plan?

The dietary eating plan DASH (Dietary Methods to Stop Hypertension) is one of the non-pharmacological therapies for controlling blood pressure. This involves dietary improvements, which include: low consumption of saturated fat, increased fruit and vegetable intakes, more replaced carbohydrate-containing foods, such as whole-grain products, increased seafood, poultry, and nuts intake. The study has shown that the nutritional plan for DASH has the highest effect on blood pressure and cholesterol reduction compared to normal diets. The result is evident within two weeks!

Downward Calory Tips Intake With DASH Eating Schedule!

1. Increase fruit

An apple holds the doctor away for one day! In the food plan for high blood pressure patients, apple and dried apricots are the best options.

2. Growth of vegetables

Burger! Yes, your blood pressure may increase, even if it's a favorite food for most people. I know it's really difficult for you to avoid eating it. However, I recommend that you weigh 3 ounces of meat rather than 6 ounces in the larger size.

The same goes for limiting chicken consumption by just 2 ounces and with a plate of raw vegetables.

3. Enhance fat-free or fat-free dairy products

For example, common ice cream can be replaced with low-fat yogurt.

Reducing Salts and Sodium

By ingesting more fruit and vegetables in the DASH food plan, the lower amount of sodium has made it possible to consume less salt and sodium. Furthermore, fruit and vegetables are rich in potassium and play a part in lowering high blood pressure. Milk products and fish are other important dietary sources.

Tips for Salt and Sodium Reduction

Restrict food high in salt. It is safer to eat no or low-salt foods.

Increased vegetable consumption.

No salted rice, pasta, or other mixed foods

Remove extra salt from preserved foods, such as tuna or beans preserved in a can.

Dash Diet Eating Plan

What is the food for DASH? The DASH diet literally means nutritional methods to avoid high blood pressure. In the early stages of high blood pressure, people are frequently put on this diet to help regulate blood pressure.

The plan is focused on 2,000 calories a day but can be changed to suit your nutritional needs. The American Heart Association recommends this diet highly because it helps to achieve excellent health in many other ways than hypertension. The most significant ingredients to naturally support hypertension are foods high in potassium, foods with calcium and magnesium.

First of all, the DASH strategy assigns great importance to crops. It is good to add whole wheat pieces of bread, wheat pastes, and whole-grain cereals with 7-8 portions per day as a daily allowance on this schedule. Your whole grain has far more nutritional qualities than those that have more refined sugars.

The DASH diet plan also encourages fruit and vegetables. You must eat four to five portions of this category every day. As you review the DASH diet guide, the author tells you several ways to include your regular servings of fruits and vegetables.

Next to this plan are non-fat and low-fat dairy products. You will have to select skim milk, or at most 1 percent, low fat or unfat cheeses and yogurts.

You have lean meat options after milk. There are small portion sizes, indicating no more than two parts. Healthy options include low-fat frankfurters, skinless chicken, and other meat.

When you come to the section where nuts and seeds are listed, they are permitted but are restricted to only five small portions a week. This included legumes as well.

The plan book on the DASH diet is complete. Since you need the plan to fit your everyday calories, it will show you how. This book will also teach you about healthy ways to eat. Eating out is a real challenge in a diet, but the DASH diet book shows you how.

The strategy contains a portion of the book on workouts and alcoholic drinks as well as ways to help you get out of smoking habits.

Additional medical issues with insulin resistance, cholesterol, and inflammation tend to be beneficial. If you have some of these other medical conditions than hypertension, you should like this meal plan very much.

What You Need To Know About The DASH Diet

Our foods will affect our overall health. A diet rich in unhealthy components such as saturated fats and cholesterol is a healthy way to achieve high blood pressure and other diseases. On the other hand, the right food option will reduce the risk of contracting these diseases.

There is a specific eating plan which has demonstrated lower blood pressure or hypertension. This diet is known as DASH or Nutritional Stop Hypertension Approaches.

The DASH diet was a product of clinical trials performed by scientists from the NHLBI. Researchers have found that a diet that is high in potassium, magnesium, calcium, protein, and fibre and low in fat and cholesterol can reduce high blood pressure significantly.

The study showed that even a diet rich in fruits, vegetables, and low-fat milk products has a major influence on hypertension reduction. It also showed that the DASH diet results easily, often in just two weeks from the beginning of the diet.

Three essential nutrients are also stressed by the DASH diet: magnesium, calcium, and potassium. These minerals are intended to minimize hypertension. A standard 2000-calorie diet includes 500 mg of magnesium, 4,7 g of potassium, and 1,2 g of calcium.

Doing the DASH Diet

It is very easy to follow the DASH diet and takes a little time to pick and prepare meals. Foods high in cholesterol and fats are stopped. Dieters should eat as much as possible of vegetables, fruits, and cereals.

Because the foods you consume in a DASH diet are high in fiber content, you can slowly increase your fiber-rich food intake to help prevent diarrhea and other digestive problems. By consuming an additional portion of fruit and vegetables with every meal, you will steadily increase your fiber intake.

Grains are also healthy sources of fiber and vitamins, and minerals of the B-complex. Whole grains, whole wheat bread, bran, wheat germs, and low-fat cereal are all grain items that you can consume to improve your intake of fiber.

You can select the food you consume by looking at processed and packaged food product labels. Check for low-fat, saturated fat, sodium, and cholesterol foods. The main source of fat and cholesterol is meat, chocolates, chips, and fast snacks, so you can limit your intake of such products.

If you wish to eat meat, limit your meal to just six ounces a day, which is close in size to a card deck. In your meat dishes, you should eat more fruits, cereals, pasta, and beans. Often a large protein source without excess fat and cholesterol is low-fat milk or skim milk.

You can taste both canned or dried fruit and fresh fruit for snacks. Snack choices are also available to those on the DASH diet, including graham crackers, unsalted nuts, and fatty yogurt.

It's Easy to DASH

It is popular with many health buffs, as no special meals and recipes are required. There are no special preparations and calorie counting as long as you eat more fruits and vegetables and reduce the consumption of foods high in fat and cholesterol. The DASH diet is the balanced diet that focuses more on the three main minerals, which are expected to have a beneficial impact on high blood pressure.

The DASH diet is perfect for people who enjoy eating comfort and convenience. The DASH diet provides tried and tested dietary systems for people who aim for good health with empirical evidence to support them.

CHAPTER TWO
5 Benefits of a DASH Diet - Proven to Lower Your Blood Pressure

Tracking your diet is a good way of life, and it helps you to check your medical condition. Many common dietary regimes can be practiced, and the DASH diet is one of them.

 DASH has been shown to reduce blood pressure levels.> It was created for hypertensive people by adopting a soft or salty food plan with minimum saturated fats and cholesterol. It is not meant for those who want to lose weight, but it is also possible to do certain workouts by decreasing calorie intake.

DASH has five advantages to deliver if strictly observed. The first is to decrease body weight, saturated fat, and cholesterol. This will avoid a heart attack, stroke, and other cardiovascular diseases.

Secondly, the increased consumption of lycopene, beta-carotene, and phytochemicals in the body is also increased by fruits, vegetables, and low-fat milk products. Phytochemicals help protect the body against cardiac cancer and disease in plants.

Third, the consumption of fiber is increased by the inclusion of whole grain items in the plan. Fiber helps to absorb food and to reduce cholesterol levels.

Fourthly, sodium decreases in one's diet to a maximum of 1.500 mg per day can be an effective hypertension treatment. The less salt ingestion, the lower the blood pressure. The risk of atherosclerosis and congestive cardiac insufficiency is thus decreased.

Fifthly, high sugar candy and drinks are avoided. This helps to reduce the consumption of calories and preserves the body's sugar balance.

In short, DASH's diet includes minerals such as magnesium, potassium, calcium, and protein. It not only decreases sodium and cholesterol in the body but also provides the main body nutrients required.

The DASH Diet: Does It Work?

Maybe you learned of the Hypertension DASH Diet.

Well, it is now one of the most well-known diet plans in the world and can be more than a trend. Built by the National Institutes of Health of the Department of Health and Human Services, this diet program is focused on nutritional facts.

DASH is an acronym for Dietary Approaches to Hypertension Stop, which essentially shows how the food you consume will reduce your blood pressure. The premise of the diet is to instruct men and women with high blood pressure and high blood pressure on how to eat much better and minimize blood pressure and connected diseases. High blood pressure is also an issue that can potentially be prevented with a safe way of living, but it can only be handled if a person has it.

Elevated blood pressure is serious and can also lead to coronary artery disease, dementia, stroke, and finally, cardiac failure. Figure that about 33% of men and women actually have high blood pressure or high blood pressure. It is one-third of the adult population, so it is possible that you or someone you know will be diagnosed as having the disease.

The DASH Hypertension Diet will help you to reduce your blood pressure and risk of affiliated diseases by laying down a few guidelines. For example, one of the key guidelines set out in the weight loss plan is to cut the intake of sodium to between 2.300 and 1.500 mg per day. This can look like you still get a lot of sodium, but not so much, in fact.

Consider some of the things that you might eat every day...

Did you know that a fourth pound of cheese contains around 1,190 milligrams of sodium? This is practically the whole daily allowance if you restrict yourself to 1,500 mg a day. Even at 2,300 a day, the proposed daily portion is still over 50 percent.

And if you believe you will be mindful of your health and receive salad, be warned... Condiments and dressings have become infamous for large sodium levels.

So, what are you going to get into the DASH Diet?

A lot of fruit and vegetables per day instead of sweets and desserts

Foods rich in fiber as an alternative to processed carbs

Low fat and fat-free milk products, not whole milk products

Water and soda club in relation to sugar soft drinks

The DASH Diet is not only a nutritional agenda; it also advises on safe lifestyles:

Join a workout, whether the blood pressure level is typical or not.

Try in doing at least 30 minutes of exercise every day.

Determine your own weight loss goals

If you take high blood pressure prescription medications, do not forget to take them every day.

It's no wonder with such common-sense recommendations that the DASH Diet is at present gaining such popularity. This is a meaningful diet that gives you the ability to lose weight and stay healthy. And people with healthy blood pressure will generally benefit from a DASH diet and adhere to a high fiber, low-fat, reduced-sodium diet. If you adopt this diet, you can not only shed pounds, and it can potentially save your lives.

The Best Diabetes Diet - The DASH Diet

Over time a large number of diabetes diets have been developed; that is to say, diets developed to enhance diabetes control have developed, have a heyday and sunny retirement. However, many remain strong and as successful as they were initially introduced. But how effective these diets are, exactly.

With the list seemingly rising by the year, a frustrated public sometimes wonders where to start. I, therefore, wanted to review the most common diets on the market at the moment, and at the conclusion of this review, two diets were established as excellent performers to support people with diabetes. One of them is the diet of DASH. The following is a short description of what I heard about this diet. But before we get into it, you might want to ask, what is a healthy diabetic diet exactly? Therefore the following are only some of these elements.

It is low in carbohydrates or at least provides a way to even out the carbohydrate during the day or to "burning" excess, as in the case of exercise.

It should be rich in dietary fiber and has demonstrated several health benefits, such as a low glycemic index and a decrease in probabilities of heart disease, etc.

Low salt. Salt low. Salt can lead to high blood pressure, so it is important to reduce it.

Low in fat. Low in fat. Since foods or fat easily converted to fat like sugar can lead to overweight of the person – a risk factor for diabetes, such foods often need low-fat content.

A healthy diabetic diet should aim to achieve the recommended daily potassium allowance. Potassium is important because it could help to reverse the adverse effects of salt on the circulatory system.

Obviously, the DASH diet has all these features and more. Yet just what the DASH diet is and how it happened. Well, the DASH Diet was created in 1992, which means nutritional methods to avoid hypertension. Under the aegis of the United States. The National Heart, Lung and Blood Institute, National Institute of Health (NIS), and five of the best-respected health centers in the United States have collaborated to study the impact of diet on blood pressure. As a result of this study, the DASH diet, the best diet for balanced blood pressure, was formulated.

But this is not as far as its advantages are concerned. The diet was also found to be as good as a diabetes diet. In reality, in the 35 diets analyzed by US News and the World report earlier this year, the Biggest Loser Diet was the best diet for diabetes. In addition to the guidance given by the American Diabetes Association, both the prevention and control qualities of diabetes were shown.

Prevention has proven that it helps people lose weight and even holds them away. As overweight is a significant risk factor for developing type 2 diabetes, it is a diabetes dietary preference.

Furthermore, a combination of the DASH diet and calorie restrictions reduces the risk factors associated with metabolic syndrome, which raises the likelihood of developing diabetes. Regarding regulation, the findings of a small study published in the 2011 edition of Diabetes Care showed that DASH type 2 diabetics had decreased A1C levels and their fasting blood sugar for eight weeks.

Moreover, the diet was found to be more versatile than most, which makes it easier to follow and adapt to encourage the patient to follow a doctor's dietary advice.

Another advantage of this diet is its compliance with dietary guidelines. Bright, as it might seem, this is actually very important since certain diets limit certain foods, leaving the person in certain nutrients and minerals potentially deficient.

A summary of this conformity reveals that the fat diet is satisfyingly below the 20 to 35% of the government-recommended daily calories. It also reaches the 10% overall saturated fat threshold, which falls just below that. The recommended amount of proteins and carbohydrates is also met.

For salt, the guideline has meal limits for this mineral. Both the recommended daily maximum of 2,300 mg and the AU maximum of 1,500 mg if you are 51 years of age or older or have hypertension, diabetes, or chronic kidney disease.

This diet also properly takes care of other nutrients. This diet offers a strong supply of the recommended daily intake of 22 to 34 grams of fiber for adults. Even potassium, a nutrient characterized by its ability to prevent salts, raises blood pressure, decreases the risk of developing renal stones, and also reduces bone loss. Impressively because of the difficulty in getting the recommended daily intake of 4,700 mg or 11 bananas a day.

The minimum daily intake of vitamin D is penciled at 15 mg for adults who are not getting enough sunlight. Although the diet is just shy of this, it is proposed that vitamin D fortified cereal can easily be made up of.

Calcium is also properly treated by the diet for healthy bones and teeth, blood vessel development, and muscle function. The guideline of the government between 1,000 mg and 1300 mg can easily be met without any air or grace. The same applies to vitamin B-12. The recommendation of the government is 2.4 mg. The supply of diets is 6.7.

From the above, it can be seen that the DASH diet is an excellent option in choosing a diet that will help you control your diabetes. While it is the second-largest loser in this diet, it has the advantage of being specially formulated to help lower blood pressure and is equally effective in this regard. So the DASH diet is highly recommended if you are searching for a great diabetes diet.

Type 2 Diabetes - The DASH Diet and Gestational Diabetes

Much as one health issue sometimes leads to another, improvements in a healthier lifestyle can often fix more than one health problem. The British Journal of Nutrition published a study on dietary approaches to avoid hypertension in gestational diabetes in November 2012.

Researchers have studied 34 female gestational diabetes diagnosed at 24 to 28 weeks of pregnancy. Seventeen women remained in daily diets of 45% to 55% carbohydrates, 15% to 20% protein, and 25% to 30% total fat, and 17 others with the DASH diet.

This diet has been similar to normal diets but has increased fruit, vegetables, whole grains, and fatty milk products and less cholesterol, saturated fat, salt, and refined grains.

After four weeks, the women showed on the DASH diet:

- •lower blood pressure
- •lowered HbA1c levels
- Improved blood sugar levels

That at the start of the analysis. The cholesterol in these women was also lower than in the normal diet.

The DASH diet has inferred from these findings that the tolerance to sugar and blood cholesterol of women with gestational diabetes is beneficial in comparison with the normal diet.

The DASH diet was intended to regulate high blood pressure by having a lifelong diet that is low in sodium chloride or table salt. Vegan diets have proven to be the best kind for diabetes, but people with diabetes will consume most of the DASH diet prescribed.

- 4 to 5 portions of fruit are recommended per day, either for desserts or between meals. Leave on the peels to provide fiber, vitamins, and texture whenever possible.
- 4 to 5 portions of vegetables on this diet are also recommended.
- Also recommended are 6 to 8 parts of whole grains.
- Tofu plates can be supplemented with 6-8 servings of DASH meat.
- We also suggest 4 to 5 portions of nuts and beans a week.
- 2 to 3 portions of oil are in the diet, with the best types of liquid oils like olive, soy, or canola.
- 5 or fewer sweet portions are recommended.

The DASH diet advises that men and women can restrict alcoholic drinks to 1 or 2 daily. Caffeine is non-commitment, but many doctors agree that caffeine is not a good option during pregnancy.

Both hypertension and gestational diabetes are conditions that can be stopped during pregnancy. Isn't it nice to help keep both health issues away from a balanced diet?

Type 2 diabetes is just not a disease with which you have to deal with. It doesn't have to get worse slowly and eventually. You can control the disease: start with a healthy diet and recover your health.

CHAPTER THREE
Dash into the DASH Diet to Solve Hypertension
What's the diet of DASH? DASH stands for Dietary Stop Hypertension Approaches. It is a common word used by doctors in the United States. It basically requires a diet composed of

nutrients that have shown lower blood pressure or hypertension. The DASH diet also needs a reduction in calories, which is well-known for leading to high blood pressure.

The DASH diet is by no means specified and, therefore, narrowly applied. However, the DASH diet recommendations have shown that hypertension patients will lower their blood pressure in a matter of weeks, which has significantly increased for six months after DASH. This dramatic change has led to increased and consistent use by doctors in the country of the DASH diet.

The DASH diet components are very basic and easy to follow. Fruits, fruits, legumes, seeds, and nuts are the primary contributors to reducing blood pressure. Good cholesterol, fiber, and negative calories are all good elements of a healthy balanced diet. Olive oil is also promoted and has demonstrated lower blood pressure through studies of olive oil consumption in Mediterranean countries and their citizens on a daily basis.

The low-fat foods are another healthy improvement that the DASH diet adds to the average American diet. The DASH diet, for example, recommends milk products with low-fat content and lean meat, such as poultry and fish. Some fish now contain more fat than others, so you must balance the consumption between them. Furthermore, the fattier fish are actually, on average, more expensive! Finally, it is critical that you take several products for whole grains every day. Breakfast oatmeal is a common alternative, along with granola bars and intermeal snacks.

The key step in the DASH diet is to eliminate food that lead to high blood pressure. Hypertension is primarily caused by inactivity, excess alcohol, excess sodium, excess weight of the body, and poor potassium, magnesium, and calcium. DASH diet items, as you also have heard, are also foods recommended for the reduction of weight diets. It is because most people with hypertension are typically overweight that these items are included in the DASH diets and in the diet of weight loss. Most doctors announce that the most effective treatment for hypertension is weight loss.

The Vegan diet is one of the nearest diets you can equate to the DASH diet. I recently wrote a paper entitled "Make the Vegetarian Diet Work For You," which describes the health benefits and uses of vegans. Many of the foods that you see recommended in the DASH diet are also foods that are part of the Vegan diet, which explains the very rare diagnosis of hypertension in Vegan.

Proper DASH diet data is available from your doctor and from other online food outlets. I would certainly recommend that you study DASH dietary foods and start preparing your regular diet immediately. The health benefits you see with lower blood pressure are important for health and well-being in the short term, but they are crucial in the longer term. The DASH diet allows you to prolong your life due to the failure of your cardiovascular system to function at a higher pressure than is intended for years. You can also receive food tips and detailed information on my website. My free membership wellness platform focuses both on dietary and fitness aspects so that people of all ages and types can contribute to a healthier lifestyle.

Dash Diet to Control Hypertension - Is it Possible?

Dash diet or dietary approaches to stop high blood pressure is a diet that restricts sodium intake. The diet supports full-grain, fruit and vegetables, fish and poultry, and snack nuts. Red meat and sweets intake is a full tabou if you adopt the dash diet correctly. The diet is also rich in magnesium, calcium, carbohydrate, magnesium, and potassium, essential for good health. The dash diet focuses primarily on maintaining your blood pressure below 120/80 mmHg.

While the dash diet is not a vegetarian diet, it advocates fruit consumption of vegetables, nutrients, and beans rather than meats. In this diet, converted foods and junk foods are not promoted at all. There are safe alternative snacks to fill this empty void by satisfying the sweet tooth. "The Guide to Lowering the Blood Pressure with Dash" shows details of diet and also lists how to get the foods you need to start. The guide also offers advice on the quantities and substitute foods to be eaten during your diet.

The diet has demonstrated a 6 mm Hg decrease in systolic blood pressure. Diastolic blood pressure of 3 mm Hg also has been shown to decrease in diets with normal blood pressure. Hypertension has also been known to decrease with diet from 11 to 6. The use of the diet in time is often believed to reduce the risk of strokes and heart disease. Therefore, the best use of the dash diet not only lowers blood pressure as well as other hypertension problems but also offers catering value beyond what anyone ever expected. In doing this, the diet also requires you to eat between 1699 and 3100 dietary calories every day!

When considering the dash diet, the calorie intake and consumption control balance are very poor. But since this diet is high in fiber, some people may feel diarrhea and flutter. To overcome this, the amount of fruit, vegetables, and whole-grain consumed can only be increased. It is important to note that excessive fiber could also cause constipation if you do not take enough water. Follow these two basic instructions, and you will successively benefit from the limitless benefits of the dash diet.

How to Lower Your High Blood Pressure and Lose Your Weight Using DASH Diet?
Recent studies show that the DASH Diet Plan and a reduced intake of salt (sodium) can reduce high blood pressure. The DASH diet also has other advantages, such as lowering LDL (bad cholesterol, which can reduce your risk for heart disease along with lowered blood pressure. However, the combination of the eating plan and a reduction in sodium intake, each method itself reduces blood pressure and prevents the development of high blood pressure.

The DASH Diet Plan is as follows:

1- Low in cholesterol, saturated fat, and total fat.
2- Rich in fat-free vegetables and fruit, low-fat in milk product.
3- Whole grain products, poultry, fish, and nuts included.

4- 4 - Poor in lean red meat, candy, added sugar, and drinks that contain sugar in contrast to the traditional US diet.

Rich in magnesium, potassium, protein calcium, and fiber (blood pressure nutrients).

Daily DASH Nutrient Goals (2.100 Calorie Plan):

- Total fat: 27% calories
- Protein: 18% calories -
- Saturated fat: 6% calories
- 150 mg of cholesterol.
- Carbohydrate: 55% calories

- Soy: 2,300 mg. Diät provides 2,300 and 1,500 milligrams of sodium daily intake per day. The highest amount appropriate to the National High Blood Pressure Education Program is 2,300 milligrams. 1.500 milligrams will help reduce blood pressure, and more recently, it has been suggested that most people aim to maintain a sufficient intake. The lower your intake of sodium, the lower your blood pressure. Studies found that a DASH menu containing 2 300 mg of sodium could reduce blood pressure and further reduce blood pressure by 1,500 mg, even lower sodium. The current intake of salt in the US is 4,200 mg daily for adult men and 3,300 mg daily for adult women.

- Calcium: 1,250 mg
- Potassium: 4,700 mg
- 500 mg magnesium.
- Fiber: 30 grams.

DASH diet and loss of weight

During the DASH diet, you will lose weight at a lower level with increased physical activity. The easiest way to lose weight is by progressively increasing physical activity and eating a healthy, lower-calorie, and fat diet.

Physical exercise can take place for a total of 30 minutes at a time or three times 10 minutes each. Take about 60 minutes a day to prevent weight gain.

How to lower the DASH food plan calories?

The DASH eating plan can be implemented for weight loss promotion. It is abundant in foods with lower calories, such as fruit and vegetables. By substituting higher calorie foods like candy with more fruits or vegetables, you can make it lower in calories, and that will help you meet your DASH goals as well. Such instances are as follows:

1- To raise fruit: instead of consuming four shortbread cookies, eat a medium apple. You're going to save 80 calories. Eat 1/4 cup of dried apricots rather than a 2-ounce bag of rinds of pork. You're going to save 230 calories.

2- To increase vegetables: have 3 ounces of meat in place of 6 ounces of hamburger. Put a 1/2 cup of carrots and a 1/2 cup of spinach. You're going to save over 200 calories. Have a stir grill with 2 ounces of chicken and 11/2 cups of raw vegetables instead of 5 ounces of chicken. Using a little vegetable oil. You're going to save fifty calories.

3- To improve fatless or fatty dairy products. Have a 1/2 tablespoon serving fatty frozen yogurt rather than a 1/2 tablespoon serving full fat ice cream. You're going to save about 70 calories.

4- Other tips to save calories:

- Use fat-free or low-fat spices. Use half as much vegetable oil, liquid or soft margarine, mayonnaise, or dressing of salad, or opt for low-fat or fat-free versions. Eat smaller servings and eventually cut back. Choose milk and milk products that are fat-free or low-fat. To compare the fat content in packaged foods, check food labeling and products marked without fat or low fat are not always lower in calories than their regular version. Simply reduce foods containing lots of added sugar, including pastries, flavored yogurts, candy bars, ice cream, sherbet, regular soft drinks, and fruit drinks.

- In their own juice or in water, eat fruit canned. Add fruit to fat-free and fat-free yogurt. Snack on fruit, sticks, and unbuttered popcorn or cakes of rice. Drink water or soda club and zest it with a lemon or lime wedge.

Foods To Eat That Lower Blood Pressure - The DASH Diet

Foods that minimize blood pressure are right in our supermarket. We just have to know what they are and want to eat them. So how do we decide what foods to choose from? The DASH diet has been saved by us. The good news for us all is that it is not easy to follow this eating plan. It makes most and many types of foods and does not require unusual or arduous dishes.

DASH diet was developed by the National Health Institutes (NIH) on the basis of the Mediterranean diet and studies from the National Heart, Lung, and Blood Institute. DASH, which means dietary approaches to avoid hypertension, is the most common diet for foods with lower blood pressure available today.

It focuses on the balanced consumption of whole grains, meat, fish, and nuts. It permits low-fat milk and lean red meats. Sweets and drinks containing sugar are reduced but not excluded. This healthy diet is high in potassium, magnesium, calcium, and fruit and vegetables. It also contains higher fiber and protein concentrations (18 percent). Also, it allows us to eliminate the salt shaker and to find delicious, healthier ways of seasoning our food.

Why We Need the DASH Diet

The medical term high blood pressure (HBT) has been measured at 73 million Americans and 1 billion people around the world. The NHLBI study found a clear correlation between hypertension and cardiovascular disease, strokes, and kidney disease. If you are between 40 and 70 years of age, your cardiovascular disease risk rises by 20mm Hg in your systolic readings or by 10mm Hg in your diastolic readings.

We recognize that an unhealthy diet is one of the risk factors for high blood pressure. With 1 in 3 Americans living with hypertension, NHLBI has launched a report on some of the country's most renowned medical facilities to discover the best diet plan to prevent or minimize high blood pressure.

The study consisted of a control diet, reflecting the standard US diet, and two other diets. The third diet, known as the DASH diet, was the most successful. Their findings: Blood pressure has been lowered with a low diet

- Cholesterol
- Saturated Fat
- Overall fat emphasizing fat-free milk and milk products

There were also plenty of vegetables and fruits in the food plan. In the two weeks following the DASH eating plan, doctors saw immediate improvements in blood pressure rates.

The importance of these results cannot be overestimated: the DASH findings mean we can now reduce the risk of the two main dietary causes of heart and stroke: cholesterol and high blood pressure.

A second study applied a sodium (salt) intake reduction to the DASH programme. A substantial additional reduction in their high blood pressure was observed among those who followed the DASH plan and consumed 1500 mg or less of salt daily.

Tips for eating at low blood pressure

- Eat fresh (fruit and vegetables).
- Make your meal centrally complicated carbohydrates (e.g., pasta)
- Make your meat a side dish, not the main one.
- Eat lean meats, fish, and poultry.
- Eat a selection of textures, colors, and tastes so that you are not bored and revert to old habits.
- Stir-fry, grill, steam, roast; don't fry.
- Eat fruit and other delicious substitutes for table sugar.
- Creates your own seasoning mix to produce food flavors and reduce salt.
- If you are eating them, cured foods and rinse off salt from canned foods.

- Modify your preferred recipes to incorporate the principles of the DASH diet.
- Allow progressive improvements.

CHAPTER FOUR
8 Advisable Foods While on a DASH Diet - Save Your Body From High Blood Pressure

The nutritional methods to avoid hypertension or DASH have been established with a set of approaches for people who want to regulate their starved behaviors in order to lessen the dangers of high anxiety levels. It is also useful for the defense of diets against osteoporosis and common human diseases such as stroke, cancer, diabetes, and heart failure. Save yourself from multiple risks of hypertension; use the eight foods you should consume for a dietary approach.

1. Grains supply healthy sources of nutrition in the body, enriched with whole grains, such as pieces of bread, cereals, oatmeal, pasta, and rice.

2. Fruits and vegetables - These two foods, eight to ten servings each, are recommended for daily consumption. Fiber, protein, carbohydrates, vitamins, and minerals are rich in tomatoes, carrots, broccoli, and sweet potatoes, as well as bananas, apes, and prunes.

3. Dairy products — The three primary dairy enterprises supplying major vitamins, calcium, and protein are milk, yogurt, and cheese. During the DASH reduction, fat-free or low-fat milk products are successful.

4. Meat, poultry, and fish—meat and fish are rich in protein, vitamin-B, iron, and zinc, whether refined or untreated. Prepare and cook correctly before broiling, roasting, or frying, taking the skin and fats.

5. The almonds, kidney beans as well as sunflower seeds, and the like are healthy magnesium, potassium, and protein source. They are also rich in fiber and help to battle cancers and cardiovascular diseases through their phytochemicals.

6. Fats and oils-fat enriched diets help the organism consume important immune vitamins; the risk of cardiovascular disease, diabetes, and obesity may be amplified by excessive fats.

7. Low-fat Sweets — In this program, jellybeans, graham crackers, and light-flavored cookies are also considered for consumption. Dark chocolate is recommended as it contains fewer hypertensive substances.

8. Snacks with low sodium—buy foods that have "no salt added" or logos of the "low sodium-rich" found in bold sections of the snack.

Now you want more energy, healthiness, look younger, weight loss, and body washing, right?

DASH Diet Plan - The Key to Lower Blood Pressure

Which ones would you prefer to regulate your high blood pressure, take costly medications with nasty side effects every day or turn to a proven diet that can help normalize your blood pressure in around two weeks?

It sounds stupid, but millions of people choose to take blood pressure medicine when they can improve their condition by adapting their DASH diet as part of their cure.

The Dietary Approach to Stop Hypertension (DASH) is a diet intended to minimize blood pressure. Contrary to fad weight-loss diets, it is not impossible to adhere to and has huge advantages not only in controlling blood pressure but also in reducing the chances of other diseases such as diabetes and cancer.

Diet plays a significant role in both developing and reducing high blood pressure. Food is the power of our body. When you take a minute to think, a bad diet is just like pouring gas into a tank, which runs unleaded. The engine will still operate, but it will run approximately and simply stop working overtime because of the build-up of fuel. A load of salt, sugar, and saturated fat on our bodies has the same effect.

There are two explanations for why the DASH diet plan works. Second, it consists of foods rich in vitamins, minerals, fibers, and antioxidants that lower pressure and reverse blood harm. Secondly, and just as critically, it substitutes for the junk that caused the problem.

Here are the types of foods you can expect from the DASH diet quickly:

- Whole grains, such as cereals, oatmeal, and whole-grain bread, deliver complex carbon and fiber products.
- Fruits such as spinach, tomatoes, bananas, beans, and berries, which supply potassium, magnesium, fibre, and antioxidants.
- No oily or fatty dairy products such as fatty milk, yogurt, and cheese that supply protein, calcium, and magnesium.
- Magnesium and Protein lean poultry, white meats, and fish.

- Nuts seeds and beans such as kidney beans, almonds and calcium, fiber, and vitamin B pistachios.
- Nice fats and oils like canola oil, olives, and our fats avocados.

It takes the diet to make it work, and it will take some plans, particularly for the food you eat. However, compare this piece of work to the prescription for drudgery and pain, and I hope you're sure that it's worth the effort.

In less than two weeks, your blood pressure reading can drop by 20 points following the DASH diet plan, combined with a bit of daily exercise and relaxation technique. Give it a chance; give it a try. Your heart's going to thank you.

The DASH diet - Foods to avoid

In this section, let us quickly look at the Dash Diet menu and see if it's all cracked up - and if our New Years' weight loss targets can be reached if we comply!

The nutritional solution to avoid a high DASH diet is a weight loss strategy tailored for moderate and sensitive eating. This method is increasingly popular as it focuses on an approach to healthy eating in the real world. Indeed, you can eat and enjoy yourself without having to count any calories in your diet if you obey their suggestion. Quick food is also OK for road warriors with this varied diet approach. Some restaurants also support dieticians using symbols on the menus to classify low-fat items. Diners are also given more room to choose how to prepare their meals.

Research suggests that this mix of nutrients can decrease blood pressure. DASH may also lead to reducing the risk of chronic disease and maintaining a balanced and healthy weight.

The DASH diet encourages cholesterol- and saturated fat-low foods. Cutting fatback is OK to retain the taste of healthy food and a choice menu. Here are some main ingredients for your success with this very common approach.

1) If you can, stay away from the bread, but when you're too hungry and the rolls on the table are too tenting - Well - just don't use butter.

2) To salad dress- ask for low fat on one side and on the other side.

3) Choose the green or spinach tossed

4) Ask your food to be prepared instead of butter with olive oil.

5) The foods that are steamed, broiled, grilled, roasted, or stir-fried should be picked.

6) Choose vegetables as the side dishes. Baked potatoes and rice are also all right.

7) Skip onion rings and French fries

8) Cut off any obvious meat fat.

9) Drinking water, soda club, juice, dietary soda, tea, or coffee is healthier

10) Say no to booze too much! (Be limited to two)

13) Skip soup and choose fruit or salad instead.

14) Always be mindful of salt consumption!

And naturally...the law of the jumbo scale is coming next!

15) Always stop too much to eat!

Other aspects the DASH diet points out are more evident pitfalls that dieters fall into the Salad paradox... Do not only assume that it has green, and it's safe or low in calories - certain dressings of salad are fat, fat, FATTENING!

A smart approach to dieting, but it won't revolutionize your figure or turn you easily into a hard body. But if you want to be just a little healthier and self-conscious, this is a small but necessary step in the correct direction!

The DASH Diet Could Help In The Fight Against Obesity

Like it or not, obesity is the first line of attacks in the conventional diet and exercise plan, and most doctors don't even recommend stomach bypass surgery until they are confident that you have actively and successfully attempted to diet and exercise. In the face of having to walk along a dietary path, it makes sense to select a diet that is at least able to function.

One potential alternative is the DASH diet, ultimately formulated to lead to lower blood pressure and endorsed by the National Heart, Lung and Blood Institute and the American Heart Association.

Many diets concentrate on foods that you should avoid, for example, that require you to cut carbohydrates or fats. Others concentrate on the nutritional properties of such foods and require you to eat massive amounts of items such as grapefruit. Without getting into the inside and outside of these diets, the real issue is that they have been shown to be unsuccessful time and time again. Simply put - they're not working.

So what is the difference in the DASH diet?

The DASH diet focuses on what to eat rather than what to eat and advises the simplest thing to eat the fruit and vegetable mix balanced with some low-fat dairy items.

Over two main factors, fruit and vegetables are excellent dietary items (as long as you eat a variety of both products and do not only limit yourself to one or two of your favorite products).

First of all, fruit and vegetables are high in water and low in calories. This means you don't have to eat huge amounts either to feel satisfied, and even relatively large amounts don't offer a high-calorie intake.

Second, fruits and vegetables not only provide your adequate daily intake of fiber but also provide essential vitamins and minerals that are necessary for healthy eating.

Whether or not the particular DASH diet is a personal preference, but when you have to try a diet and practice a solution to obesity, it could be an excellent route to take a diet which complies with the concepts outlined in the DASH diet and which mainly focuses on fruit and vegetables.

Heart Healthy Foods

The National Heart, Lung, and Blood Institute and the American Heart Association support DASH's heart-healthy diet. DASH stands for (Dietary Hypertension Avoid Approaches). It is also the base of the current USDA MyPyramid. The basis of the DASH diet is obviously nothing new for you. This includes berries, vegetables, whole grains, and fats that are low in saturation. "It's not glamorous" Learn more about the new and improved diet that is safe at heart, and did I mention it will help to protect against cancer and undesired weight?

The basis of a balanced heart diet is:

Total fat: 27%

Saturated fat: 6%

Protein: 18%...

Carbohydrates: 55%

It also contains not more than 2300 mg (1500 mg is better) of sodium per day and at least 30 g of fiber. This means very little for you if you're like me and you'd rather only know what foods to consume and which foods to avoid. So, I'm going to put the DASH diet on your base shelf.

Eating Foods:

It is essential for oily fish and/or lean protein. Salmon, tuna, and mackerel are plentiful in omega-3 fatty acids, which have been shown to enhance the elasticity of your blood vessels. Chicken and turkey breast are always good protein choices if fish isn't your solid.

Fruit and vegetables were high in antioxidants that protect the blood vessels from heart disease through neutralizing damaging free radicals. It is an established way to help protect the body from atherosclerotic cardiac disease. Fruits and vegetables are naturally also rich in cleansing fiber.

Nuts and seeds are rich in healthy (non-saturated) fats and more essential in vitamin E that protects against "bad" (saturated/trans fats. Nuts fill you and are a perfect choice for a balanced snack.

Foods To Avoid:

The fried foods are among the heart's worst foods. They are rich in cholesterol-related saturated fats. Most people were aware of the health dangers of fast food, but the food in the restaurant can be just as bad for you.

For a good cause, Red Meat has earned a poor reputation. The marbled cuts are worse and have a higher fat percentage. Try restricting your consumption to as much fat as you can once a week or less before cooking.

I assume most people are not shocked by the above guidance but have trouble applying these activities in their everyday lives. Here are some tips for a superfood that make it easy to eat healthily.

Purchase whole-grain cereals and bread.

Get to know safe recipes and try new stuff.

Replace butter or shortening with olive oil.

Leave on the counter new fruit.

Buy 1% milk or skim

The investigation is definitive. Hypertension and cholesterol have been correlated with our diet. Heart safe food is not rocket science, but some discipline is important. You can be shocked how easy it is to eat healthier, and thank you for your heart. Using the DASH diet to protect yourself against heart disease.

CONCLUSION

Everything you eat will affect your brain's way of functioning because food gives your body the raw materials to create, rebuild, repair, and function efficiently. For example, oatmeal is highly recommended both for the health of your heart and brain. Oatmeal also contains ferulic acid, a germ and grain bran antioxidant. Ferulic acid seems to be a general protector of the brain cells, and eliminating toxins keeps them supple and responsible. I suppose we'll see more research on this antioxidant.

However, too much fat is not good in your diet, particularly the saturated fats found in whole milk and cream and animal products. Trans fats can be prevented from being found usually in processed foods and margarine and can block blood vessels and reduce circulation. In general, refined foods, processed foods, and junk foods won't help your brain. They often contain excessive salt, contain incorrect fat types, and contain sugar and preservatives. They lack a great deal of nutritional value, including healthy fiber, antioxidants, and essential nutrients.

There is also too much sugar to be avoided. Too much sugar and fatty sweets may cause metabolic and diabetes syndrome. Both conditions are linked to a higher risk of high blood pressure, cardiovascular diseases, and cognitive problems. You can do nothing for genetic factors that can raise the risk of heart attacks but reduce the risk of creating issues for your brain by maintaining a healthier lifestyle and eating well-nourished.

Snacks & Appetizers

Hummus Dip
Ingredients:

- 2 (15-ounce) cans chickpeas, drained and rinsed
- 1/2 cup extra-virgin olive oil, or more as needed, plus more for garnish
- 1/2 lemon, juiced
- 2 tablespoons roughly chopped fresh parsley leaves, plus more for garnish
- 2 cloves garlic, peeled
- 1 1/2 teaspoon salt
- 1/2 teaspoon dark Asian sesame oil
- 1/2 to 1 teaspoon ground cumin
- 12 to 15 grinds black pepper
- 1/4 cup water
- Paprika, for garnish

Instructions:

- Blend together everything but parsley and paprika. Blend until smooth on a low
- setting. Add garnish.
- Chill

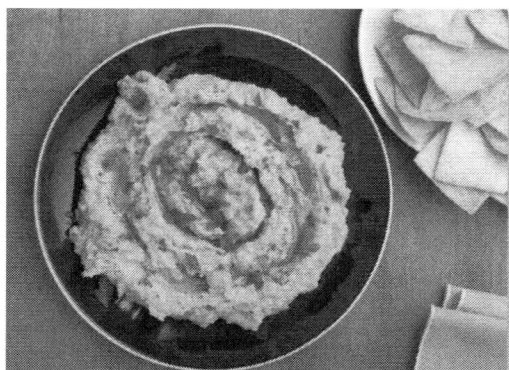

Sweet and spicy snack mix
Ingredients:

- 2 cans (15 ounces each) garbanzos, rinsed, drained and patted dry

- 2 cups Wheat Chex cereal
- 1 cup dried pineapple chunks
- 1 cup raisins
- 2 tablespoons honey
- 2 tablespoons reduced-sodium Worcestershire sauce
- 1 teaspoon garlic powder
- 1/2 teaspoon chili powder

Instructions:

- Turn on oven to 350. Grease a large baking sheet with low fat oil or cooking spray.
- Put garbanzo beans in pan and cook until brown or for about 10 minutes. Put
- beans on cooking sheet. Add cooking spray. Bake until crisp or for about twenty minutes.
- Spray roasting pan with cooking spray. Add cereal, raisins, and pineapple. Add beans and stir.
- In a large glass bowl add honey, spices, and Worcestershire sauce. Mix. Back an additional 15 minutes. Remove and cool.

Spiced carrot raisin bread
Ingredients:

- 1 1/2 cup whole-wheat pastry flour
- 1/2 teaspoon baking soda
- 1 1/2 teaspoons baking powder
- 1/2 teaspoon salt
- 1 tablespoon cinnamon
- 1/2 teaspoon nutmeg
- 1/4 teaspoon cloves
- 1/4 teaspoon paprika or cayenne
- 1 tablespoon grated lemon zest
- 1/4 cup ground flaxseed
- 2 eggs
- 1/2 cup brown sugar

- 1/4 cup honey
- 1/2 cup unsweetened applesauce
- 1/4 cup olive oil
- 3/4 teaspoon almond extract
- 2 cups shredded carrots (about 4 carrots)
- 2/3 cup raisins

Instructions:

- Combine dry ingredients. In a different bowl, combine wet ingredients. Add carrots and raisins. Mix wet to dry ingredients until moist. Pour into a greased bread pan. Bake at 375 for about an hour.

Fruit Salad
Ingredients:

- 1 large mango, peeled, diced
- 2 cups fresh blueberries
- 2 bananas, sliced
- 2 cups fresh strawberries, halved
- 2 cups seedless grapes
- 2 nectarines, unpeeled, sliced
- 1 kiwi fruit, peeled, sliced
- Honey Orange Sauce
- ⅓ cup unsweetened orange juice
- 2 Tbsp lemon juice
- 1½ Tbsp honey
- ¼ tsp ground ginger
- 1 dash nutmeg

Instructions:

- Prepare the fruit.
- Combine all ingredients for sauce and mix.
- Pour honey–orange sauce over fruit.

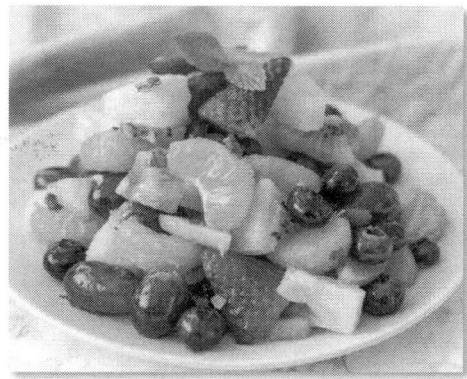

Trail mix
Ingredients:

- 1/4 cup whole shelled (unpeeled) almonds
- 1/4 cup unsalted dry-roasted peanuts
- 1/4 cup dried cranberries
- 1/4 cup chopped pitted dates
- 2-ounce dried apricots, or other dried fruit
- Smoothie
- 1 medium banana, peeled
- 1 orange, peeled
- 1 cup berries (I like to use 1/2 cup blueberries, 1/4 cup raspberries and 1/4 cup
- strawberries)
- 1/4 avocado, pitted
- 2 to 3 cups or large handfuls of fresh, baby spinach (or other leafy green)
- 1 tablespoon of ground flax seed
- 4 ounces of filtered water

Instructions:

- Add liquid to blender then the soft fruit. Add the greens to blender last. Blend on high for 30 seconds or until the smoothie is creamy.

Bean Dip and Olive Athens
Ingredients:

- 2 15-oz. cans, rinsed and drained, or 3 1/2 cups cooked garbanzo or navy
- beans 2/3 cup fat-free sour cream
- 2 tsp minced garlic

- 4 tbsp balsamic vinegar
- 1/4 cup chopped sun-dried tomatoes (not in oil) 1/4 cup finely chopped fresh
- or dried parsley 2 tbsp chopped Kalamata or ripe olives Kalamata olives, as garnish
- Assorted vegetables and crackers for serving

Instructions:

- Place the beans, garlic, sour cream and vinegar in the food processor and process until smooth.
- Mix in the tomatoes, parsley, olives and combine well.
- Transfer the mixture into a bowl and add a few olives for garnishing.
- Can be served with vegetables and crackers.
- The dip can be made about 2 to 3 hours ahead or refrigerated overnight.

Stuffed Quesadillas
Ingredients:

- 2 small green and/or red sweet peppers, cut into thin strips 1 small red onion, cut into thin 1-inch-long strips 2 tsps. olive oil or cooking oil
- 1/2 tsp. ground cumin
- 1/2 tsp. chili powder
- 2 Tbsps. snipped fresh parsley or cilantro 1/3 cup reduced-fat cream cheese
- (tub style)
- 5 6-to 7-inch flour tortillas
- Salsa (optional)

Instructions:

- Preheat the oven to 425F.
- Place 1 tsp of oil in a nonstick skillet and heat well.
- Add the sweet peppers and strips of onions and sauté until tender.
- Toss in the chili powder and cumin and leave for about another minute.
- Mix in the parsley and leave aside.

- Place cream cheese on half of each tortilla on one side.
- Spread the pepper mix on top and place the tortillas on a baking sheet.
- Rub the balance oil on each tortilla and bake in a preheated oven for about 5-6
- minutes.
- Slice into 4 wedges and serve warm.
- If required serve with the salsa.

Summer Melon Fresh Cooler
Ingredients:

- 2 cups cubed cantaloupe
- 1 cup low-fat lemon yogurt
- 1 cup orange juice

Instructions:

- Place all the ingredients in a blender.
- Process until smooth.
- Place the leftovers in the refrigerator within about 3 hours.

Triple Muffins
Ingredients:

- Nonstick cooking spray
- 1-1/3 cups all-purpose flour 3/4 cup buckwheat flour
- 1/4 to 1/3 cup sugar
- 1-1/2 tsp. baking powder
- 1 tsp. ground cinnamon
- 1/2 tsp. baking soda
- 1/2 tsp. salt
- 2 eggs, slightly beaten
- 1 cup mashed cooked butternut squash
- 1/2 cup fat-free milk
- 2 Tbsps. cooking oil
- 1/2 tsp. finely shredded orange peel 1/4 cup orange juice
- 3/4 cup fresh or frozen blueberries Rolled oats

Instructions:

- Preheat the oven to 400F.
- Insert paper liners into a 12 x 2 ½" muffin cups and leave aside.

- In a bowl, place the flours, baking powder, baking soda, sugar and salt and mix well.
- Dig a well in the middle of the mixture and keep aside for a while.
- Mix the eggs milk, squash, oil, orange juice and the peel in another bowl.
- Fold the flour mixture into the egg mixture and mix until moist.
- Mix in the blueberries.
- Fold the batter mixture into the lined muffin cups and top up each cup with oats.
- Bake for about 20 minutes until the muffins are a light brown in color.
- Allow to cool for 5-6 minutes.
- Take out from the muffin cups and serve.

Sesame Hummus
Ingredients:

- 1/3 cup toasted sesame seeds or ¼ cup tahini
- 1/8 tsp crushed red chilies
- 1 15-oz. can garbanzo beans, rinsed and drained, or 2 cups cooked garbanzo
- beans
- 1/8 cup lime, lemon or orange juice
- ½ tsp garlic, minced
- ½ tsp salt
- 2 tbsp olive oil

Instructions:

- Preheat the oven to 350F.
- Place the seeds on a baking tray and bake for about 8 – 10 minutes until slightly toasted.
- Place the sesame seeds in a food processor and process well into a puree.
- Mix in the chilies, beans, juice, minced garlic and salt.
- Process until smooth in consistency.
- Transfer the mixture into a bowl.
- Cover and leave it for about 1 hour or more for better blending of flavors.

Roasted Almonds with Rosemary
Ingredients:

- 1 Tbsp. finely chopped fresh rosemary 1 Tbsp. extra-virgin olive oil
- 1 tsp. Chile powder
- 3/4 tsp. kosher salt
- Dash of ground red pepper
- 1 (10-oz.) bag whole almonds (about 2 cups)

Instructions:

- Preheat the oven to 325F.
- Mix all the ingredients in a bowl.
- Spread the mixture on a lined baking sheet.
- Bake for about 20-25 minutes until slightly toasted.
- Leave to cool in room temperature.

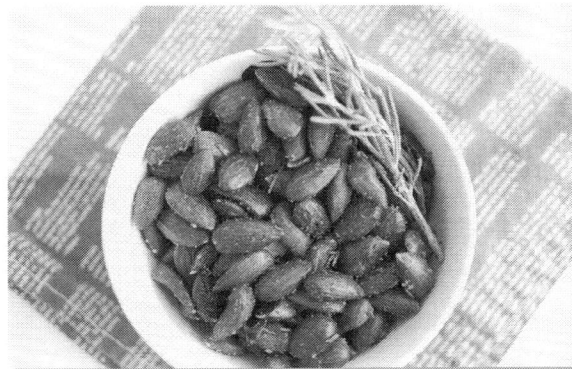

Yellow Pick-Me-Up Smoothie
Ingredients:

- 3 milk ice cubes, cracked
- 1 container (6 oz) plain fat-free yogurt
- 2 Tbsps. granulated sugar
- 1 tsp. fresh or from concentrate lemon juice
- ½ tsp. finely grated lemon zest (yellow part of peel only)
- optional: additional lemon zest for garnish

Instructions:

- Pour about 1 to 1 ½ cups of the milk into an ice cube tray.

- Leave in the freezer for about 3 hours or more until ice is formed.
- Place all the ingredients in a food processor.
- Process until smooth and serve into dishes.
- Serve garnished with lemon zest and milk ice cubes.

White Bean and Nut Dip
Ingredients:

- 1/4 cup soft whole wheat bread crumbs 2 Tbsps. fat-free milk
- 1 15-oz. can white kidney beans (cannellini beans) or Great Northern beans,
- rinsed and drained 1/4 cup fat-free or light dairy sour cream 3 Tbsps. pine
- nuts, toasted
- 1/4 tsp. salt-free garlic and herb seasoning blend or other salt-free seasoning
- blend 1/8 tsp. cayenne pepper
- 2 tsps. chopped fresh oregano or basil or 1/2 tsp. dried oregano or basil,
- crushed Pine nuts, toasted (optional)
- Fresh oregano or basil leaves (optional) Assorted vegetable dippers

Instructions:

- Place the bread crumbs in a bowl and add the milk.
- Ensure to cover and leave for about 5 to 6 minutes.
- In the meantime, place the beans, toasted pine nuts, sour cream, seasoning blend and pepper in a food processor.
- Process until the texture is smooth in consistency.
- Spoon the bread crumb mixture and blend again.
- Toss in the oregano or basil.
- Pour the mixture into a container with lid, cover and refrigerate for over 2 hours.

- Garnish with pine nuts, basil or oregano as desired.
- Can be served with vegetable dippers.
- Enjoy!

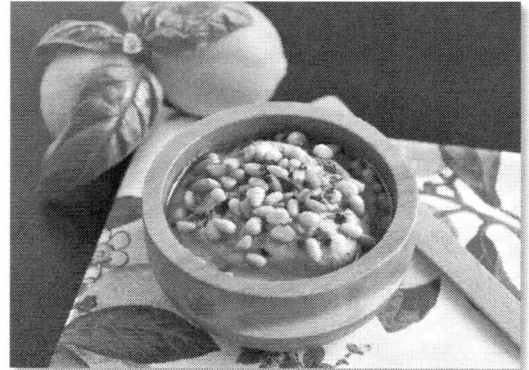

Peach and Raspberry Mixed "Lassi"
Ingredients:

- 1 cup fresh or frozen peaches
- ½ medium ripe banana
- ½ cup fresh or frozen raspberries
- 1 cup low fat buttermilk
- 2-3 ice cubes

Instructions:

- Place all the ingredients in a blender.
- Process until smooth in consistency.
- Serve and enjoy!

Wafers and Cinnamon Snack Mix
Ingredients:

- 3 cups NILLA Wafers
- 1 cup PLANTERS Pecan Halves
- 1 cup pretzel sticks
- 3 Tbsp. butter or margarine, melted 2 Tbsp. sugar
- 1 tsp. ground cinnamon
- 1/4 tsp. Kosher salt
- 1/2 cup yogurt-covered raisins

Instructions:

- Heat the oven to 375F.
- Place the wafers, pecans and pretzel sticks in a bowl and combine well.

- In a separate bowl, mix the butter, cinnamon, salt and the sugar.
- Spread over the wafer mixture.
- Place in a lined baking pan of about 15 x 10 x 1" in size.
- Place in the oven for about 10-12 minutes until slightly toasted to light brown.
- Allow to cool and mix in the raisins.
- Serve.

Pumpkin Vanilla Smoothie
Ingredients:

- 1 cup milk
- 2 Tbsps. unsweetened instant tea (optional)
- ½ tsp. pumpkin pie spice
- ¼ tsp. ground cardamom
- 1 banana
- ¾ cup fat-free vanilla yogurt
- ½ cup canned pumpkin
- 1 Tbsp. pure maple syrup
- 1 cup ice cubes (about 10 cubes)

Instructions:

- Place the instant tea and the spices in a food processor.
- Mix in the milk and process until the tea is well dissolved.
- Toss in the balance ingredients excluding the ice cubes and blend until smooth.
- Depending on the thickness keep on adding ice cubes to get into the right consistency.
- Transfer the mixture into individual glasses and serve.

Nectarine and Blueberry Gratin
Ingredients:

- 1 cup Almond-Fruit Granola
- 4 medium nectarines, sliced 1/2 cup fresh blueberries 2 Tbsps. orange liqueur
- (such as Grand Marnier) or orange juice 2 Tbsps. packed brown sugar

Instructions:

- Place sliced nectarines, fresh blueberries and orange liqueur in a bowl.
- Mix well and spoon the mixture into 6 dishes.
- Sprinkle brown sugar on the surface of each dish.
- Bake in a preheated oven (450F) for about 8 minutes until the sugar is completely dissolved.
- Make the Almond-Fruit Granola and splash about ¼ cup of the mixture over each dish.
- Serve and enjoy!

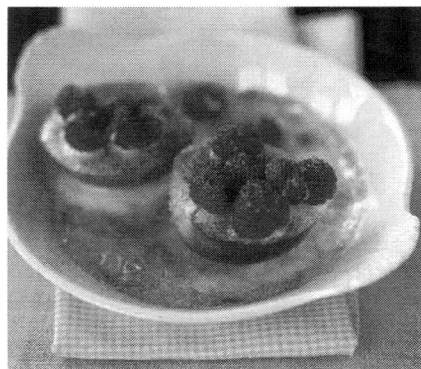

Vanilla Granola Skillet
Ingredients:

- 1/3 cup vegetable oil
- 3 Tbsps. honey
- ¼ cup powdered milk
- 1 tsp. vanilla
- 4 cups uncooked, old-fashioned rolled oats
- ½ cup sunflower seeds
- 1 cup raisins

Instructions:

- Prepare a lined baking tray and keep aside.
- Pour the oil and honey into a skillet and heat for about 1 minute.
- Mix in the vanilla, powdered milk, oats, sunflower seeds and mix well.

- Heat the mixture until the oatmeal becomes a light brown in color.
- Remove from heat and toss in the raisins.
- Spread the mixture into the baking tray.
- Allow the mixture to cool.
- The mixture can be stored in air tight jars for some time.

Cereal Snack Mix
Ingredients:

- 6 cups Frosted Cheerios cereal
- 1/2 cup animal crackers
- 1 1/2 cups small pretzel twists 1 1/2 cups cheese-flavored snack crackers 5
- pouches Betty Crocker Shark Bites chewy fruit snacks (from 9-oz. box)

Instructions:

- Mix all the ingredients in a bowl.
- Store the mix in airtight containers for future use.

Golden Potato Pancakes
Ingredients:

- 6 potatoes, peeled, cooked, and mashed
- 2 eggs
- ¼ cup seasoned whole wheat bread crumbs
- 1 Tbsp parsley
- ¼ cup flour
- 1/3 cup canola oil

Instructions:

- Mix the potatoes with eggs, parsley and bread crumbs in a bowl.
- Form the mixture into oval shapes and coat each shape with flour.
- Heat the oil and fry the shapes for about 5-6 minutes until golden in color.
- Serve warm and enjoy!

Healthy Chicken Wings Honey
Ingredients:

- 2 tbsps. olive oil
- 2 tbsps. catsup
- Half tsp. garlic, minced
- 1 One-Fourth pounds chicken wings
- 2 tbsps. honey
- Half mug low sodium soy dip sauce

Instructions:

- Soak chicken wings; pat dry. Cut off and discard wing tips and then cut each wing at the joint to make two sections. Put wings on a broiler pan sprayed with nonstick vegetable oil Sprinkle. Broil about 4 inches (10 cm) from the Warm up for 5 minutes on each side or until chicken wings are nicely browned.
- Shift chicken wings to baking dish. In a dish, Merge left-over ingredients. Spill dip sauce over chicken wings. Cover and Prepare at 350°F until chicken is done, about 20 minutes.

Chinese Chicken Wing Starters
Ingredients:

- Half mug brown Lactose alternative,
- 1 tsp. ground ginger
- Half tsp. garlic, minced
- 1 One-Fourth pounds chicken wings
- Half mug onion, Diced
- One-Fourth mug low sodium soy dip sauce
- One-Fourth mug sherry

Instructions:

- Soak chicken wings; pat dry. Cut off and discard wing tips then cut each wing at the joint to make two sections.
- Put wings on a broiler pan sprayed with nonstick vegetable oil Sprinkle. Broil about 4 inches (10 cm) from the Warm up for 5 minutes on each side or until chicken wings are nicely browned.

- Shift chicken wings to baking dish. In a dish, Merge Diced onion, soy dip sauce, brown Lactose, ginger, garlic, and sherry. Spill dip sauce over chicken wings. Cover and Prepare at 350°F until chicken is done, about 20 minutes.

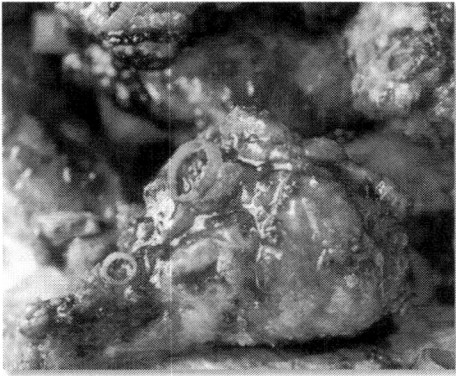

Low Calories Broccoli and Tomato Salad
Ingredients:

- 1 tbsp. white wine lemon juice
- 1 tbsp. lemon juice
- 2 tbsps. fresh bay leaf, Diced
- One-Fourth mug green onion, minced
- One-Fourth tsp. garlic, minced
- 1-pound broccoli
- One-Fourth-pound mushrooms
- Third-Fourth mug (105 g) olives, drained
- 8 ounces cherry tomatoes
- One-Fourth mug olive oil
- One-Fourth tsp. black pepper, fresh ground

Instructions:

- Crop florets from broccoli. You should have about 1 quart (1.1 kg). Reserve stems for another use. Drop broccoli florets into boiling mineral water for 1 minute or just until they turn bright green; drain. Crop mushroom stems to Half inch (1.3 cm).
- Merge broccoli, mushrooms, olives, and cherry tomatoes in dish. Measure

oil, lemon juice, lemon juice, bay leaf, onion, garlic, and black pepper into small dish. Whip until blended. Spill dressing over vegetable mixture. Turn gently to Cover veggies. Cover and freeze 3 hours or more until ready to serve.

Black Pepper Garbanzo and Macaroni Salad
Ingredients:

- One-Third mug (41 g) carrot, diced
- One-Fourth mug green onion, Diced
- 3 tbsps. Balsamic lemon juice
- 2 tbsps. Low fat mayonnaise
- 4 ounces whole warm up macaroni, unprepared
- 2 mugs garbanzo beans,
- Half mug Poblano pepper, Diced
- One-Third mug celery, diced
- 2 tsps. Mustard
- Half tsp. black pepper
- One-Fourth tsp. parched seasoning
- 4 mug (188 g) leaf green lettuce leaf, torn into bite-sized pieces

Instructions:

- Prepare macaroni according to directions, omitting salt. Drain and Soak well under cold mineral water until macaroni is cool; drain well.
- Merge macaroni, garbanzo beans, red bell pepper, celery, carrot, and green onion in medium-sized dish. Whip together lemon juice, mayonnaise, mustard, black pepper, and seasoning in small dish until blended. Spill over salad; Roll to Cover evenly. Cover and freeze up to 8 hours. Sort green lettuce leaf on individual plates. Serve salad over green lettuce leaf.

Baked Vegetable Orzo Salad
Ingredients:

- 1 mug cucumber, cut into pieces

- Half tsp. garlic, minced
- 1 tbsp. olive oil
- 8 ounces whole warm up orzo
- One-Third mug lemon juice
- Half mug Poblano pepper, cut into pieces
- Half mug yellow bell pepper, cut into pieces
- Half mug red onion, cut into pieces
- 1 tsp. black pepper, fresh ground, Cut up
- One-Fourth mug pine dry fruits, Heat upped

Instructions:

- Prepare the Roast. Roll cucumber, red and yellow bell pepper, onion, and garlic with the olive oil and Half tsp. black pepper in a big dish. Shift to a Roast basket. Roast for 15 to 20 minutes, until browned, whisking from time to time.
- Meanwhile, Prepare the orzo in boiling mineral water according to package directions. Drain and Shift to a big serving dish. Add the roasted veggies to the macaroni. Merge the lemon juice and black pepper and Spill on the macaroni and veggies. Let cool to. Whisk in the pine dry fruits and serve.

Mexican Tomatoes Bean Salad
Ingredients:

- Third-Fourth mug (89 g) cucumber, Peel offed and Diced
- 2 tbsps. Onion, chopped
- Half mug guacamole
- 1 Half mugs no-salt-added kidney beans, drained
- 1 Half mugs no-salt-added garbanzo beans, drained
- 1 mug tomatoes, Diced
- Half mug low fat plain curd
- 4 mugs (288 g) iceberg green lettuce leaf, cut into small pieces

Instructions:

- In a big dish, Roll together the kidney beans, garbanzo beans, tomatoes, cucumber, and onion. In a small dish, combine the guacamole and curd.
- If dressing seems thick, whisk in a little fat free milk. Whisk into the bean mixture and cool down. Serve on Cover of cut into small pieces green lettuce leaf.

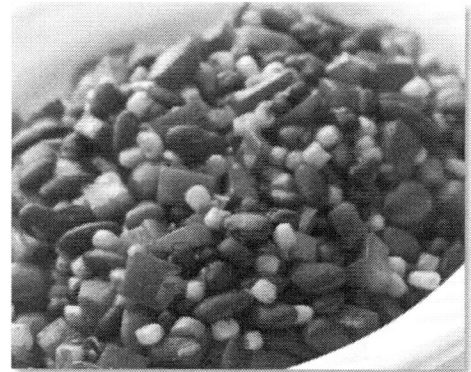

Low Calorie Yukon Golds with Buttermilk
Ingredients:

- ⅓ mug buttermilk
- 2 pounds Yukon Gold potatoes,
- 1 tbsp. Without salt butter
- 2 scallions, white and green parts, finely Diced
- One-Fourth tsp. freshly ground black pepper

Instructions:

- Put the potatoes in a medium-sized dip saucepan and add enough cold mineral water to cover by 1 inch. Cover the dip saucepan and bring to a boil over high Warm up. Decrease the Warm up to medium-sized and set the lid ajar.
- Prepare until the potatoes are ripe when pierced with the tip of a sharp knife, about 25 minutes. Drain well and put back to the dip saucepan. Do not Peel off the potatoes. Defrost the butter

in a small nonstick dip saucepan over medium-sized-high Warm up. Add the scallions and Prepare, whisking from time to time, until they begin to brown, about 3 minutes. Add to the potatoes.

- Using a potato masher or a big slotted Serve, coarsely mash the potatoes, adding the buttermilk. Season with the salt and pepper. Shift to a serving dish and serve warm.

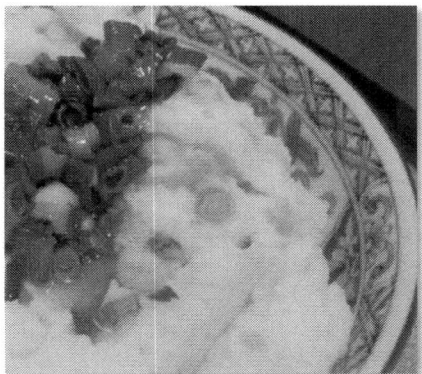

Macaroni and Kidney Bean Salad
Ingredients:

- 1 mug tomato, Diced
- One-Third mug (47 g) green olives, Diced
- Half mug low fat mayonnaise
- Half tsp. chili powder
- Half tsp. coriander
- 4 ounces whole warm up rotini, or other small macaroni
- 2 mugs red kidney beans, prepared
- 1 mug cucumber, chopped
- 1 mug Poblano pepper, chopped
- Half tsp. paprika
- One-Fourth tsp. parched sage

Instructions:

- Prepare macaroni until al dente. Soak and drain. Put in big dish and add rest of the ingredients. Combine thoroughly and serve cool downed or at. Garnish with green chili and mint. Serve immediately.

Sugary and Low Pineapple Slaw
Ingredients:

- 3 mugs cabbage, cut into small pieces
- 1 mug carrot, cut into small pieces
- Half mug crushed pineapple, drained
- 2 tbsps. (19 g) Poblano pepper, Diced
- Half mug apple, chopped
- 1 tsp. Lactose alternative One-Fourth mug cider lemon juice

Instructions:

- Merge Poblano pepper, apple, Lactose alternative, and lemon juice. Spill over veggies and pineapple and whisk to Merge. Garnish with honey and dry fruits. Serve immediately.

Fresh Warm sauce
Ingredients:

- 1 jalapeño pepper, seeded and Diced
- 1 avocado, chopped
- 1 mug plum tomatoes, seeded and finely Diced
- One-Fourth mug red onion, chopped
- 2 tbsps. lime juice
- 1 tbsp. cilantro

Instructions:

- Put all the ingredients in to a dish. Whisk to combine. Serve immediately.

Fresh Veggie Medley
Ingredients:

- Half pound green beans
- One-Fourth tsp. garlic powder
- 4 tomatoes, Diced
- 1 cucumber, chopped
- 1 tsp. parched basil

Instructions:

- Wash, Crop, and Prepare beans until almost ripe. Drain. Put back to pan with other ingredients and Prepare to if you want doneness. Garnish with green chili and mint. Serve immediately.

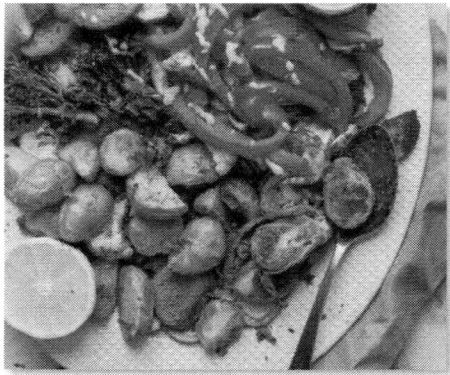

Calorie Free Curried Fresh Veggies
Ingredients:

- 1 mug Poblano pepper, Diced
- One-Fourth tsp. garlic powder
- 3 mug (540 g) tomatoes, Diced
- 1 mug onion, coarsely Diced
- 1 Half mugs cucumber, chopped
- 1 tbsp. curry powder

Instructions:

- Merge all ingredients in a dip saucepan. Prepare and whisk until veggies are softened. Garnish with green chili and mint. Serve immediately.

Indian Carrots and Green lettuce
Ingredients:

- One-Fourth mug celery, grind
- Half mug low sodium vegetable broth
- 1 tsp. ginger root, grind
- Half tsp. coriander
- Half mug coconut, grind
- Half mug green onion, diced
- 2 cloves garlic, minced
- Half tsp. turmeric
- 1 tbsp. olive oil
- 3 mugs (330 g) carrot, coarsely grind
- 1 One-Fourth mugs (195 g) frozen green lettuce, softened and drained

Instructions:

- Deep-fry green onion, garlic, and turmeric in oil until scallions are soft. Add left-over ingredients, simmer for 10 minutes. Garnish with green chili and mint. Serve immediately.

Low Sodium Sesame Green Beans
Ingredients:

- Half mug low sodium chicken broth
- 1 tsp. sesame seeds
- 1-pound green beans, softened if frozen
- 2 tsps. lemon juice

Instructions:

- Heat up sesame seeds in a heavy nonstick frying pan over medium-sized Warm up, about 3 minutes, shaking pan constantly until seeds are browned and have popped. Add green beans and broth. Cover frying pan and Prepare 7 to 8 minutes or until green beans are ripe and liquid is evaporated. Whisk in lemon juice before serving.

Healthy Cheesy Corn and Cucumber Bake
Ingredients:

- 10 ounces frozen corn, prepared
- Half mug low fat Cheddar Cheese, cut into small pieces
- Half mug egg alternative
- 3 mugs cucumber, diced
- One-Fourth mug onion, Diced
- 1 tbsp. olive oil
- 2 tbsps. Parmesan cheese

Instructions:

- Prepare cucumber in boiling mineral water until soft. Drain and mash with fork. Deep-fry onion in oil until soft.
- Merge cucumber, onion, corn, cheese, and egg alternative. Turn into a 1-quart (950 ml) casserole Sprinkled with

nonstick vegetable oil Sprinkle. Sprinkle Parmesan cheese over Cover. Put on a baking sheet and bake Unwrapped at 350°F until a knife inserted near the center comes out wipe, about 40 minutes.

Sweet Steamy Brown rice
Ingredients:

- 3 One-Third (780 ml) mugs mineral water One-Fourth mug coconut
- 1 tsp. ground ginger
- Third-Fourth mug (178 g) tropical fruit cocktail
- 1 Half mugs (285 g) brown rice, unprepared

Instructions:

- Process the fruit cocktail in a food processor or blender until finely Diced. Put all ingredients in a dip saucepan with a tightly fitting lid.
- Bring to a boil, decrease Warm up to low, cover, and simmer until brown rice is soft, about 20 minutes. Whisk before serving.

Amazing Barley Mushroom Pilaf
Ingredients:

- 3 mugs low sodium chicken broth
- 2 tbsps. (13 g) green onion, Diced
- 1 tsp. olive oil
- Half mug mushrooms, diced
- 1 mug pearl barley
- One-Fourth tsp. parched rosemary

Instructions:

- Warm up olive oil in dip saucepan; add mushrooms and Deep-fry until limp. Add barley, broth, green onion, and rosemary.
- Bring to a boil. Decrease Warm up to low, cover, and Prepare 45 minutes or until barley is ripe and liquid is absorbed.

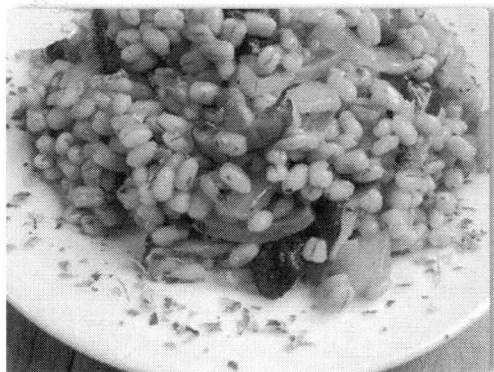

Spice Up Your Dinner with Bulgur Warm up with Pecans
Ingredients:

- One-Eighth tsp. black pepper
- 2 mugs (475 ml) mineral water, boiling
- 1 mug bulgur, unprepared
- Half tsp. parched basil
- One-Fourth mug pecans, Diced

Instructions:

- Switch on oven to 350°F. Lightly Sprinkle a 1-quart (950 ml) baking dish with a nonstick vegetable oil Sprinkle. Put bulgur, basil, and black pepper in prepared baking dish. Add boiling mineral water and combine well.
- Cover tightly and bake 20 minutes. Fluff with a fork, add pecans, and combine well. Serve warm.

Onion and Butternut with Squash
Ingredients:

- 1 mug butternut squash, Peel offed and chopped
- Half mug bulgur
- 1 tbsp. Without salt butter
- Half mug onion, Diced
- 2 whole cloves Half tsp. parched rosemary 2-inch (5 cm) cinnamon stick
- 1 bay leaf

- 1 mug low sodium chicken broth

Instructions:

- Defrost butter over medium-sized Warm up. Add onion and squash. Prepare until onion is soft. Add warm up, cloves, rosemary, cinnamon, and bay leaf. Whisk until bulgur is brown. Whisk in chicken broth. Cover and bring to a boil.
- Decrease Warm up and Prepare 15 minutes. Take away bay leaf before serving.

Teriyaki Garlic Chicken Nibbles
Ingredients:

- Half tsp. gingers
- 1-pound boneless skinless chicken breast
- Half mug mineral waters
- One-Fourth tsp. garlic powder
- 1 tsp. Lactose
- 1 Half mugs (175 g) bread crumbs

Instructions:

- Merge mineral water, soy dip sauce, garlic powder, and ginger. Cut chicken into pieces. Marinate in soy dip sauce mixture for 2 hours.
- Cover pieces with bread crumbs. Deep fat fry in vegetable oil at 375°F (190°C) for about 1 minute. Drain on absorbent towels.

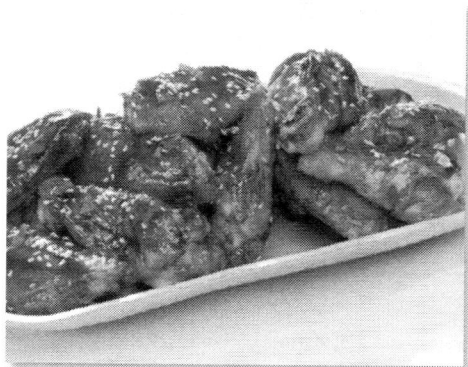

Low Fat Japanese Chicken Wings
Ingredients:

- 3 tbsps. Sodium Soy Dip sauce
- 1 tsp. gingerroot, grind
- 1-pound chicken wings
- One-Third mug sake or sherry
- One-Fourth mug cornstarch

Instructions:

- Cut chicken wings at joints. Discard the wing tips. In a dish, Merge sake or sherry, soy dip sauce, and gingerroot to make a marinade. Put chicken in a resealable plastic bag. Spill marinade over the chicken in the bag. Close the bag.
- Marinate in the fridge several hours or overnight, turning from time to time. Drain chicken; pat it dry with paper towels. Cover chicken wings with cornstarch. Fry, 3 or 4 pieces at a time, in deep warm fat for about 5 minutes. Drain on paper towels.

Healthy Chicken Drumettes
Ingredients:

- 2 tbsps. Olive oil
- 2 tbsps. Honey
- 1 tsp. oregano
- 2 chicken wings
- 3 tbsps. Lemon juice
- 1 garlic clove, minced

Instructions:

- Set apart chicken wings into sections. Discard wing tips. Merge all ingredients except chicken in a big resealable plastic bag. Combine well.
- Add chicken, seal, and turn to Cover. Freeze 8 hours or overnight. Take away chicken from marinade and Put in baking pan. Bake at 400°F for 30 to 40 minutes until golden brown.

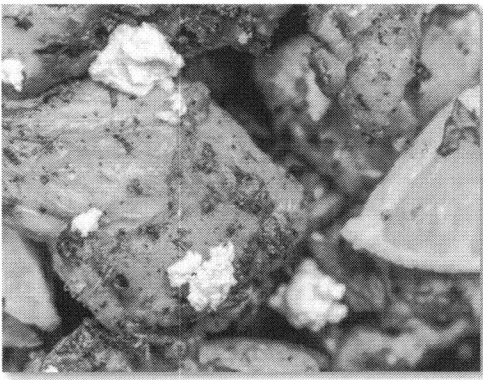

Carnitas Tequila Bites
Ingredients:

- 1 tbsp. molasses
- One-Fourth tsp. black pepper
- 2 cloves garlic, finely Diced
- 1 Half pounds pork loin, cut into (2Half cm) cubes.
- 2 tbsps. brown Lactose, packed
- 1 tbsp. tequila
- One-Third mug mineral water
- One-Fourth mug green onion with Cover, diced

Instructions:

- Put pork cubes in single layer in 1 0-inch (25 cm) frying pan. Cover with left-over ingredients except green onion. Warm up to boiling.
- Decrease Warm up and simmer Unwrapped, whisking from time to time, until the mineral water has evaporated and the pork is slightly caramelized, about 35 minutes. Sprinkle with green onion and serve with wooden picks.

Scotch Eggs with Bread Crumbs
Ingredients:

- 1 Half pounds (675 g) sausage
- 1 2 eggs, hard prepared and Peel offed
- 1 egg, Siren
- Half mug dry bread crumbs

Instructions:

- Switch on oven to 450°F. Cut up sausage into 12 equal portions; shape into patties. Wrap each sausage patty completely around 1 hard prepared egg, pressing edges together to seal. Dip sausage wrapped eggs in Siren egg; roll in bread crumbs until completely Covered.
- Put in unlubricated jelly roll pan. Bake at 450°F for 30 minutes or until meat is thoroughly browned and prepared.

Cheddar Cheese Quesadillas
Ingredients:

- 2 flour waffles, 7-inch (18 cm))
- One-Fourth mug black olives, drained
- One-Fourth mug Cheddar Cheese cut into small pieces
- 2 tbsps. Warm sauce
- One-Fourth mug fresh cilantro

Instructions:

- Switch on oven to 425°F. Put waffle flat on baking sheet. Merge olives, cheese and dip sauce in dish. Add cilantro to cheese mixture.
- Evenly Expand mixture over waffle. Cover with other waffle; pressing down firmly. Bake 8-10 minutes or until Covers are lightly browned. Take away from oven and cool 5 minutes. Cut quesadilla into 8 pieces.

Chicken Carrots Wontons
Ingredients:

- 1 tbsp. sherry
- 2 tsps. cornstarch
- 8 ounces ground chicken
- Half mug carrots, cut into small pieces
- One-Fourth mug celery, finely Diced
- 2 tsps. ginger root
- 8 ounces wonton wrappers

- 2 tbsps. Without salt butter, Defrosted

Instructions:

- In a medium-sized frying pan Prepare and whisk ground chicken until no pink remains; drain. Whisk in carrots, celery, soy dip sauce, sherry, cornstarch, and ginger root; combine well. Serve 1 rounded tsp. of the filling a Cover a wonton wrapper.
- Lightly brush edges with mineral water. To shape each wonton, carefully bring 2 opposite points of the square wrapper up over the filling and pinch together in the center. Carefully bring the 2 left-over opposite points to the center and pinch together. Pinch together edges to seal. Put wontons on a lubricated baking sheet. Brush the wontons with Defrosted butter. Bake in a 375°F oven for 8-10 minutes or until lightly brown and crisp.

Fried Cheddar Cheese Cubes
Ingredients:

- 1 Half mugs baking combine (such as Bisques), Cut up
- 1-pound Cheddar Cheese
- Half mug fat free milk
- 1 egg

Instructions:

- Cut cheese into 3-4-inch (2 cm) cubes. Warm up oil in deep fryer or dip saucepan to 375°F Stir 1 mug baking combine, milk, and egg with hand Stirrer (or fork) until smooth. Cover cheese cubes lightly with left-over baking combine and insert round wooden pick in each cube.
- Dip into batter, covering cheese completely. Fry several cubes at a time, turning carefully until golden brown (1 to 2 minutes). Drain on paper towels.

Fresh Green Beans and Tomatoes
Ingredients:

- 1 mug onion, Diced
- Half tsp. parched oregano
- 1 tsp. lemon juice
- 2 pounds fresh green beans, cut into lengths
- Half tsp. garlic, crushed
- 2 mugs tomatoes, Diced
- black pepper, fresh ground, to taste

Instructions:

- Merge all ingredients in a big covered dip saucepan and simmer until beans are ripe, about 30 minutes. Garnish with green chili and mint. Serve immediately.

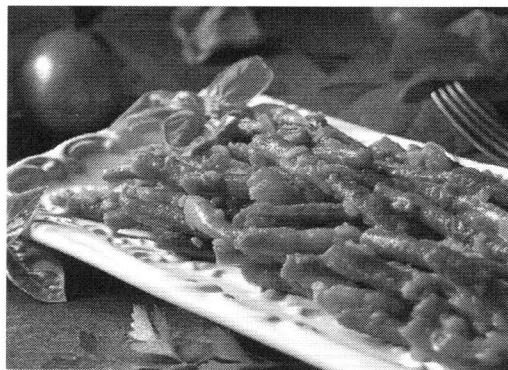

Spicy Potato Skins
Ingredients:

- Half tsp. black pepper
- 1 Half 62spas. Chili powder
- 4 potatoes
- 1 Half 62spas. Coriander
- 1 Half 62spas. Curry powder

Instructions:

- Switch on the oven to 400°F. Bake the potatoes for 1 hour. Take away the potatoes from the oven but keep the oven on. Slice the potatoes in half longitudinally and let them cool for 10 minutes. Scoop out most of the potato flesh, leaving about One-Fourth inch (2 cm) of flesh against the potato skin (you can save the potato flesh for another use, like mashed potatoes).

- Cut each potato half crosswise into 3 pieces. Cover with olive oil Sprinkle. Merge the spices and sprinkle the mixture over the potatoes. Bake the potato skins for 15 minutes or until they are crispy and brown.

Salted Stuffed Mushrooms
Ingredients:

- 2 tbsps. minced fresh bay leaf
- 1 tbsp. horseradish
- 2 cloves garlic, pressed
- One-Fourth mug minced scallions
- 2 tsps. Without salt butter
- 1 can (4 ounces or 115 g) crabmeat, drained
- One-Fourth tsp. warm pepper dip sauce
- 2Half mugs mushroom caps (24), stems Take away
- Ground red pepper for Decorate

Instructions:

- Merge scallions and butter in 2-mug measure. Microwave on high 2 minutes; whisk in crabmeat, bay leaf, horseradish, garlic, and pepper dip sauce. Whisk well. Put half the mushrooms, stemmed sides up, in a pie plate.
- Fill each mushroom cap with 1 tsp. crab mixture. Microwave on high 3 to 4 minutes, turning plate once. Take away mushrooms to serving plate; repeat with left-over mushrooms and filling. Let stand 2 to 3 minutes before serving. To Decorate, sprinkle with ground red pepper. Each serving contains 4 mushrooms.

Healthy Apple Cheese Snack
Ingredients:

- 1-ounce cheddar
- 1 apple
- 1 tsp. cinnamon Lactose

Instructions:

- Wash apple. Pat dry. Cut apple into quarters. Take away seeds. Cut quarters in half. Sort apple slices on a plate to resemble a pinwheel.
- Sprinkle slices with cinnamon-Lactose. Cut slice of cheese into 8 pieces. Put a piece of cheese on each apple slice. Warm in the microwave on high for 10-20 seconds until cheese Defrosts.

Herbed Cheese
Ingredients:

- 2 cloves garlic, pressed
- Half tsp. basil
- Half tsp. oregano
- 8 ounces cream cheese
- One-Fourth mug nonfat evaporated milk
- Half mug minced bay leaf

Instructions:

- Combine all the ingredients together and let stand 1 day in Fringe. Garnish with green chili and mint. Serve immediately.

Garlic Shrimp with Lemon Juice
Ingredients:

- 2 tbsps. Shallots, finely minced
- One-Fourth tsp. black pepper, freshly ground
- 2 tbsps. Lemon juice
- 1 Third-Fourth pounds (800 g) shrimp, big
- 2 tbsps. Without salt butter
- 1 tbsp. olive oil
- 1 tbsp. garlic, finely minced
- 2 tbsps. Fresh dill, finely Diced

Instructions:

- Peel off and devein shrimp. In a big frying pan over low Warm up, Defrost butter with olive oil. Add garlic and shallots and Deep-fry for 2 minutes without browning. Add shrimp, increase Warm up slightly, and Prepare shrimp for 3 minutes or until just done to taste. Add pepper to taste and Roll well.
- Take away to a dish, scraping in all the dip sauce. Add lemon juice and dill; Roll together well. Cover and freeze 3 to 4 hours before serving. Serve on the ends of bamboo skewers as an appetizer.

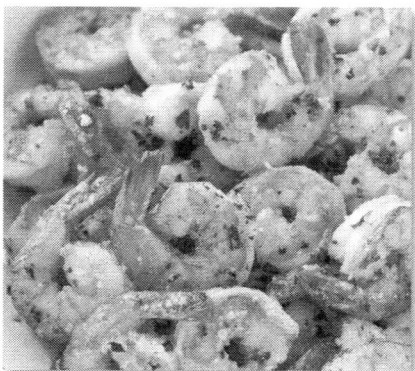

Vegetable Cheese Ball with Dip Sauce
Ingrediens:

- Half tsp. minced garlic
- 1 tsp. Worcestershire dip sauce
- 1 Half mugs (165 g) cut into small pieces carrot
- 8 ounces cream cheese, softened
- 2 mugs cut into small pieces Cheddar cheese
- Half tsp. Tabasco dip sauce
- 3 tbsps. Diced fresh bay leaf
- Half mug Diced pecans

Instructions:

- Press carrot between paper towels to Take away excess moisture; set aside.

Merge cream cheese and Cheddar cheese in a medium-sized dish; whisk well. Add carrot and garlic; whisk well. Cover and cool down 1 hour. These ingredients may also be Merged in a food processor and combined.

- Shape cheese mixture into a ball; roll in bay leaf and pecans. Wrap in waxed paper and cool down at least 1 hour.

Curried Cheese Chutney
Ingredients:

- 1 mug cheddar cheese, cut into small pieces
- 2 tbsps. tomato chutney
- 1 tsp. curry powder
- 1 tbsp. sherry
- One-Fourth mug onions, Diced
- 1 tbsp. olive oil
- 6 ounces cream cheese

Instructions:

- Deep-fry onions in oil until softened. Combine all ingredients and cool down. Garnish with green chili and mint. Serve immediately.

Roasted Red Pepper
Ingredients:

- 1 garlic clove
- 2 tbsps. olive oil
- 1 slice whole warm up bread, crusts Cropped
- 12 ounces roasted red peppers, drained

Instructions:

- In a covered food processor canister, process bread until crumbly; set aside. Add red peppers and garlic to canister. Cover and process until smooth.
- With the processor running, slowly add oil through feed tube. Add bread crumbs; cover and process until smooth. Shift to small dish. Serve cool

downed or at with crackers or Heat upped bread.

Apple Pecan Lemon Log
Ingredients:

- 1 tsp. fresh lemon juice
- 1 mug apple, Diced
- 8 ounces cream cheese, softened
- 1 tbsp. apple juice
- Half tsp. ground nutmeg
- 1 mug pecans, Diced

Instructions:

- Merge cream cheese, apple juice, and nutmeg in combiner dish and blend until smooth. Spill lemon juice over Diced apples and add to the creamed cheese mixture.
- Gently fold in mug of the pecans and then shape into a log and roll in the left-over Diced dry fruits. Wrap it in plastic and freeze until ready to serve.

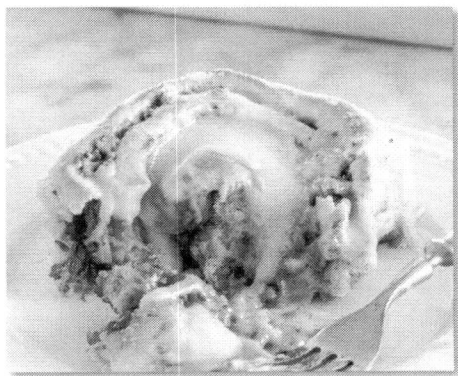

Green Onion Cheese Dip
Ingredients:

- One-Fourth mug Diced green onion
- 1 mug cottage cheese
- 2 tsps. lemon juice

Instructions:

- Merge ingredients in a blender or food processor and process until smooth. Freeze for at least an hour to give the flavors time to develop. Garnish with green chili and mint. Serve immediately.

Bean Chili Dip
Ingredients:

- 1 jalapeno pepper, finely Diced
- 1 tsp. chili powder
- 2 mugs prepared kidney beans
- 2 tbsps. olive oil
- Half tsp. crushed garlic
- 1 mug finely Diced onion
- Half mug (58 g) cut into small pieces Cheddar cheese

Instructions:

- Warm up oil in a frying pan. Add garlic, onion, jalapeno, and chili powder and Prepare gently 4 minutes. Drain kidney beans, reserving juice. Process beans in a blender or food processor to a puree. Add to onion mixture and whisk in 2 tbsps. of bean liquid; combine well.
- Whisk in cheese. Prepare gently about 2 minutes, whisking until cheese Defrosts. If mixture becomes too thick, add a little more bean liquid. Serve into serving dish and serve warm with waffle chips.

Tofu Avocado Dip Sauce
Ingredients:

- 2 tsps. minced fresh ginger
- Half mug fresh bay leaf leaves
- 2 tbsps. lemon juice
- 1 tbsp. peanut butter
- 8 ounces tofu
- Half mug avocado
- 2 garlic cloves, Diced
- 1 tbsp. apple dip sauce

Instructions:

65

- Blend all ingredients in a food processor until very smooth. Garnish with green chili and mint. Serve immediately.

Spicy Cheese Dip Sauce
Ingredients:

- 3 ounces cream cheese,
- 3 ounces blue cheese
- 8 ounces sour cream
- 2 Half tsps. (5.8 g) unflavored gelatin
- One-Fourth mug mineral water
- 2 tbsps. lemon juice
- 2 jalapeno peppers, minced
- 1 One-Fourth mugs pecans, Heat upped, Diced
- 2 ounces pimento, drained and minced

Instructions:

- Combine cheeses with sour cream until smooth. Add gelatin that has been softened in mineral water and Warm upped to dissolve.
- Add lemon juice and let stand until slightly thickened. Add jalapenos, pecans, and pimentos. Spill into mold that has been Covered with nonstick vegetable oil Sprinkle and cool down.

Bread Dish Dip
Ingredients:

- Half mug Diced green onion
- Half mug Diced fresh bay leaf
- 1 round bread loaf, homemade
- 1 mug mayonnaise
- One-Fourth mug plain curd

Instructions:

- Slice off the Cover of the loaf and scoop out as much of the interior of the loaf as possible while leaving about 2 inches (1 cm) of the crust.
- Slice the Cover and the interior into bite-size pieces. Merge the rest of the

ingredients in a big dish and combine together. Serve the mixture into the hollowed loaf and Sort the bread pieces around.

Indian Dipping Dip sauce
Ingredients:

- One-Fourth tsp. chili oil
- One-Fourth tsp. honey
- 1 tbsp. Sodium Soy Dip sauce
- 1 tsp. sesame oil
- 1 tsp. brown rice lemon juice
- 1 tbsp. mineral water

Instructions:

- Merge all ingredients in a jar with a lid. Shake to Merge. This will keep indefinitely if stored in the fridge. Garnish with green chili and mint. Serve immediately.

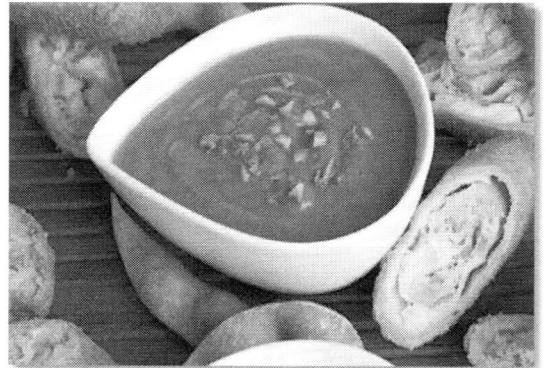

Parched Beef Appetizer Dip Sauce
Ingredients:

- 2 tbsps. minced onion
- 2 tbsps. (19 g) green pepper, finely Diced
- One-Eighth tsp. pepper
- 8 ounces cream cheese, softened
- 2 tbsps. milk
- 2 Half ounces diced parched beef, finely snipped
- Half mug sour cream
- One-Fourth mug dry fruits, coarsely Diced

Instructions:

- Blend cream cheese and milk. Whisk in parched beef, onion, green pepper, and pepper; combine well. Whisk in sour cream.
- Serve into pie plate or small shallow baking dish. Sprinkle dry fruits over Cover. Bake at 350°F for 15 minutes. Serve warm with assorted crackers.

Black Bean and Apple Warm sauce
Ingredients:

- 3 tbsps. Diced fresh cilantro
- Juice of Half big lime
- Juice of Half big orange
- 1 (15-ounce) can black beans, Soaked and drained
- Half big Granny Smith apple, chopped
- One-Fourth mug finely Diced red onion
- Half medium-sized serrano chile pepper, unseeded and finely Diced
- One-Eighth tsp. cracked black pepper
- One-Eighth tsp. sea salt

Instructions:

- Merge all the ingredients in a big dish. Before serving, freeze for at least 20 minutes so that the flavors blend. Serving Suggestion: Serve a Cover a chicken breast, or as a snack or appetizer with Without salt, baked waffle chips.

Broccoli Rabe with Pine Dry fruits
Ingredients:

- 2 tsps. olive oil
- 2 cloves garlic, minced
- 1 bunch broccoli rabe, coarsely Diced into ¾-inch-wide pieces
- One-Fourth mug pine dry fruits
- 2 tsps. red wine lemon juice
- One-Fourth tsp. kosher salt

Instructions:

- Soak the broccoli rabe well in a big dish of cold mineral water, then lift the pieces out of the mineral water, leaving any grit behind in the dish, and Shift to another dish; do not drain. Warm up a nonstick medium-sized frying pan over medium-sized Warm up. Add the pine dry fruits and Prepare, whisking from time to time, until Heat upped, about 2 minutes.
- Shift the dry fruits to a small plate. Prepare the oil and garlic in the frying pan over medium-sized Warm up, whisking often, until the garlic softens, about 1 minute. In batches, add the broccoli rabe and any clinging mineral water to the frying pan. Cover and Prepare, whisking from time to time, until ripe, about 15 minutes.
- Whisk in the lemon juice. Season with the salt, and whisk in the pine dry fruits. Shift to a serving dish and serve warm.

Tropical Tomatoes sauce
Ingredients:

- Half mug chopped red onion
- 3 tbsps. Diced fresh cilantro
- Half big jalapeño chile pepper, finely Diced (seeded for less Warm up)
- Juice of 1 lime
- One-Eighth tsp. sea salt
- 1 big mango, Peel offed, pitted, and chopped
- 2 big avocados, Peel offed, pitted, and chopped
- 1 small Poblano pepper, chopped
- 2 big Roma tomatoes, chopped
- One-Eighth tsp. cracked black pepper

Instructions:

- Merge all the ingredients in a big dish. Before serving, freeze for at least 20 minutes so that the flavors blend. Garnish with green chili and mint. Serve immediately.

French Chives Onion Dip
Ingredients:

- 1 mug low-fat sour cream
- 2 tbsps. Worcestershire dip sauce
- One-Eighth tsp. sea salt
- 2 tbsps. extra virgin olive oil
- 1 small white onion, Diced
- 2 cloves garlic, minced
- 1 mug low-fat plain Greek curd
- One-Eighth tsp. cracked black pepper
- Minced chives, for Decorate

Instructions:

- Warm up the oil in a small pan over low Warm up. Add the onion and garlic, and Deep-fry until the onion becomes brown and ripe. Take away from Warm up.
- In a set apart dish, Merge the curd, sour cream, Worcestershire dip sauce, and salt and pepper to taste. Add the onion and garlic mixture, and combine well. Decorate with minced chives. Serving Suggestion: Serve with flaxseed chips, Diced bell pepper, cucumber, and baby carrots.

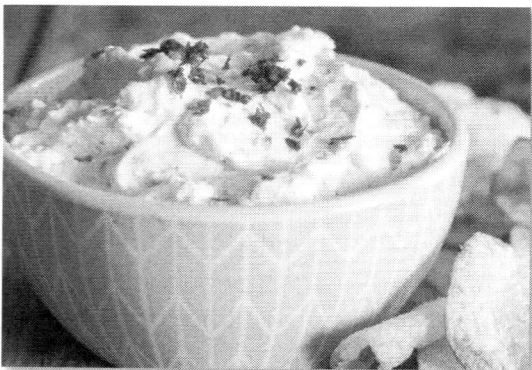

Sweet Potato Fillet-steak Fries
Ingredients:

- Half tsp. cayenne pepper
- One-Fourth tsp. cracked black pepper
- One-Fourth tsp. sea salt
- 1 pound (about 4 medium-sized) sweet potatoes, unpeel offed
- 4 tbsps. extra virgin olive oil
- Half tsp. ground cumin

Instructions:

- Fill a big pot with mineral water, and bring it to a boil. Add the sweet potatoes, and boil 10 to 12 minutes, or until an inserted fork glides in easily but the potato is slightly firm in the center. Strain the potatoes, and let them cool.
- Once cooled, cut them in half longitudinally and then into Half-inch-thick pieces longitudinally. The skin may Peel off a bit, but keep it on as it provides nutritious fiber. Brush oil onto each slice, and sprinkle with cumin, cayenne, and black pepper. Sort on the Roast, and Prepare 1 to 2 minutes per side. Take away from the Warm up, season with salt, and serve.

Roasted Garlic Asparagus
Ingredients:

- Juice of Half lemon
- 3 big cloves garlic, minced
- One-Fourth tsp. sea salt
- 1-pound asparagus
- 5 tbsps. extra virgin olive oil
- Grind zest of 1 big lemon
- One-Eighth tsp. cracked black pepper

Instructions:

- Cut off and discard the fibrous thick ends of the asparagus spears. In a big baking dish or rimmed Prepare sheets, lay the spears in a single, even layer, and Sprinkle with oil. Roll the spears in the oil to Cover evenly.

- Add the lemon zest, lemon juice, garlic, salt, and pepper over the Cover. Roll the spears again, to Cover all sides with the seasonings. Put on a warm Roast, and rotate the spears constantly so they do not burn. Roast for about 2 minutes, and put back to marinating pan to serve.

Roasted Lemon Collard Greens
Ingredients:

- 5 tbsps. extra virgin olive oil
- One-Fourth tsp. sea salt
- 1-pound collard greens
- 4 tbsps. red wine lemon juice
- One-Fourth tsp. cracked black pepper

Instructions:

- Cut off the thick ends of the stems, and then wash the greens and pat them completely dry. Lay each leaf directly on a warm Roast. After 30 seconds, flip each leaf over. When they start to wither and blacken, take away the leaves, Put them in a big pot, and cover with a lid. After all the leaves have been Roasted, let them sit in the covered pot for about 5 minutes to continue Brewing.
- Take away the leaves from the pot, and cut them into 2- inch-wide pieces. Put them back in the pot, cover with the lemon juice, oil, salt, and pepper to taste. Serve warm or cool downed.

Brussels Black Pepper Sprouts Casserole
Ingredients:

- 2 tbsps. Diced shallot
- 2 big cloves garlic, finely minced
- Half mug Heat upped pine dry fruits, Cut up

- 1 Half pounds (6 mugs) Brussels sprouts
- 2 thick slices pancetta, chopped
- Half tsp. cracked black pepper

Instructions:

- Switch on the oven to 400°F. Bring a big pot of mineral water to a boil. Peel off up and discard the outer leaves of the Brussels sprouts and Crop the stems. Halve the Brussels sprouts, and add to the boiling mineral water. Boil 10 to 15 minutes, or until the sprouts are easily pierced with a fork. Drain and set aside.
- Crop the fat from the pancetta before dicing. Warm up a big dip saucepan over medium-sized Warm up, and add the pancetta. Deep-fry until brown and crispy, about 4 to 5 minutes. Shift the pancetta to paper towels to drain.
- Add the garlic and shallots and half the pine dry fruits to the same pan. Prepare until the dry fruits turn light brown, about 1 to 2 minutes, and then add the Brussels sprouts. Prepare them for an additional 2 to 3 minutes so they absorb the pancetta and garlic flavors.
- Spill the mixture into an 8-by 8-inch baking dish, season with pepper, and bake for 10 to 15 minutes, or until the Covers of the Brussels sprouts brown. Take away from the oven, and Cover with the left-over pine dry fruits before serving.

Roasted Fresh Basil Cauliflower
Ingredients:

- Half tsp. chile pepper flakes
- Grind zest of 1 big lemon
- One-Eighth tsp. sea salt
- 4 mugs cauliflower florets (1 small head cauliflower)
- 4 tbsps. extra virgin olive oil
- 3 big cloves garlic, minced

- One-Eighth tsp. cracked black pepper
- 3 tbsps. Diced fresh basil

Instructions:

- Switch on the oven to 400°F. Take away and discard the stems and core of the cauliflower. Put the cauliflower head in an 8- by 8-inch baking dish. Sprinkle with oil, and then sprinkle on the garlic, chile pepper flakes, lemon zest, salt, and pepper.
- Shake the pan a bit so that the oil Expands and the ingredients cover the cauliflower. Bake 15 to 20 minutes, shaking the pan after 10 minutes to prevent the cauliflower from sticking. Take away from the Warm up, cover with fresh basil, and serve instantly.

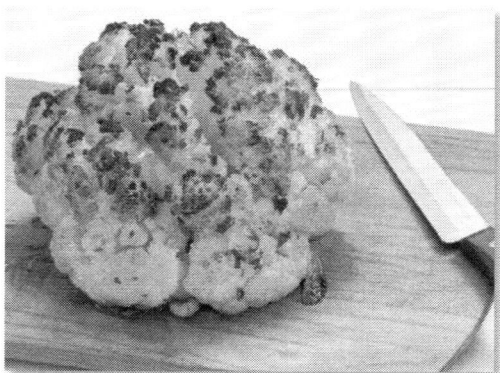

Salty Corn and Vegetable Pudding
Ingredients:

- 1 clove garlic, minced
- Half jalapeño, seeded and minced
- 2 mugs fresh corn kernels (cut from 3 big ears of corn)
- 2 tsps. Cornstarch
- 2 tsps. canola oil, plus more in a pump Sprinkler
- 1 medium-sized Poblano pepper, cored and cut into Pieces
- 2 scallions, white and green parts, finely Diced
- 1 mug low-fat (1%) milk

- 1 big egg plus 2 big egg whites
- Half tsp. kosher salt
- One-Fourth tsp. freshly ground black pepper

Instructions:

- Switch on the oven to 350°F. Sprinkle a 1 Half-quart or 2-quart round baking dish with canola oil. Warm up the 2 tsps. oil in a medium-sized nonstick frying pan over medium-sized Warm up. Add the bell pepper, scallions, garlic, and jalapeño and Prepare, whisking often, until the bell pepper is ripe, about 5 minutes. Add the corn kernels and Prepare, whisking often, until Warm upped through, about 5 minutes.
- Shift to a medium-sized dish and let cool slightly. Sprinkle the cornstarch over the milk in a medium-sized dish and Whip to dissolve. Add the egg, egg whites, salt, and pepper and Whip together. Spill over the corn mixture and whisk well. Spill into the baking dish. Bake just until a knife inserted in the center of the pudding comes out wipe, about 30 minutes. Let stand for 5 minutes, then serve warm.

Roasted Eggplant and Cucumber
Ingredients:

- One-Fourth tsp. parched oregano
- 1 big eggplant, diced into Half-inch rounds
- 2 cucumbers, diced longitudinally
- One-Eighth tsp. cracked black pepper
- One-Fourth tsp. parched bay leaf
- One-Fourth tsp. parched basil
- One-Fourth tsp. sea salt, Cut up
- 6 tbsps. balsamic lemon juice
- 4 tbsps. extra virgin olive oil

Instructions:

- Lay the diced eggplant on paper towels, and sprinkle each slice with a pinch of salt to pull out excess moisture. After 10 to 15 minutes, pat the slices dry with paper towels. Sort the eggplant and cucumber on a Prepare sheet with edges on it.
- Sprinkle pepper and parched herbs over the herbs, and Sprinkle with lemon juice and oil. Roast the herbs on a warm Roast or Roast pan for 4 to 6 minutes, flipping halfway through. Take away from the Roast or Roast pan and serve.

Barley and Herbs
Ingredients:

- One-Fourth mug Diced red onion
- 1 small clove garlic, minced
- 1 mug unprepared Barley
- 2 mugs vegetable broth
- 2 tbsps. extra virgin olive oil
- 1 big cucumber, Diced into small cubes
- One-Eighth tsp. chile pepper flakes
- 3 mugs green lettuce

Instructions:

- Soak the Barley (if not presoaked). Put the Barley and broth in a big pot, and bring to a boil. Decrease Warm up to low, and cover with lid slightly ajar. Simmer on low for about 15 to 20 minutes, or until liquid is absorbed and the Barley has uncoiled and is al dente. Warm up the oil in a set apart pan over medium-sized Warm up.
- Add the onion, garlic, and cucumber, and Prepare until the onion is translucent. Season with chile flakes, and Shift the herbs to the pot with the prepared Barley. Add the green lettuce, whisk, and cover the pot. Let sit for 5 minutes. Serve warm.

Black Beans and Brown rice
Ingredients:

- Half mug long-grain brown rice
- 1 Half mugs mineral water
- Half tsp. kosher salt
- 1 (15-ounce) can decreased-sodium black beans,
- 2 tsps. olive oil
- 1 small yellow onion, finely Diced
- 1 clove garlic, minced
- 2 tbsps. finely Diced fresh cilantro

Instructions:

- Warm up the oil in a small dip saucepan over medium-sized Warm up. Add the onion and garlic and Prepare, whisking from time to time, until ripe, about 5 minutes. Add the brown rice and whisk well. Whisk in the mineral water and salt and bring to a boil. Decrease the Warm up to low and cover tightly.
- Simmer until the brown rice is ripe and almost all the liquid has been absorbed, about 40 minutes. Add the beans, but do not whisk them into the brown rice. Cover the dip saucepan again and Prepare until the liquid is absorbed and the beans are warm, about 5 minutes. Take away from the Warm up and let stand for 5 minutes. Whisk in the cilantro with a fork, fluffing the brown rice as you do so. Shift to a serving dish and serve warm.

Rapid "Baked" Beans
Ingredients:

- 1 small Poblano pepper, cored and cut into Pieces
- 1 Granny Smith apple, cored and cut into Pieces
- 1 (15-ounce) can no-salt
- 1 shred decreased-sodium bacon, coarsely Diced

- 1 tsp. canola oil
- 1 small yellow onion, Diced
- no-salt-added tomato ketchup
- 1 tbsp. amber agave nectar, maple syrup, or honey
- 1 tbsp. cider lemon juice

Instructions:

- Prepare the bacon and oil together in a medium-sized dip saucepan over medium-sized Warm up, whisking from time to time, until crisp and browned, about 6 minutes.
- Add the onion, bell pepper, and apple and Prepare, whisking from time to time, until the onion softens, about 5 minutes. Whisk in the beans, ketchup, agave, and lemon juice. Prepare, whisking from time to time, until the dip sauce has thickened slightly, about 10 minutes. Serve warm.

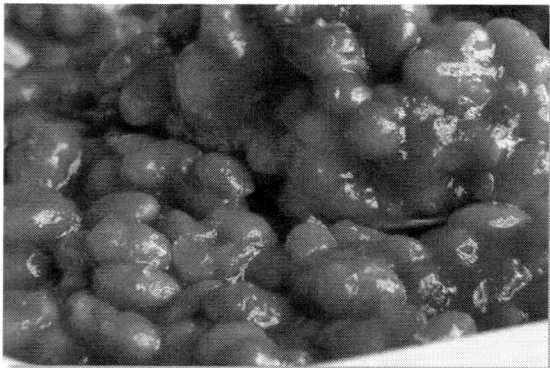

Choy and Shiitake Mushrooms
Ingredients:

- 1 tbsp. unpeel offed finely cut into small pieces fresh ginger
- 2 cloves garlic, minced
- 6 baby book choy (6 ounces), well Soaked
- 2 tsps. canola or corn oil
- 8 shiitake mushrooms, stems discarded, cut in half vertically
- 1 scallion, white and green parts, finely Diced

- Half mug Homemade Chicken Broth or canned low-sodium chicken broth One-Fourth mug
- plus 1 tbsp. mineral water
- 2 tsps. decreased-sodium soy dip sauce
- One-Eighth tsp. crushed warm red pepper flakes 1 tsp. cornstarch

Instructions:

- Warm up the oil in a big nonstick frying pan over medium-sized-high Warm up. Add the mushrooms and Prepare, whisking from time to time, until lightly browned, about 6 minutes. Add the scallion, ginger, and garlic and whisk until fragrant, about 30 seconds. Sort the book choy in the frying pan.
- Add the broth, the One-Fourth mug mineral water, soy dip sauce, and warm pepper and bring to a simmer. Decrease the Warm up to low and cover. Simmer until the book choy is just ripe when pierced with the tip of a small, sharp knife, 7 to 10 minutes. Using a slotted Serve, Shift the vegetable mixture to a serving dish. Spill the left-over 1 tbsp. mineral water into a ramekin or custard mug, sprinkle in the cornstarch, and whisk until dissolved.
- Whip into the frying pan and bring to a simmer to thicken the dip sauce. Spill any juices from the serving dish into the frying pan and Whip. Spill the dip sauce over the veggies and serve warm.

Broccoli Olive Ziti
Ingredients:

- 1 tbsp. olive oil
- 1 Half mugs ziti or other tubular macaroni
- Pinch of kosher salt
- 1 clove garlic, minced
- 1 broccoli head (about 14 ounces)
- Pinch of freshly ground black pepper

- Bring a big pot of mineral water to a boil over high Warm up.

Instructions:

- Warm up the oil and garlic together in a small frying pan over medium-sized Warm up, whisking often, until the garlic is softened and fragrant, but not browned, about 2 minutes. Take away from the Warm up and set aside.
- Crop the broccoli, cutting the florets from the stalks. Peel off the stalks with a vegetable Peel offer (don't worry about getting every bit of the Peel off off) and cut crosswise into One-Fourth-inch-thick slices. Cut the florets into bite-sized pieces. Add the broccoli to the boiling mineral water and Prepare until crisp-ripe, about 5 minutes. Using a wire sieve or a skimmer, Shift the broccoli to a dish. Leave the mineral water boiling.
- Add the ziti and Prepare according to the package directions until al dente. During the last minute, put back the broccoli to the mineral water. Drain the ziti and broccoli and Shift to a serving dish. Whisk in the garlic-oil mixture, salt, and pepper. Serve warm.

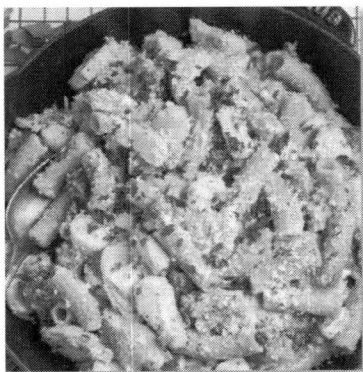

Brussels Sprouts with Heat upped Almonds
Ingredients:

- One-Fourth mug diced almonds; Heat upped 1 tbsp. sherry

- Lemon juice
- Olive oil in a pump Sprinkler
- 10 ounces Brussels sprouts, Cropped and halved
- One-Eighth tsp. freshly ground black pepper

Instructions:

- Switch on the oven to 400°F. Sprinkle a big baking sheet with oil. Expand the Brussels sprouts on the baking sheet and Sprinkle them with oil.
- Bake, whisking from time to time, until barely ripe with browned edges, 30 to 40 minutes. Shift to a serving dish. Sprinkle with the almonds, lemon juice, and pepper and Roll. Serve warm.

Carrots with Ginger-Lime Butter
Ingredients:

- 2 tsps. Peel offed and minced fresh ginger
- Freshly grind zest of Half lime
- 1 tbsp. fresh lime juice
- 8 ounces baby-cut carrots
- 1 mug softened frozen edamame
- 2 tsps. Without salt butter
- Pinch of kosher salt
- Pinch of freshly ground black pepper

Instructions:

- Bring a medium-sized dip saucepan of mineral water to a boil over high Warm up. Add the carrots and Prepare until almost ripe, about 6 minutes. Add the edamame and Prepare until Warm upped through, about 2 minutes more.
- Drain in a colander. Prepare the butter and ginger together in the dip saucepan over medium-sized Warm up, whisking often, until the ginger softens, about 2 minutes. Add the veggies, lime zest and juice, salt, and pepper and combine well. Shift to a serving dish and serve warm.

Healthy Collard Greens with Bacon
Ingredients:

- 2 cloves garlic, minced

- 1 (1-pound) bag Diced collard greens, Soaked, but not parched
- Half mug mineral waters
- Half tsp. crushed warm red pepper
- 2 slices decreased-sodium bacon, coarsely Diced
- 1 tsp. vegetable oil
- 1 medium-sized yellow onion, Diced
- 2 tsps. cider lemon juice

Instructions:

- Prepare the bacon and oil in a big dip saucepan over medium-sized Warm up, whisking often, until the bacon is crisp and browned, about 6 minutes. Add the onion and Prepare, whisking from time to time, until golden, about 5 minutes.
- Whisk in the garlic and Prepare until fragrant, about 30 seconds. In batches, whisk in the collard greens with any clinging mineral water and cover, letting the first batch wilt before adding another. Add the mineral water and warm pepper. Decrease the Warm up to medium-sized-low and cover.
- Prepare, whisking from time to time, until the collard greens are very ripe, about 30 minutes. Whisk in the lemon juice. Shift the collard greens and any Preparing liquid to a serving dish and serve warm.

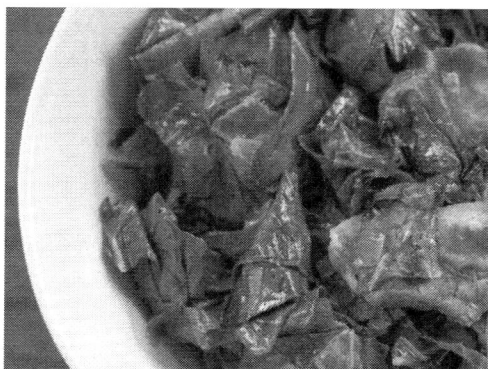

Corn and Tomato Deep-fry
Ingredients:

- 1 tbsp. finely Diced shallot
- Half tsp. finely Diced fresh thyme, or One-Fourth tsp. parched thyme One-Fourth tsp.

- kosher salt
- Olive oil in a pump Sprinkler
- 1 Half mugs fresh corn kernels (from 3 ears of corn)
- 1 mug cherry or grape tomatoes, cut in halves crosswise
- One-Eighth tsp. freshly ground black pepper

Instructions:

- Sprinkle a big nonstick frying pan with oil and Warm up over medium-sized-high Warm up. Add the corn and Prepare, whisking from time to time, until the kernels begin to brown, about 5 minutes. Whisk in the tomatoes, shallot, thyme, salt, and pepper and Prepare, whisking often, until the tomatoes are Warm upped through, about 3 minutes. Serve warm.

Lemon Garlic Herb Brown rice
Ingredients:

- One-Fourth tsp. garlic powder
- Half tsp. onion powder
- 1 tbsp. fresh bay leaf, Diced
- 2 mugs brown rice, prepared
- One-Fourth mug low sodium chicken broth
- 2 tbsps. lemon juice
- One-Fourth tsp. black pepper

Instructions:

- Whisk all ingredients together in a dip saucepan or microwave safe dish and Warm up through. Garnish with green chili and lettuce. Let stand for 5 minutes, then serve warm.

Asian Cale and White Beans
Ingrediens:

- 1 Pound Dark kalte
- Ohne-Forth kalte koscher spalt
- 1 nbsp. Olive Oliv
- 1 medium-sized yellow onion, Diced
- 3 cloves garlic, minced
- One-Eighth tsp. crushed warm red pepper
- 1 (15-ounce) can no-salt-added cannellini beans, 1 tbsp.
- red wine lemon juice

Instructions:

- Warm up the oil in a big dip saucepan over medium-sized Warm up. Add the onion and garlic and Prepare, whisking often, until the onion is translucent, about 5 minutes. Meanwhile, pull off and discard the thick stems from the kale. Taking a few pieces at a time, stack the kale and coarsely slice crosswise into Half-inch-thick shreds.
- Shift to a big dish of cold mineral water and agitate to loosen any grit. Lift the kale out of the mineral water, leaving behind any dirt. Do not dry the kale. Add the kale, salt, and warm pepper to the dip saucepan.
- Cover and Prepare, whisking from time to time, until the kale is almost ripe, about 10 minutes. Whisk in the beans and Prepare, whisking from time to time, until the kale is ripe and the beans are Warm upped through, about 5 minutes. Take away from the Warm up and whisk in the lemon juice. Serve warm.

Mushrooms with Thyme and Garlic
Ingredients:

- Half tsp. kosher salt
- One-Fourth tsp. freshly ground black pepper
- 2 (10-ounce) canisters white mushrooms
- 1 tsp. finely Diced fresh thyme
- 2 garlic cloves, thinly diced

Instructions:

- Combine the mushrooms, oil, thyme, salt, and pepper in a big dish to Cover the mushrooms. Expand on a big rimmed baking sheet. Bake the mushrooms, whisking from time to time, until they are ripe and beginning to brown, about 25 minutes.
- Tuck the garlic slices under the mushrooms (where they will be protected and not burn) and Prepare until the garlic softens, about 5 minutes more. Serve warm.

Bay Leaf Brown rice
Ingredients:

- 1 parched bay leaf
- 1 mug brown rice
- 2 mugs mineral water

Instructions:

- Bring the brown rice, bay leaf, and 2 mugs of mineral water to a boil in a small heavy-based dip saucepan over high Warm up. Decrease the Warm up to medium-sized-low and tightly cover the dip saucepan. Simmer, without whisking the brown rice, until it is ripe and has absorbed the mineral water, about 40 minutes.
- If the mineral water evaporates before the brown rice is ripe, add 2 tbsps. warm mineral water to the dip saucepan (do not whisk it in). Take away from the Warm up and let stand for 5 minutes. Fluff the brown rice with a fork. Discard the bay leaf. If any mineral water remains in the dip saucepan when the brown rice is ripe, drain the brown rice in a wire sieve. Serve warm.

Indian Brown rice with Cashews, Raisins, and Spices
Ingredients:

- Two-third mug basmati brown rice
- One-Fourth tsp. ground turmeric
- 1 (2-inch) piece cinnamon stick
- One-Eighth tsp. ground coriander
- 2 tsps. canola oil
- 1 small yellow onion, finely Diced
- 1 tsp. Peel offed and minced fresh ginger
- 1 small clove garlic, minced
- One-Eighth tsp. freshly ground black pepper

Instructions:

- Warm up the oil in a medium-sized dip saucepan over medium-sized Warm up. Add the onion, ginger, and garlic and Deep-fry, whisking often, until softened, about 3 minutes. Add the brown rice, turmeric (if using), cinnamon, coriander, and pepper and whisk for 30 seconds. Add the broth and bring to a simmer.

- Decrease the Warm up to medium-sized-low and tightly cover the dip saucepan. Prepare until the liquid is absorbed and the brown rice is ripe, about 20 minutes. Take away the dip saucepan from the Warm up.
- Add the cashews and raisins, but do not whisk them in. Cover the dip saucepan and let stand for 5 minutes. Fluff the brown rice with a fork, whisking in the cashews and raisins. Shift to a serving dish and serve at once.

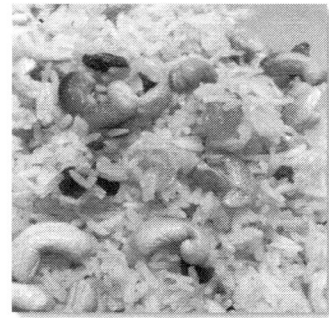

Open-Faced Breakfast Sandwich
Ingredients:

- ½ whole-wheat English muffin
- 1 slice reduced-fat (2% milk) Swiss cheese, torn into pieces to fit the muffin
- Olive oil in a pump sprayer
- ½ cup seasoned liquid egg substitute
- 1½ teaspoons finely chopped scallion (green part only)

Instructions:

- Toast the English muffin in an oven toaster or broiler. Turn off the toaster (or broiler). Top the muffin with the cheese pieces and let stand until the cheese is melted by the residual heat, about 30 seconds.
- Transfer to a plate.
- Meanwhile, spray a small nonstick skillet with the oil and heat over medium heat. Add the egg
- substitute and cook until the edges are set, about 15 seconds. Using a heatproof spatula, lift the edges of the egg substitute so the uncooked liquid can flow underneath. Continue cooking, lifting the edges about every 15 seconds, until the egg mixture is set, about 1½ minutes total. Using the spatula, fold the edges of the egg mixture into the center to make a rough-shaped "patty" about 3 inches across.
- Transfer the egg patty to the muffin and sprinkle with the scallion. Serve hot.

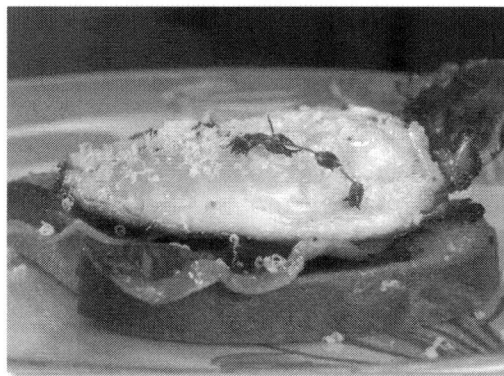

Tartine with Cream Cheese and Strawberries
Ingredients:

- 1 slice whole-grain bread
- 2 tablespoons spreadable fat-free cream cheese
- 2 large strawberries, hulled and sliced
- 1 teaspoon honey (optional)

Instructions:

- Toast the bread in a toaster. Spread with the cream cheese, and top with the strawberries. Drizzle with the honey, if using.

Applesauce and Oatmeal Squares
Ingredients:

- 1 egg
- ½ cup applesauce, sweetened
- 1 ½ cups non-fat or 1% milk
- 1 tsp. vanilla
- 2 Tbsps. oil
- 1 apple, chopped (about 1 ½ cups)
- 2 cups rolled oats
- 1 tsp. baking powder
- ¼ tsp. salt
- 1 tsp. cinnamon

Topping:

- 2 Tbsps. brown sugar
- 2 Tbsps. chopped nuts

Instructions:

- Preheat the oven to a temperature of 375 degrees.
- Prepare a baking tray of about 8"x8", lightly oil the tray and leave aside.
- Place the rolled oats in a bowl and add the baking powder, cinnamon and salt.
- Mix all ingredients well and leave aside.
- In a separate bowl, beat the egg and mix in the milk, applesauce and vanilla.
- Finally mix in the oil and mix well.
- Pour the egg mixture into the rolled oats mixture and mix once again until all ingredients are well combined.
- Pour this mixture into the prepared baking tray and place in the oven.
- Leave for 25-30 minutes until well browned and remove from the oven.
- Sprinkle the 2 tbsps. of the brown sugar on the surface.
- Place the tray once again in the oven and leave for 4 minutes.
- Remove from oven and cut into squares of your preference.
- Serve to guests and the balance squares could be refrigerated for future use.
- Enjoy!

Sweet and Sour Almond Muffins
Ingredients:

- 1 3/4 cups
- all-purpose flour
- 2 tsp baking powder
- ½ tsp salt 1 cup sugar 4 large eggs 2 tsp grated orange zest 2 tsp grated lemon
- zest 2 Tbsp balsamic vinegar
- 2 Tbsp whole milk
- 3/4 cup extra-virgin olive oil 2/3 cup sliced almonds, toasted and crushed

Instructions:

- Preheat the oven to a temperature of 350F.

- Prepare a muffin pan consisting of 12 cups and insert paper lines in each cup.
- Sift flour, baking powder together and place in a bowl.
- Add the salt and leave aside.
- In a separate bowl, place the eggs and beat well.
- Mix in the sugar, orange zest, lemon zest and beat until pale in color.
- Pour the vinegar, milk and oil into the mixture.
- Fold in the flour mixture and mix with the hand until all ingredients are well combined.
- Toss in the almonds.
- Pour the mixture into muffin cups.
- Place in the oven and bake for 25 minutes.
- Allow to cool for a few minutes.
- Enjoy!

Onion and Asparagus Frittata
Ingredients:

- 1 tsp olive oil
- 1 medium onion, thinly sliced
- 2 tsp balsamic vinegar
- 2 cups (about 1 bunch) asparagus, cut into 1-inch sections
- 3 green onions, sliced
- ¼ cup fresh basil, thinly sliced
- 6 large eggs
- ¼ cup plus 1 tbsp parmesan cheese, grated
- ½ tsp kosher salt
- Fresh ground pepper to taste

Instructions:

- Preheat the broiler to a high temperature.
- Heat an oven proof dish for a few minutes.
- Pour the olive oil and heat well.
- Toss in the sliced onion and cook for about 5 minutes until soft and tender.

- Pour the vinegar into the onion mixture.
- Toss in the cut asparagus and water (about 2 tbsps.), cover and steam for about 5 minutes.
- In the meantime, place the eggs in a bowl and whisk well.
- Toss in the ¼ cup of the parmesan, ¼ tsp salt and a dash of pepper.
- Mix in the sliced green onions, sliced basil and the balance salt to the asparagus mixture.
- Spoon the whisked egg mixture to the asparagus and mix well.
- Use a spatula to bring the cooked egg to the surface.
- Leave for about 2-3 minutes for the ingredients to cook through.
- Leave the pan for about 3-4 minutes just under the broiler and add the balance cheese.
- Allow the pan to be kept under broiler for about 3 minutes until the mixture is a slight brown.
- Take out from the broiler and add the 1 tbsp of parmesan
- Leave for 5 minutes and remove the frittata from the pan to a wooden cutting board.
- Cut into 4 portions and serve.

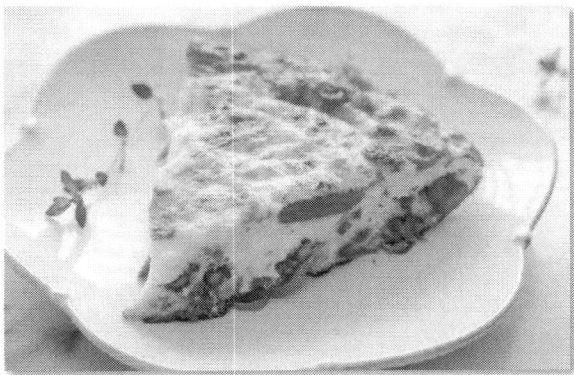

Strawberries and Orange Swirl
Ingredients:

- 2 (10-oz.) packages frozen strawberries in light syrup
- 1 (6-oz.) container plain low-fat yogurt

- 1 cup fresh orange juice
- 1 cup fat-free milk

Instructions:

- Place all ingredients in a blender.
- Process until the mixture is smooth in consistency.
- Serve and enjoy!

Nutty Pancakes
Ingredients:

- 1 cup whole wheat flour
- 2 tsp baking powder
- 1/4 tsp salt
- 1/4 tsp cinnamon
- 1 large banana, mashed
- 1 cup 1% milk
- 3 large egg whites
- 2 tsp oil
- 1 tsp vanilla
- 2 tbsp chopped walnuts

Instructions:

- Place all the dry ingredients in a bowl.
- Pour the milk into another bowl.
- Separate the eggs and add the egg whites to the milk.
- Mix in the vanilla, mashed banana and oil and combine well ensuring not to over mix.
- Heat a pan on a medium temperature.
- Use a cooking spray slightly.
- Start on the pancakes and pour about 1/4 the of a cup of the batter onto the pan.
- Once the pancake is firm and lightly browned on one side, flip each pancake to the other side.
- Remove the cooked pancake from the pan.
- Cook the pancakes until the batter is over.
- Serve warm

Breakfast Fruit Split
Ingredients:

- 1 small banana, peeled
- ½ cup oat, corn, or granola cereal
- ½ cup low fat vanilla or strawberry yogurt
- ½ tsp. honey, optional (skip for children under the age of one)
- ½ Cup Canned Pineapple Tidbits or Chunks

Instructions:

- Cut the peeled banana lengthways.
- Place each piece in two bowls, preferably cereal bowls.
- Add a dash of granola over the banana pieces and leave a little of the granola for further use.
- Spread the yogurt on top of the granola.
- Add a bit of honey over the yogurt.
- Top up with the extra granola and pineapple chunks.
- Serve and enjoy!
- Leftover could be refrigerated within a 2-hour frame.

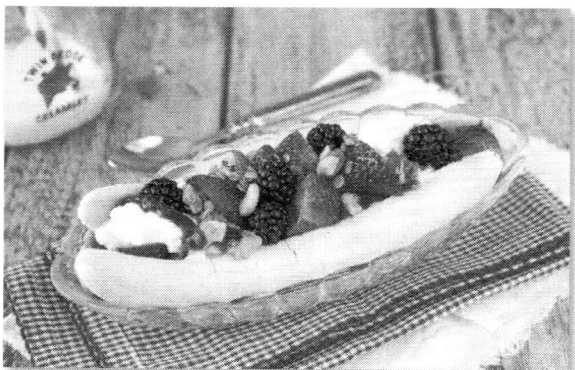

Early Morning Fruit Crunch
Ingredients:

- 4 cups assorted fresh fruit, such as orange or grapefruit sections, chopped
- apple or pear, seedless grapes, cubed fresh pineapple and/or peeled and sliced
- kiwi fruit 2 6-oz. carton low-fat vanilla yogurt 2 Tbsps. honey

- 1/2 cup low-fat granola or Grape Nut cereal (wheat and barley nugget cereal)
- 1/4 cup coconut, toasted (optional)

Instructions:

- Take 6 parfait glasses and insert the fresh fruits into the glasses.
- Spread the yogurt on top of the fruits.
- Sprinkle with a bit of honey, granola and toasted coconut (Optional).
- Enjoy!

Fruit Green Smoothie
Ingredients:

- 1 medium banana
- 1 cup baby spinach, packed
- 1/2 cup fat-free milk
- 1/4 cup whole oats
- 3/4 cup frozen mango
- 1/4 cup plain nonfat yogurt
- 1/2 tsp. vanilla

Instructions:

- Place the oats in a blender.
- Mix in the yogurt and milk and process on for about 15 seconds on high.
- Mix in the spinach, mango, banana and a bit of vanilla.
- Process until the mixture is smooth in consistency.
- If you prefer the smoothie to be a bit thicker in consistency freeze the peeled banana overnight.

Stuffed Peach Halves
Ingredients:

- 4 peaches, halved and pitted
- 1/2 cup dried tropical mixed fruit (such as Sunkist brand) 1/4 cup slivered
- almonds, toasted 2 Tbsps. graham cracker crumbs 2 Tbsps. brown sugar
- 1/4 tsp. ground allspice
- 1 (12-oz.) can peach nectar
- 1/2 cup vanilla yogurt, divided

Instructions:

- Preheat the oven to a temperature of 350F.
- Remove the pulp from each peach half leaving about 2" cavity in the middle.
- Leave the scooped-out pulp aside.
- Chop the pulp into very fine pieces.
- Mix the chopped pulp, dried fruit, almonds, cracker crumbs, all spice and the brown sugar together.
- Spread the pulp mixture on each peach half.
- Place the fruits in a baking dish.
- Pour the contents of the peach nectar into the pan.
- Bake for about 35-40 minutes until the fruits are soft and tender.
- Use a spoon and sprinkle the nectar from the pan on the fruits.
- Spread each fruit with yogurt.
- Serve

Stuffed French Toast
Ingredients:

- 1/2 cup fat-free cream cheese (about 5 oz.) 2 Tbsps. strawberry or apricot
- spreadable fruit 8 1-inch slices whole wheat French bread
- 2 egg whites
- 1 egg, slightly beaten
- 3/4 cup fat-free milk
- 1/2 tsp. vanilla
- 1/8 tsp. apple pie spice
- Nonstick cooking spray
- 1/2 cup strawberry or apricot spreadable fruit

Instructions:

- Place cream cheese in a bowl.
- Add the 2 tbsp of strawberry or apricot spreadable fruit and mix well.
- Take the bread slices and make a horizontal slit in the middle of each slice.
- Stuff a little of the cream cheese mix into each slit.

- Place the egg whites, slightly beaten egg, vanilla, milk and apple spice in a bowl and mix well.
- Insert the slices of bread into the egg mix and ensure to coat both sides.
- Heat a lightly sprayed griddle and place the coated bread on the griddle.
- Allow the bread slices to turn a slight brown for about 3-4 minutes.
- Place the balance ½ cup of strawberry or apricot spreadable fruit and heat until well melted.
- Spread the melted spreadable fruit over the toast.
- Serve and enjoy.

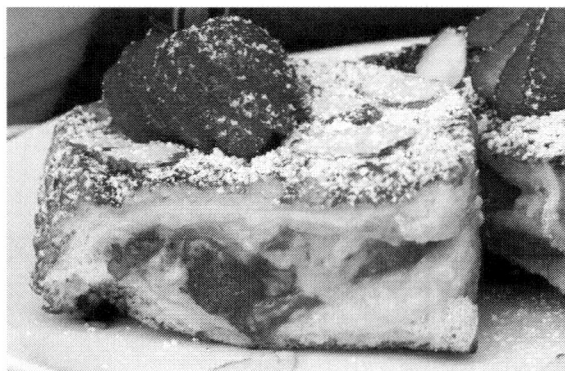

Breakfast Triple Strata
Ingredients:

- 8 oz. whole wheat bread,
- cut into 1-inch cubes
- 6 oz. low sodium turkey or chicken breakfast sausage
- 1 medium russet potato (peel optional) cut into ¼-inch slices
- 2 cups fat-free milk
- 1 ½ cup (4 oz.) reduced fat shredded sharp cheddar cheese
- 3 large eggs
- 12 oz. egg substitute (such as Egg Beaters)
- ½ cup chopped green onions
- 1 cup sliced mushrooms
- ½ tsp. paprika
- Dash of Ground Black Pepper

Instructions:

- Preheat the oven to a temperature of 400F.
- Place the 1" bread cubes on a baking tray.
- Bake for about 8-10 minutes until the cubes are slightly toasted.
- Place the sausages in a pan and cook for 7-8 minutes until slightly browned.
- Add the cheese, eggs, milk, egg substitute, spices in a separate bowl and stir using a whisk.
- Toss in the bread cubes, potatoes, sausage, mushrooms and scallions and mix well.
- Place the mixture in a baking tray.
- Cover with lid and refrigerate for 8 hours.
- Subsequently, preheat the oven temperature to 350F.
- Remove cover and bake for about 350F.
- Cut into pieces

Easy Spanish Scramble
Ingredients:

- Cooking spray
- 3/4 cup chopped seeded tomato 1/4 cup chopped green bell pepper 1/4 cup
- sliced green onions
- 3 large eggs
- 1 1/2 cups egg substitute 1/4 cup fat-free milk
- 1/4 tsp. salt
- 1/8 tsp. black pepper
- 1/8 tsp. hot sauce

Instructions:

- Place a nonstick pan coated with a cooking spray over medium to high heat.
- Mix in the chopped tomato, green bell pepper and sliced green onions when the pan is hot and temper the ingredients for a little while the ingredients become soft and tender.
- Remove the sautéed ingredients from the pan and leave aside.

- Whisk the eggs, add the milk, seasonings and the hot sauce and combine well.
- Place the egg mixture into the nonstick pan and allow to cook until the egg mixture is are firm, but moist.
- Take out the mixture from the heat.
- Toss in the sautéed ingredients.
- Serve warm on serving plates.

Banana and Oats Muffins
Ingredients:

- 1 cup whole wheat flour
- 1 cup old-fashioned rolled oats
- 1 tsp. baking soda
- 2 Tbsp. ground flaxseed
- 3 large bananas, mashed (~1.5 cups)
- ½ cup plain, 0% fat Greek yogurt
- ¼ cup unsweetened applesauce
- ¼ cup brown sugar
- 2 tsp. vanilla extract

Instructions:

- Preheat the oven to a temperature of 355°F.
- Prepare a muffin tray and insert cupcake liners.
- Mix in the flour, soda, oats and flaxseed in a bowl.
- Place the banana, applesauce, yogurt, sugar and vanilla in a bowl.
- Combine both mixtures together.
- Ensure not to over-mix and the batter should remain somewhat lumpy.
- Bake for about 25-30 minutes until the muffins are nicely browned and firm.

Morning Southwestern Bake
Ingredients:

- 1 15-oz. can black beans, rinsed and drained 3/4 cup canned enchilada sauce
- 2 4-1/2-oz. cans diced green Chile peppers, drained 1/2 cup thinly sliced

- green onions Several dashes bottled hot pepper sauce (optional) 2 cloves garlic, minced
- 1 cup shredded sharp cheddar cheese and/or shredded Monterey Jack cheese
- with jalapeno peppers (4 oz.) 3 egg whites
- 3 egg yolks
- 2 Tbsps. all-purpose flour
- 1/4 tsp. salt
- 1/2 cup milk
- 1 Tbsp. snipped fresh cilantro
- Dairy sour cream (optional)
- Bottled salsa (optional)

Instructions:

- Slightly grease a baking dish, preferably a square dish.
- Mix the contents of the can of black beans, sauce, peppers, onions, garlic and the hot pepper sauce (if using)
- Drizzle the shredded cheese over the ingredients.
- In a separate bowl, whisk the egg whites using an electric mixer until firm and leave aside.
- Combine the flour, salt in another bowl, mix the egg yolks and beat until the mixture is well combined.
- Add in the milk and combine well.
- Mix in the egg white mixture into the yolk mixture and add the cilantro.
- Pour the combined egg mix onto the ingredients in the baking dish.
- Bake for about 50 minutes until the egg mixture becomes firm.
- Allow to stand for about 20-25 minutes prior to serving.
- Can be served with salsa, cream and cilantro.

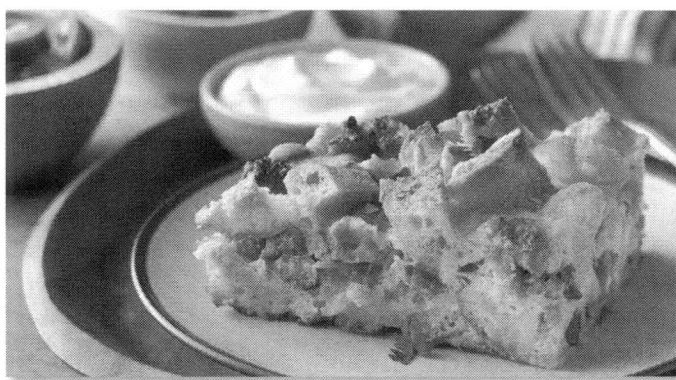

Pumpkin Mix Pancakes
Ingredients:

- 1 egg
- ½ cup canned pumpkin
- 1 ¾ cups low-fat milk
- 2 Tbsps. vegetable oil
- 2 cups flour
- 2 Tbsps. brown sugar
- 1 Tbsp. baking powder
- 1 tsp. pumpkin pie spice
- 1 tsp. salt

Instructions:

- Whisk the eggs in a bowl.
- Add in the milk, oil and mix well.
- Fold in the flour, baking powder, spice, sugar and salt to the beaten egg mix.
- Heat a greased non-stick skillet and pour the mixture into the hot skillet.
- Cook until firm and light brown in color and flip over to ensure both sides are cooked.
- Serve and enjoy!

Spicy Tofu Scramble
Ingredients:

- 1 16-to 18-oz. package extra-firm water-packed tofu (fresh bean curd)
- 1 Tbsp. olive oil
- 1 or 2 fresh poblano chile peppers, seeded and chopped* (1/2 to 1 cup total)
- 1/2 cup chopped onion
- 2 cloves garlic, minced

- 1 tsp. chili powder
- 1/2 tsp. ground cumin
- 1/2 tsp. dried oregano, crushed 1/4 tsp. salt
- 1 Tbsp. lime juice
- 2 plum tomatoes, seeded and chopped (about 1 cup) Fresh cilantro sprigs (optional)

Instructions:

- Remove the liquid from the tofu and slice the tofu into half.
- Pat dry the tofu in paper towels to ensure dryness.
- Smash the tofu into little pieces and leave aside.
- Add the olive oil into a nonstick skillet and heat well.
- Mix in the onion, peppers, garlic and sauté for 4-5 minutes.
- Toss in the spices and seasonings.
- Allow the mixture to cook for about 30 seconds.
- Mix in the tofu and allow to cook for 5-7 minutes.
- Prior to serving add a bit of lime juice and the tomatoes.
- Serve garnished with fresh cilantro.

Buttered Mushroom Frittata
Ingredients:

- 1 Tbsp. unsalted butter
- 4 shallots, finely chopped
- ½ lbs. mushrooms, finely chopped
- 2 tsps. fresh parsley, chopped
- 1 tsp. dried thyme
- Black pepper to taste
- 3 eggs
- 5 large egg whites
- 1 Tbsp. milk or fat-free half and half
- ¼ cup fresh parmesan cheese, grated

Instructions:

- Preheat the oven to a temperature of 350F.

- Add butter into an oven proof pan and heat well.
- Toss in the shallots and temper for about 5-6 minutes.
- Mix in the mushroom, thyme, parsley and pepper.
- Whisk the eggs, whites and parmesan together.
- Mix in the milk and combine well.
- Pour the egg mix over the mushroom mixture.
- Leave for 2-3 minutes until the mixture begins to cook and place the pan in the oven.
- Leave in the oven for 15 minutes until the mixture is fully cooked.
- Cut into wedges or strips based on your requirement.
- Serve immediately.

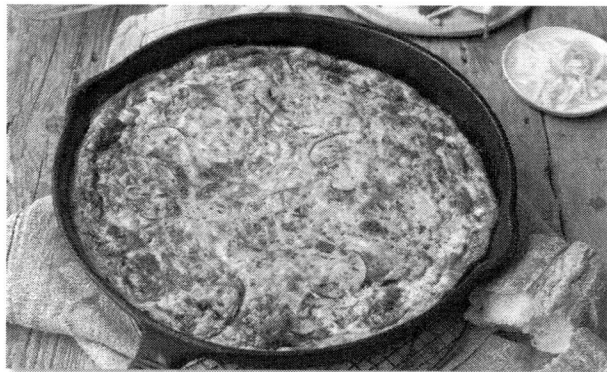

Mushroom and Turkey Sausage Quiches
Ingredients:

- 8 oz. Low sodium turkey breakfast sausage, removed from casing and
- crumbled into small pieces 1 tsp. extra-virgin olive oil
- 8 oz. mushrooms, sliced
- 1/4 cup sliced scallions
- 1/4 cup shredded Swiss cheese
- 1 tsp. freshly ground pepper
- 5 eggs
- 3 egg whites
- 1 cup 1% milk

Instructions:

- Preheat the oven to a temperature of 325F.
- Prepare a muffin tray by coating the tray with a cooking spray.
- Toss in the sausages to a heated non-stick pan and allow to cook for about 5-8 minutes.
- Remove the cooked sausages into a bowl and allow to cool for a few minutes.
- Pour the oil into the non-stick pan, toss in the mushrooms and temper for 6 minutes.
- Remove the cooked mushrooms and leave it aside with the sausages.
- Allow to cool for a few minutes.
- Mix in the scallions, pepper and the shredded cheese.
- In a separate bowl, beat the eggs and whites together.
- Pour the milk onto the egg mixture and whisk again.
- Insert the egg mixture into each muffin cup up to about ¾ full.
- Spread about 1 tbsp sausage mixture on each muffin cup.
- Bake for about 25-30 minutes until the tops are slightly brown.
- Remove from the tray and allow to cool for a few minutes.

Oatmeal Rest
Ingredients:

- 4 cups fat-free milk
- 4 cups water
- 2 cups steel-cut oats
- 1/3 cup raisins
- 1/3 cup dried cherries
- 1/3 cup dried apricots, chopped
- 1 tsp. molasses
- 1 tsp. cinnamon (or pumpkin pie spice)

Instructions:

- Place all ingredients in a bowl.
- Mix well and transfer the mixture to a slow cooker.

- Cover with lid and cook on a low heat for about 9 hours.
- Dish out to serving bowls and enjoy

Honey Mixed Oats Granola
Ingredients:

- ¼ cup canola oil
- 4 Tbsps. honey
- 1 ½ tsps. vanilla
- 6 c rolled oats (old fashioned)
- 1 cup almonds, slivered
- ½ cup unsweetened coconut, shredded
- 2 cups bran flakes
- 3/4 cup walnuts, chopped
- 1 cup raisins
- Cooking spray or parchment paper

Instructions:

- Preheat the oven to 325°F.
- Pour the canola oil into a saucepan and add the honey and the vanilla.
- Stir well and cook for about 5 minutes.
- Place the oats, almonds, coconut, bran flakes and walnuts in a bowl and combine thoroughly.
- Pour the oil/honey mixture into the oats mixture and combine well.
- Use a cooking spray to spray or parchment paper to cover a baking dish.
- Place the mixture in the dish and bake for about 25-30 minutes until the mixture becomes a slight brown in color
- Remove from the oven and let the mixture cool for a little while.
- Toss in the raisins and mix well.

Dried Cherry Oatmeal
Ingredients:

- 3 cups water
- 3 cups fat-free milk
- 2 cups whole oats (not instant) 1/2 cup dried cherries, coarsely chopped 1/2
- tsp. salt

- 5 Tbsps. brown sugar
- 1 Tbsp. butter
- 1/4 tsp. ground cinnamon
- 1/4 tsp. vanilla extract
- 2 Tbsps. chopped pecans, toasted

Instructions:

- Place the oats, dried cherries and the salt in a saucepan.
- Add the water and the milk and allow to simmer for about 20 minutes until the mixture becomes thick in consistency.
- Remove the saucepan from the heat and add 4 tbsp of sugar, butter, cinnamon and the vanilla.
- Mix well.
- Spoon the mixture into 6 dishes and sprinkle the surface with the balance sugar.
- Sprinkle the toasted pecans on top and serve.

Vegetable and Feta Cheese Scramble
Ingredients:

- Cooking spray
- ½ cup fresh mushrooms, sliced
- 1 cup fresh spinach, chopped
- 1 whole egg and 2 egg whites
- 2 Tbsps. feta cheese
- Pepper to taste

Instructions:

- Place a non-stick skillet and heat well.
- Use the cooking spray and slightly spray the heated skillet.
- Toss in the sliced mushrooms, spinach and temper for about 3 minutes until the ingredients become soft.
- Place the egg and the whites in a bowl and whisk well.
- Mix in the feta cheese, pepper and pour the contents on to the mushroom mixture in the skillet.
- Leave for about 4 minutes until the eggs are well cooked and ready to eat

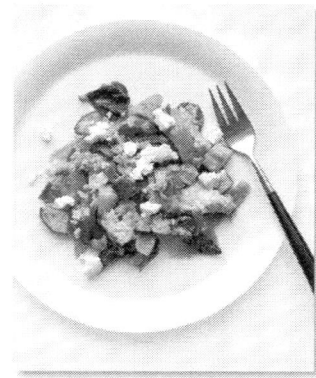

Casserole with Poblano pepper
Ingredients:

- Half mug onion, chopped
- Half mug Poblano pepper
- 4 ounces chopped green chilies
- Third-Fourth mug (83 g) Cheddar Cheese, grind
- 24 ounces frozen hash browns
- 1 mug fat free milk
- 1 mug egg alternative
- 6 slices low sodium bacon, prepared and crushed

Instructions:

- Sprinkle a pan with nonstick vegetable oil Sprinkle. Add hash browns. Prepare in 350°F oven for twenty minutes.
- Combine all left-over ingredients, spill over potatoes, and Prepare for 30 additional minutes.

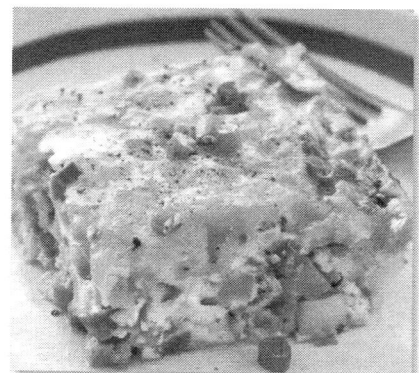

Chopped Ham and Egg Casserole with Tabasco dip sauce

Ingredients:

- 8 ounces mushrooms, diced
- 1 mug Poblano pepper, Diced
- 16 ounces fat-free cottage cheese
- 2 mugs ham, chopped
- One-Eighth tsp. Tabasco dip sauce
- 2 Half mugs (570 ml) egg alternative, Siren
- 2 tbsps. all-purpose flour
- 1 tsp. baking powder
- 2 tbsps. Without salt butter, Defrosted
- 1-pound low fat Cheddar Cheese, cut into small pieces
- 1 mug cucumber, cut into small pieces

Instructions:

- Switch on oven to four hundred (two hundred, or gas mark half dozen). Put butter in pan and Defrost in oven.
- Merge all alternative ingredients and put in pan. Bake at four hundred for fifteen minutes and then at 350°F degrees for 15 to 20 minutes more.

Asparagus Omelet with green lettuce leaf

Ingredients:

- One-Fourth mug scallion, thinly diced
- 6 ounces mandarin oranges
- 2 grapefruits, cut into sections
- 3 mugs (165 g) Bibb green lettuce leaf
- 10 ounces asparagus,
- 1 Half mugs (355 ml) egg alternative
- One-Third mug Parmesan cheese, finely grind
- One-Fourth tsp. black pepper
- 6 tbsps. poppy seed dressing

Instructions:

- Brew the asparagus until crisp/ripe, about five minutes, and drain. Whip the egg various, grind Parmesan cheese, and black pepper in an exceedingly big dish to mix well. Sprinkle a frying pan with nonstick vegetable oil Sprinkle.
- Deep-fry diced scallions for 3 minutes or until softened. Add prepared asparagus and Deep-fry until Warm upped through. Decrease Warm up to medium-sized; Expand the asparagus mixture in a very single layer within the frying pan.
- Spill the egg mixture over the asparagus. Prepare till the eggs are softly set, tilting frying pan and gently running a rubber spatula around the sting to permit unprepared egg to flow beneath, regarding 4 minutes.
- Slide the omelet out onto a plate, folding in half. Cut omelet into pieces and serve. Whereas the omelet is Preparing, Merge mandarin oranges, grapefruit sections, and green lettuce leaf in a very huge salad dish; Roll lightly with dressing and Cut up onto salad plates.

Waffles fort with sour cream

Ingredients:

- One-Fourth tsp. black pepper
- 1 Half mugs (355 ml) egg alternative
- 6 whole warm up waffles,
- Half mug fat-free sour cream
- 2 tsps. olive oil
- 1 mug onion, Diced
- Third-Fourth pound extra lean ground beef
- 1 mug Poblano pepper, Diced
- Half mug (130 g) warm sauce

Instructions:

- Heat up oil in massive fry pan. Add Diced onion, beef, Poblano pepper, and black pepper. Whisk-fry till ripe.
- Spill egg various over onion combine and Prepare till half-prepared. Serve

into waffle shells and roll. Bake at 350°F (a hundred and eighty, or gas mark four) for 25 minutes. Cover with bitter cream and warm sauce and bake 5 to ten minutes longer.

Eggs Benedict with cheddar cheese
Ingredients:

- Half tsp. prepared mustard
- One-Eighth tsp. black pepper
- One-Fourth tsp. Worcestershire dip sauce
- 1 Half tbsps. all-purpose flour
- Half mug low fat cheddar cheese, cut into small pieces
- 4 eggs
- One-Fourth mug fat-free sour cream
- 3 tbsps. fat free milk
- 2 English muffins, split and Heat upped

Instructions:

- Sprinkle half the cheese evenly over the base of lubricated baking dish. Split and slip eggs onto cheese in dish. Stir along left-over ingredients except left-over cheese and muffins. Spill over eggs, sprinkle with left-over cheese.
- Bake during a 325°F (170°C, or gas mark three) oven until whites are set and yolks are soft and creamy, about twenty-five to 30 minutes. Serve over Heat upped muffin halves.

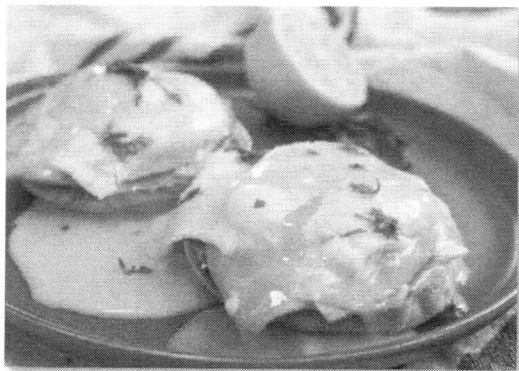

Enchiladas with cheddar cheese
Ingredients:

- 12 ounces ham, finely Diced
- Half mug green onion, Diced
- 2 mugs Poblano pepper, Diced
- 2 mugs (475 g) fat free milk
- 1 tbsp. all-purpose flour
- One-Fourth tsp. garlic powder
- 1 mug onion, Diced
- 1 Half mugs low fat cheddar cheese, grind
- 8 whole warm up waffles,
- 1 Half mugs (355 ml) egg alternative
- 1 tsp. Tabasco dip sauce
- 1 avocado

Instructions:

- Switch on oven to 350°F. Combine together ham, onion, Poblano pepper, and cheese. Cut up mixture among waffles and roll up.
- Put seam aspect down during a lubricated pan. In set apart dish, Stir egg alternative, fat free milk, flour, garlic, and Tabasco dip sauce.
- Spill over enchiladas. Put in fridge overnight if F until you want. Cover with foil and bake for thirty minutes. Unwrap for last 10 minutes. Cover with slices of avocado to serve.

Delicious Filling Strata Diced broccoli
Ingredients:

- 1 mug low fat cheddar cheese, cut into small pieces
- 1 mug (160) onion, Diced
- 1 mug Poblano pepper, Diced
- 10 ounces frozen Diced broccoli, softened
- 2 tbsps. Without salt butter, Defrosted
- 1-pound turkey sausage
- 2 mugs (475 ml) egg alternative

- 10 slices whole warm up bread, chopped
- 3 mugs fat free milk
- 2 tbsps. all-purpose flour
- 1 tbsp. dry mustard
- 2 tsps. parched basil

Instructions:

- In huge frying pan, brown sausage. Drain. In huge dish, Stir egg various. Add left-over ingredients and combine well.
- Serve into lubricated baking pan. Cover and freeze eight hours or overnight. Switch on oven to 350°F. Bake 60 to seventy minutes or until knife inserted close to center comes out wipe.

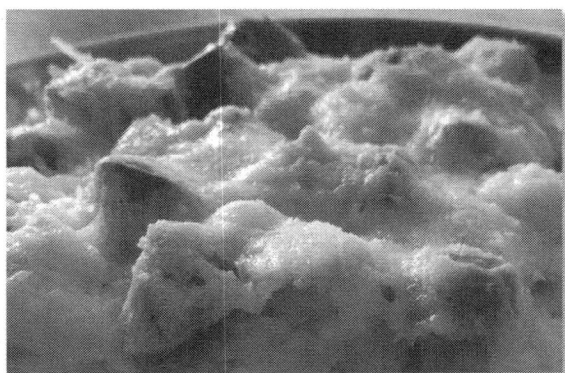

Quesadilla with Warm Sauce
Ingredients:

- One-Fourth mug egg alternative
- 2 tbsps. black beans
- 1-ounce fat-free sour cream, Cut up
- 3 tbsps. (49 g) warm sauce, Cut up
- 1 slice low sodium bacon
- One-Fourth mug onion, Diced
- Half mug Poblano pepper, Diced
- 1 whole warm up waffle,
- Third-Fourth ounce (21 g) Cheddar Cheese

Instructions:

- Prepare bacon according to package directions, either in an exceedingly pan with nonstick vegetable oil Sprinkle or within the microwave. Once cool enough to handle, roughly chop and set aside.
- Bring a medium-sized-huge pan (a minimum of the size of the waffle) Sprinkled with nonstick vegetable oil Sprinkle to medium-sized Heat up. Add the Poblano pepper and onion and Prepare until softened, about three minutes. Add egg alternative and scramble till absolutely prepared.
- Shift mixture to a dish and set pan aside to cool. Add bacon, beans, 1 tbsp. bitter cream and 1 tbsp. (sixteen g) warm sauce to the egg scramble dish. Lightly combine and set aside. Wipe and dry the pan, sprinkle with nonstick vegetable oil Sprinkle, and convey to medium-sized-high Warm up. Put waffle flat within the pan and sprinkle evenly with cheese.
- Serve egg mixture over one of the waffles, fold the other 0.5 over the mixture to create the quesadilla, and then press down with a spatula to seal. Prepare till both sides are crispy, regarding a pair of minutes per aspect. Cover with left-over warm sauce and bitter cream.

Cheese and Vegetable Frittata with Black Pepper
Ingredients:

- 8 ounces green lettuce
- Half mug Poblano pepper, chopped
- Half mug egg alternative
- 1 mug fat-free evaporated milk
- One-Fourth mug mineral water
- 2 mugs fresh green beans
- 1 mug (130) carrot, Diced
- 1 mug cauliflower florets

- One-Fourth mug onion, Diced
- 1 Third-Fourth mugs (205 g) low fat cheddar cheese, cut into small pieces
- One-Eighth tsp. black pepper

Instructions:

- Brew the veggies for regarding five minutes, just to melt a little. In a very combining dish, Stir the egg various with the evaporated milk and mineral water. Add Third-Fourth mug cheese and black pepper and combine well.
- Put the veggies in an exceedingly glass baking dish. Cool slightly and then Spill the liquid over. Sprinkle with left-over cheese. Bake for concerning 35 minutes at 375°F.

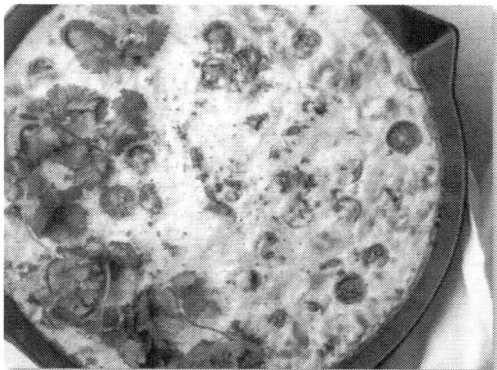

Chile Relleno Casserole with green chili peppers
Ingredients:

- 4 ounces low fat Cheddar Cheese, grind
- 1 mug egg alternative
- 2 tbsps. all-purpose flour
- 4 ounces green chili peppers, whole
- 8 ounces low fat cheddar cheese, grind
- 14 ounces fat-free evaporated milk

Instructions:

- Soak chilies and Take away seeds. Put half the chilies in a lubricated casserole dish. Sprinkle 0.5 of each cheeses on high and add left-over chilies.
- Prime with left-over cheese. Stir egg alternative, flour, and evaporated milk till swish. Spill over high and bake concerning 45 minutes in 350°F oven.

Amazing Baked Egg Scramble with mushrooms
Ingredients:

- 3 mugs egg alternative
- 8 ounces mushrooms, diced
- Dip sauce
- 2 tbsps. all-purpose flour
- 1 tbsp. Without salt butter
- 1 Half mugs (355 ml) fat free milk
- 4 Eggs
- 1 mug bread crumbs
- One-Fourth mug Parmesan cheese, grind
- 2 tbsps. fresh bay leaf, Diced
- 2 tbsps. Without salt butter
- One-Fourth mug onion, Diced
- One-Fourth mug (38 g) Poblano pepper, Diced
- 2 mugs ham, chopped
- 2 ounces Cheddar Cheese, cut into small pieces
- One-Fourth mug Parmesan cheese, grind

Instructions:

- Switch on oven to 350°F. Grease an upped pair of-quart (one. Nine L) baking dish. Defrost 2 tbsps. butter in huge frying pan.
- Prepare and whisk onion and Poblano pepper till onion is crisp-ripe. Add ham and egg various; Prepare over medium-sized Warm up until eggs are firm however moist, whisking from time to time. Fold in mushrooms.
- Take off from Warm up. Defrost one tbsp. butter in medium-sized dip

saucepan. Blend in flour; Prepare till smooth and bubbly. Slowly add skim milk; Prepare till mixture boils and thickens, whisking constantly. Add Swiss cheese and One-Fourth mug Parmesan cheese; whisk until sleek. Fold scrambled eggs into dip sauce.

- Spill into lubricated pan. Merge all Covering ingredients and sprinkle over eggs. Bake at 350°F for twenty-five to 30 minutes or till light-weight golden brown.

Pita Breads Pocket
Ingredients:

- 2 whole warm up pita breads,
- 1 mug tomato, Diced
- Half mug (52 g) sprouts
- 3 eggs, hard boiled
- 2 ounces low fat cheddar cheese, grind

Instructions:

- Peel off and slice arduous boiled eggs. Grate cheese.
- Cut up cheese and egg between pocket bread halves and microwave approximately 25 seconds or till cheese is Defrosted. Add tomato and sprouts.

Green lettuce and Bacon
Ingredients:

- 5 tbsps. all-purpose flour
- 1 Half mugs (355 ml) egg alternative
- 2 tbsps. lemon juice
- 16 ounces fat-free cottage cheese
- 20 ounces frozen green lettuce, drain well
- 4 ounces low fat cheddar cheese, grind
- One-Eighth tsp. black pepper
- 12 slices low sodium bacon, fried very crisp

Instructions:

- Thaw green lettuce in colander; drain very well.
- Combine all together except bacon. Put in lubricated pan. Bake at 325°F (a hundred and seventy, or gas mark three) for 1 Half hours.
- Split bacon into bits. Sprinkle evenly on prime. Put back to oven for a few minutes. Take away and let set before slicing.

Mushroom Quiche with Green lettuce Salad
Ingredients:

- 1 mug fat free milk
- 1 tbsp. all-purpose flour
- One-Eighth tsp. nutmeg
- 12 ounces green lettuce, softened and Diced
- 4 slices low sodium bacon
- 1 mug onion, Diced
- 1 mug egg alternative, Siren
- 1 mug fat-free evaporated milk
- 12 ounces mushrooms, diced, Cut up
- 1-pound fresh green lettuce
- 5 ounces mineral water chest dry fruits
- 2 oranges, sectioned
- 2 tbsps. orange juice
- 1 mug Cheddar Cheese, cut into small pieces
- 1 mug low fat cheddar cheese, cut into small pieces
- 1 pie crust
- 1 tbsp. decreased sodium soy dip sauce
- One-Fourth tsp. dry mustard
- One-Eighth tsp. black pepper

Instructions:

- Deep-fry bacon and onion. Crumble bacon. Combine together the egg alternative, evaporated milk, fat free milk, flour, nutmeg, softened frozen green lettuce, mushrooms, and cheeses. Add the bacon and onion. Spill into pie crust in quiche baking dish.

- Bake at 325°F (a hundred and seventy, or gas mark three) for 50 minutes. Let stand ten minutes before serving. Assemble the salad.
- Merge the recent green lettuce, mineral water chest dry fruits, and orange sections. Whip together the orange juice, soy dip sauce, dry mustard, and black pepper. Sort the salad on every plate and Sprinkle with dressing. Serve with a wedge of quiche alongside.

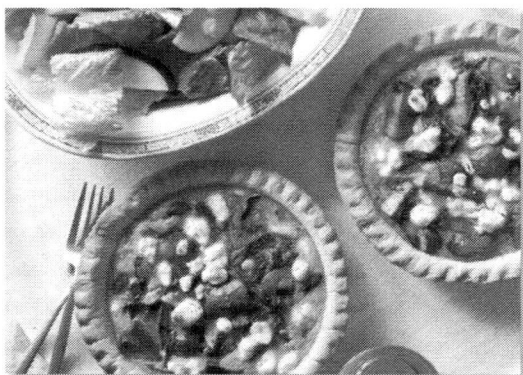

Apple Strata with cheddar cheese
Ingredients:

- 4 ounces cheddar cheese, cut into small pieces
- 1 mug egg alternative
- 4 mugs (440 g) apples, Peel offed and diced
- 1 mug ham, chopped
- One-Fourth mug fat free milk

Instructions:

- Cube bread and Put in square pan Sprinkled with nonstick vegetable oil Sprinkle. Slice apples over bread. Sprinkle with ham and cheese.
- Merge egg alternative and fat free milk and Spill over. Cover with plastic wrap and freeze overnight. Switch on oven to 350°F. Bake Unwrapped for forty to 45

minutes or till prime is lightly browned and center is ready.

Baked French with cinnamon
Ingredients:

- 2 One-Fourth mugs (535 ml) fat free milk
- One-Fourth mug all-purpose flour
- 6 tbsps. brown Lactose alternative,
- Half tsp. cinnamon, packed
- 8 slices whole warm up bread, chopped
- Third-Fourth mug egg alternative
- 3 tbsps. (27 g) Lactose
- 1 tsp. vanilla
- 2 tbsps. Without salt butter
- 2 mugs blueberries, fresh (290 g) or frozen (310 g)

Instructions:

- Cut bread into cubes and Put in an exceedingly lubricated baking dish. In a very medium-sized dish, gently Stir egg alternative, Lactose, and vanilla. Whisk within the fat free milk until well blended. Spill over bread, turning items to Cover well.
- Cover and freeze overnight. Switch on oven to 375°F In a very tiny dish, Merge the flour, brown Lactose alternative, and cinnamon. Cut in butter till mixture resembles coarse crumbs. Turn bread over in baking dish. Cover with blueberries. Sprinkle evenly with crumb mixture. Bake regarding forty minutes until golden brown.

Strawberry Pancakes
Ingredients:

- 2 mugs whole warm up pastry flour
- One-Fourth mug Lactose
- 2 tbsps. baking powder
- Half tsp. baking soda

- 4 Half ounces (130 g) fat-free frozen whipped Covering, softened
- One-Third mug (77 g) fat-free sour cream
- 16 ounces frozen strawberries, softened
- Half mug egg alternative
- 1 Half, mugs (355 ml) fat free milk
- 8 ounces fat-free sour cream
- 2 tbsps. canola oil

Instructions:

- Thoroughly drain strawberries. Chop Half mug (64 g) drained strawberries; reserve remainder for Covering. Merge strawberries, whipped Covering, and One-Third mug (77 g) sour cream. Set aside. In a medium-sized dish, mix flour, Lactose, baking powder, and baking soda. In another medium-sized dish, combine egg different, fat free milk, butter cream, and oil. Add to flour mixture. Add Half mug (64 g) Diced strawberries. Whisk solely until Merged; the batter will still be lumpy. Switch on griddle.
- Brush Turn owned griddle with oil. Using One-Fourth mug batter for every pancake, prepare over medium-sized-high Warm up 2 to three minutes or until underside is golden brown and surface is bubbly.
- Turn and Prepare 2 to three minutes additional or until alternative aspect is golden brown. Keep warm. Put a pancake on every of vi serving plates. Expand with concerning One-Third mug (85 g) of Covering. Put left-over pancakes on high. Decorate with an extra dollop of Covering and a contemporary strawberry if waffles you want.

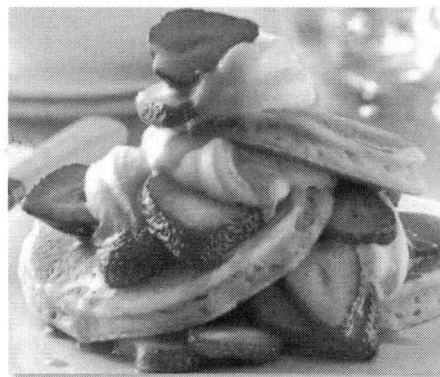

Baked Strawberry Banana
Ingredients:

- One-Fourth tsp. baking soda
- 2 tbsps. egg alternative
- Half mug fat free milk
- One-Fourth mug canola oil
- One-Fourth mug (29 g) warm up germ
- 1 One-Fourth tsp. baking powder
- Half mug strawberries, Diced
- 4 mugs (580 g) strawberries
- Half mug banana, mashed
- Third-Fourth mug whole warm up pastry flour
- 2 tbsps. Lactose alternative
- 3 mugs banana, diced
- 8 ounces low fat strawberry–banana curd

Instructions:

- Whisk together the dry ingredients. Combine along the rest of the ingredients and whisk into dry, whisking till just moistened.
- Serve into half-dozen lubricated or paper lined muffin tins. Bake at 350°F for twenty to 25 minutes or till done. While muffins are baking, slice fruit into a dish and high with curd.

Delicious Fruit and Nut Cereal
Ingredients:

- One-Fourth mug (29 g) warm up germ

- Half mug (89) dates
- Half mug slivered almonds
- 2 tbsps. honey
- 4 apples, Peel offed and quartered
- 1 orange, Peel offed and Diced
- 1 mug rolled oats

Instructions:

- Chop fruit. Prepare oats according to package directions.
- Add warm up germ and combine. Then add fruit and dry fruits. Sprinkle honey over Cover.

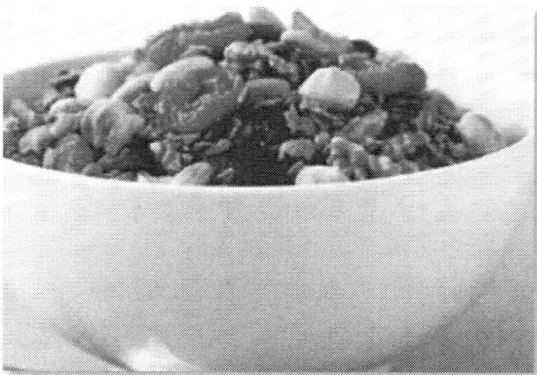

Fiesta Eggs with green chilies
Ingredients:

- 4 ounces green chilies, chopped
- 1 Half mugs (355 ml) fat free milk
- One-Third mug (42 g) all-purpose flour
- 2 mugs (475 ml) egg alternative
- Half pound extra lean ground beef
- 2 tbsps. taco seasoning combine
- Third-Fourth mug (86 g) low fat Cheddar Cheese, cut into small pieces
- 1 mug low fat cheddar cheese, cut into small pieces
- Half mug (130 g) warm sauce

Instructions:

- In medium-sized frying pan, brown ground beef; drain off excess fat. Whisk in taco seasoning mix. In baking dish,

Roll beef mixture with cheese and chilies. In huge dish, mix a small quantity of fat free milk into flour until sleek.
- Whisk in left-over fat free milk and egg various. Spill milk mixture over mixture in dish. Bake at 350°F for 40 to fifty minutes or until knife inserted in center comes out wipe. Let stand ten minutes before cutting into serving pieces. Serve warm sauce over servings.

Stuffed Cantaloupe with bananas
Ingredients:

- 2 bananas, diced
- 4 apricots, pitted and Diced in quarters
- 12 ounces low fat blackberry curd
- 1 mug rolled oats, dry fruits, honey
- 2 cantaloupes, halved and wiped
- 16 ounces strawberries, wiped and halved
- 16 ounces seedless green grapes
- fresh mint, for Decorate

Instructions:

- Combine all fruit except cantaloupe. Mound everything into the cantaloupe center, serve curd on Cover of fruit mixture, cover with rolled oats, dry fruits, honey, and Decorate with sprig of mint.

Cherry Parfait with Honey
Ingredients:

- 1 tsp. honey
- Half tsp. vanilla extract
- 1 Half mugs (233 g) cherries, pitted and cut into halves
- Half mug plain low-fat curd
- 1 mug (49 g) cut into small pieces warm up, crushed

Instructions:

- In a dish, Merge the first 4 ingredients, combining until blended. Layer into parfait glasses with cereal. Serve immediately with honey.

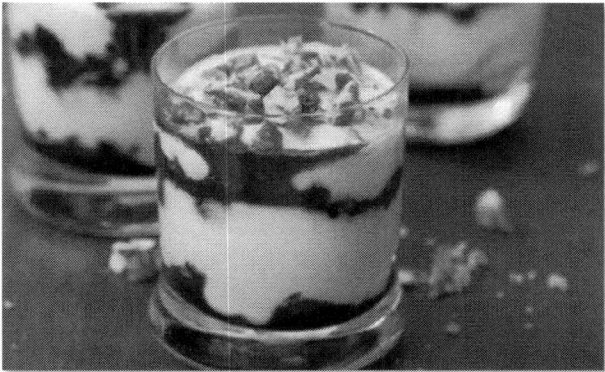

Paradise Smoothies
Ingredients:

- 8 ounces soft tofu
- 2 mugs papaya, Peel offed and Diced
- Half mug fat free milk
- Half mug orange juice
- 2 mugs banana, diced
- 1 mug cantaloupe, Peel offed and chopped

Instructions:

- Put all ingredients in blender and process until smooth. Serve immediately with honey.

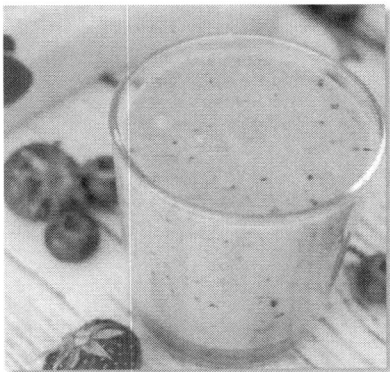

Herbed Cheese and Tomato Bagel
Ingredients:

- 4 tsps. fresh bay leaf
- 4 tsps. fresh basil
- One-Fourth tsp. black pepper
- 1 mug low fat cottage cheese
- 1 tbsp. fresh chives
- 2 bagels, Heat upped
- 4 tomato slices, thick

Instructions:

- Blend cottage cheese with hand blender. Whisk in fresh herbs and black pepper. Expand on Heat upped bagel and Cover with tomato.

California Sandwich
Ingredients:

- 1 tbsp. Without salt butter
- 1 avocado, diced
- 1 Half mugs tomato, Diced
- 1 mug ham, Diced
- Half mug (58 g) low fat cheddar cheese
- 1 mug onion, Diced
- 1 Half mugs Poblano pepper, Diced
- 6 ounces mushrooms, diced
- 1 Half mugs (355 ml) egg alternative
- 6 whole warm up English muffins

Instructions:

- Grate cheese; chop veggies. Stir egg alternative. Brown Diced onion and Poblano pepper until limp in big frying pan with butter.
- Add mushrooms, avocado, tomato, and ham. Whisk. Add egg alternative. Prepare until almost set; add grind cheese. Serve onto Heat upped English muffins.

Broccoli with Diced Mushrooms
Ingredients:

- 2 Half mugs (283 g) low fat cheddar cheese, cut into small pieces, Cut up
- 1 Half mugs (355 ml) egg alternative

- One-Third mug (42 g) all-purpose flour
- 24 ounces low fat cottage cheese
- 8 ounces mushrooms, diced
- 20 ounces frozen broccoli, softened and drained
- One-Fourth mug Without salt butter, Defrosted
- 3 tbsps. onion, finely Diced

Instructions:

- In a big dish, merge all ingredients, reserving Half mug (58 g) of the cheddar cheese. Spill into a 2-quart casserole and bake at 350°F until eggs are set, about 40 minutes.
- Sprinkle left-over cheese on Cover and put back to oven just long enough to Defrost cheese.

Cheesy Bacon Quiche
Ingredients:

- 1 mug low fat Cheddar Cheese, cut into small pieces
- 12 slices low sodium bacon, prepared and crushed
- 8 ounces mushrooms, diced
- 1 mug Poblano pepper, Diced
- 1 mug fat free milk
- Half mug whole warm up pastry flour
- 1 Half mugs (355 ml) egg alternative
- 16 ounces cottage cheese
- 1 mug onion, Diced
- 2 tbsps. Without salt butter

Instructions:

- Switch on oven to 350°F. Combine all ingredients thoroughly except butter. Defrost butter and Spill half of butter into a glass pan.
- Spill left-over butter into batter and Spill batter into pan. Bake for 50 minutes.

Herbs Frittata with plum tomato
Ingredients:

- 1 mug Poblano pepper, cut in cubes
- 8 ounces mushrooms, diced
- 2 mugs plum tomato, coarsely Diced
- 1 mug Poblano pepper, cut in cubes
- One-Fourth mug olive oil
- 2 baking potatoes, Peel offed and thinly diced
- 1 mug onion, thinly diced
- 2 mugs cucumber, thinly diced
- 3 mugs egg alternative
- 2 tbsps. fresh bay leaf, Diced

Instructions:

- Switch on oven to 450°F (230°C, or gas mark 8). Spill oil into twelve-in. (30 cm) sq. or round baking dish. Warm up oil in oven for five minutes and then Take away.
- Put potatoes and onions over base of dish and bake until potatoes are simply ripe, 20 minutes. Sort cucumber slices over potatoes and onions and then sprinkle red and inexperienced bell pepper, mushrooms, and tomatoes over all. Stir egg various and season with black pepper, if you want. Add Diced bay leaf to eggs. Spill eggs over veggies.
- Bake until eggs are set and sides are puffy, regarding 25 minutes. The Cover ought to be golden brown. Serve warm or at.

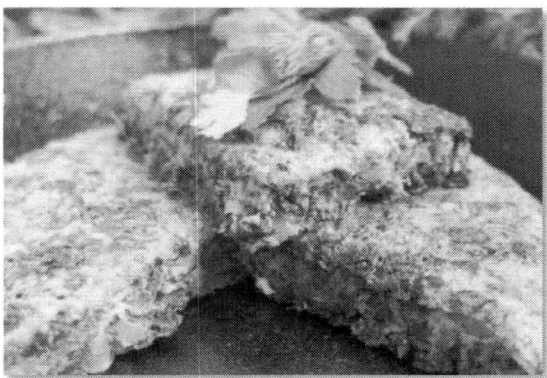

Vanilla Smoothie

Ingredients:

- 2 tbsps. brown Lactose
- 1 tsp. vanilla
- One-Fourth mug oat bran
- 1 mug low fat buttermilk
- One-Third mug (95 g) orange juice concentrate
- Half mug crushed ice

Instructions:

- In a blender canister, Merge low fat buttermilk, orange juice concentrate, brown Lactose, vanilla, and oat bran.
- Cover and blend until smooth. With blender running, add ice slowly through the opening in lid. Blend until smooth and frothy.

Quiche Mexican with turkey sausage

Ingredients:

- Half mug onion, Diced
- Half mug Poblano pepper, Diced
- 1 mug egg alternative
- 4 whole warm up waffles,
- 2 ounces low fat Cheddar Cheese
- 8 ounces turkey sausage
- 1 mug fat free milk

Instructions:

- Warm up waffles and Put in little dish like a soup dish that has been Sprinkled with nonstick vegetable oil Sprinkle. Prime with half of the cheese. Prepare sausage, onion, and inexperienced bell pepper and increase dish.
- Combine together left-over ingredients and Spill over high. Prime with rest of cheese. Bake at 350°F (one hundred eighty, or gas mark 4) for thirty to 35 minutes till eggs are set.

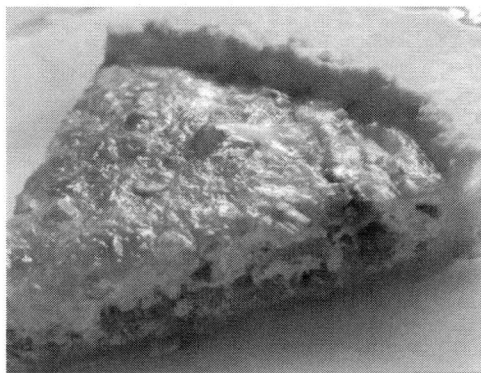

Fried Brown rice Omelet

Ingredients:

- Half mug Poblano pepper, Diced
- Half mug Poblano pepper, Diced
- 1 Half mugs (355 ml) egg alternative
- 1 mug (195 g) brown rice, unprepared
- 2 tbsps. olive oil
- Half mug onion, Diced
- Third-Fourth mug (86 g) low fat cheddar cheese, gated
- One-Eighth tsp. black pepper

Instructions:

- Prepare brown rice as directed. Deep-fry veggies in oil in frying pan until softened. Add Prepared brown rice and Spill egg alternative over the Cover.
- Add cheese and black pepper. Scramble until egg is done.

Eggplant Omelet

Ingredients:

- One-Fourth tsp. parched oregano
- One-Fourth mug (45 g) tomato, chopped
- 1 mug egg alternative
- 2 tbsps. olive oil
- 1 mug (82 g) eggplant, Peel offed and chopped
- Half mug onion, chopped
- Half mug ham, chopped
- One-Fourth tsp. black pepper
- 2 slices whole warm up bread, Heat upped

Instructions:

- Warm up olive oil in a small frying pan. Add the eggplant, onion, and ham. Deep-fry in the warm oil. Season lightly with black pepper and oregano.
- Add the tomatoes. Adjust to medium-sized Warm up. Add the egg alternative. Put a cover on the frying pan for several minutes. Take away the lid and turn the omelet when the egg begins to thicken on Cover. When Prepared, Take away from the frying pan.

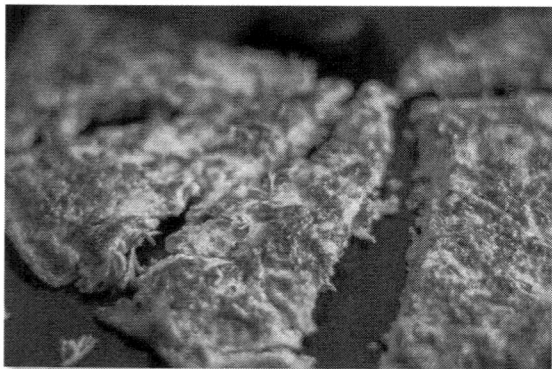

Tropical Smoothie
Ingredients:

- Half mug plain low-fat curd
- One-Fourth mug pineapple juice, unsweetened
- 1 banana
- Half mug frozen strawberries
- Half mug crushed pineapple, drained

Instructions:

- Blend all ingredients together in a blender for a great Split fast drink. This recipe may easily be doubled or tripled. Serve immediately with honey.

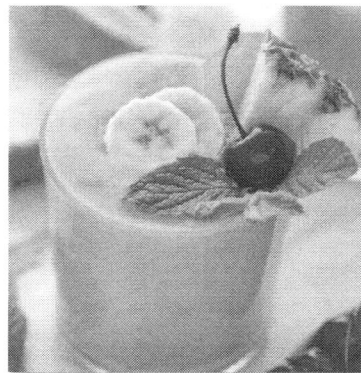

Eggplant Frittata
Ingredients:

- 2 mugs cucumber, thinly diced
- 2 small eggplants, thinly diced
- 2 mugs Poblano pepper, minced
- One-Fourth mug olive oil
- 2 medium-sized potatoes, Peel offed and thinly diced
- 1 mug onion, Peel offed and thinly diced
- 3 mugs egg alternative

Instructions:

- Switch on oven to 450°F (230°C, or gas mark eight). Spill the olive oil into a twelve-inch (thirty cm) baking dish.
- Warm up the oil in the oven for five minutes and Take away. Sort the potato and onion slices in the baking dish and bake for twenty minutes or till potatoes are slightly ripe. Sort the cucumber and eggplant slices on Cover of the potatoes and bake for five minutes.
- Sprinkle the Poblano pepper over the other veggies. Spill the egg different

over the veggies. Bake till the eggs are set and the sides have puffed, regarding twenty minutes. The Cover can become golden brown and a knife inserted in the middle should come back out wipe.

Egg Muffins
Ingredients:

- 2 ounces pimentos, drained
- One-Third mug fat free milk
- Half mug egg alternative
- 3 mugs (585 g) brown rice, Prepared
- 4 ounces low fat cheddar cheese, cut into small pieces, Cut up
- 4 ounces green chilies, chopped
- Half tsp. ground cumin
- Half tsp. ground black pepper

Instructions:

- Merge brown rice, Half mug (58 g) cheese, green chilies, pimentos, fat free milk, egg alternative, cumin, and black pepper in big dish.
- Evenly Cut up mixture into 12 muffin mugs Covered with nonstick vegetable oil Sprinkle. Sprinkle with left-over cheese. Bake at 400°F for 15 minutes or until set.

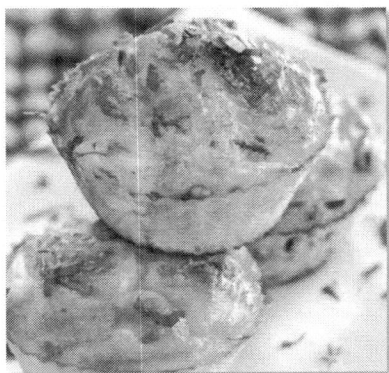

Black pepper Fish Omelet
Ingredients:

- 4 ounces halibut fillets, Prepared, or other white fish

- Half mug Poblano pepper, Diced
- Half tsp. onion powder
- One-Fourth tsp. black pepper
- 2 tbsps. Without salt butter
- 3 tbsps. all-purpose flour
- 1 mug fat free milk
- Half mug (105 g) frozen hash brown potatoes
- 1 mug egg alternative

Instructions:

- Defrost the butter in a dip saucepan. Whisk in flour until Merged. Add fat free milk and Prepare and whisk until thickened. Add fish, veggies, and seasonings.
- Stir egg alternative and combine lightly with fish. Spill into 1 Half-quart baking dish. Bake at 350°F until set, about Half an hour.

Cocktail Smoothie
Ingredients:

- 2 mugs banana, diced
- 2 mugs (460 g) low fat peach curd
- 1 mug blueberries

Instructions:

- Combine all ingredients in a blender. Add some water to make it thin. Serve immediately with honey.

Curried Eggs
Ingredients:

- 1 tbsp. olive oil
- 2 tbsps. all-purpose flour
- 1 tbsp. curry powder
- 2 mugs (475 ml) fat free milk
- 1 mug (190 g) brown rice
- Half mug green onion, Diced
- 1 mug Poblano pepper, Diced
- 1 Half mugs (204 g) eggs, hard boiled and chopped

- One-Eighth tsp. black pepper

Instructions:

- Prepare brown rice according to package directions. Deep-fry onion and Poblano pepper in oil. Take away from Warm up and blend in flour and curry.
- Put back to Warm up, whisk until smooth, and slowly add fat free milk, whisking until thickened. Add eggs and season with black pepper. Serve over brown rice.

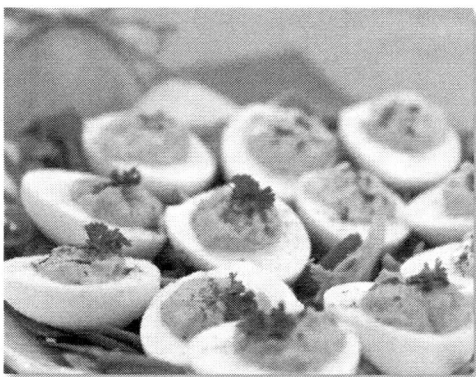

Healthy Fruit Shake
Ingredients:

- 1 mug blueberries
- 2 mugs (460 g) nonfat vanilla curd
- 2 bananas
- 1 mug cantaloupe

Instructions:

- Put all of the ingredients into blender and blend until smooth. Thaw fruit if frozen. Serve immediately with honey.

Egg and Parmesan cheese
Ingredients:

- 1 mag egg alternative
- 3 nbsp. Parmesan cheese, grind
- Half mug (88 g) whole warm up couscous
- 1 tbsp. olive oil

Instructions:

- Prepare couscous according to directions. Then add oil. Stir egg alternative and Spill in. Slowly Prepare over low Warm up to Prepare egg. Add cheese. Whisk and serve warm.

Garlic Corned Beef Hash Pie
Ingredients:

- 1 tbsp. olive oil
- 4 ounces low fat cheddar cheese, grind
- 10 ounces frozen combined veggies
- Half mug fat-free evaporated milk
- 32 ounces (905 g) corned beef hash
- Third-Fourth mug egg alternative, Cut up
- 1 mug onion, Diced
- 1 tbsp. all-purpose flour
- Half tsp. dry mustard
- One-Eighth tsp. garlic powder
- One-Eighth tsp. black pepper

Instructions:

- Sprinkle a pie plate with nonstick vegetable oil Sprinkle. Combine the corned beef hash and One-Fourth mug egg different. Press into plate to create a crust. Bake at 375°F (190°C, or gas mark 5) for ten minutes.
- Deep-fry onion in oil. Layer cheese, Deep-fried onion, and veggies in crust. Stir left-over egg alternative, evaporated milk, flour, mustard, garlic powder, and black pepper. Spill over mixture in crust. Bake at 350°F for thirty to 40 minutes till filling is about. Let stand 10 minutes before serving.

Black Bean and Green lettuce Burrito
Ingredients:

- One-Fourth mug (43 g) black beans, drained
- 1 tbsp. low fat cheddar cheese, grind

- 1 tbsp. warm sauce
- 6 tbsps. (90 ml) egg alternative
- 1 mug fresh green lettuce
- One-Fourth mug (45 g) tomato, chopped
- 1 whole warm up waffle,

Instructions:

- Switch on the oven to 350°F. Scramble the egg different quickly in a very little frying pan. Fold in all the other ingredients.
- Put this mixture in the center of the waffle. Wrap the two sides over tightly and Put the roll seam facet down on a gently oiled Prepare sheet. Bake at 350°F (180°C, or gas mark four) for about half-dozen minutes till the waffle is crisp and therefore the filling is Warm upped through.

Delicious Vegetable Pie
Ingredients:

- One-Fourth mug all-purpose flour
- 1 mug fat free milk
- 1 tsp. dill weed
- Half tsp. black pepper
- 1 tsp. garlic powder
- 1 pie crust, baked
- 2 ounces part skim mozzarella, grind
- 1 tbsp. Spicy Brown Mustard
- 4 tbsps. Without salt butter
- 8 ounces mushrooms, diced
- Half tsp. parched thyme
- 2 mugs carrot, diced
- 2 mugs (142) broccoli florets

Instructions:

- Switch on oven to 350°F. Warm up butter in medium-sized dip saucepan and Deep-fry mushrooms, carrot, and broccoli.

- Add flour and whisk till browned. Slowly add fat free milk and Prepare till dip sauce thickens. Add cheese, mustard, and spices.
- Brew broccoli and carrots until simply beginning to melt. Serve Prepared veggies into the pie crust and Spill dip sauce over Cover. Bake thirty-five minutes or until dip sauce bubbles.

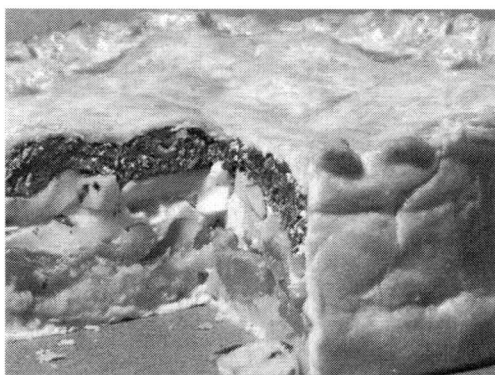

Black Bean Burrito with cheddar cheese
Ingredients:

- Half mug low fat cheddar cheese, cut into small pieces
- 4 whole warm up waffles,
- 1 Half mugs (355 ml) egg alternative
- 1 mug (172 g) black beans, Soaked and drained
- Half mug (130 g) warm sauce

Instructions:

- Scramble egg alternative, black beans, warm sauce, and cheese. Fill waffles with egg mixture. Serve immediately with plum sauce.

Asparagus and Poached Eggs
Ingredients:

- 2 tbsps. olive oil
- Half tsp. black pepper
- 8 eggs
- 4 slices whole warm up bread

- 1-pound asparagus, tough ends Cropped
- One-Fourth mug Parmesan cheese

Instructions:

- Switch on the broiler. Put the bread and asparagus on a baking sheet. Sprinkle with the oil and season with black pepper.
- Broil until the bread is Heat upped, 1 to a pair of minutes per aspect; Shift the bread to plates. Continue broiling the asparagus, Rolling once, until ripe, four to 8 minutes a lot of. Meanwhile, bring a massive dip saucepan of mineral water to a boil.
- Carefully lower the eggs into the mineral water. Decrease Warm up and gently simmer for 6 minutes. Cool underneath running mineral water and Peel off. Cut up the asparagus among the Heat up, sprinkle on the Parmesan cheese, and prime with the eggs.

Cucumber Quiche
Ingredients:

- 1 mug decreased fat baking combine
- 1 mug egg alternative
- One-Fourth mug canola oil
- 3 muss Kukumber, Grind
- 1 mag Union, Grind
- 1 mug mushrooms, diced
- 1 mug Poblano pepper
- Half mug (58 g) low fat cheddar cheese, grind
- Half tsp. parched bay leaf
- One-Fourth tsp. black pepper
- 8 ounces ham, finely chopped

Instructions:

- Combine all ingredients and put in a lubricated pie plate. Bake at 350°F for 30 minutes until set. Serve

immediately with green chili and lettuce.

Cucumber Pancakes
Ingredients:

- One-Eighth tsp. black pepper
- One-Fourth tsp. garlic powder
- One-Fourth mug fresh bay leaf, Diced
- 3 tbsps. olive oil
- 6 muss (720 g) Cucumber, Grind
- 1 mug egg alternative
- Half mug all-purpose flour
- 6 ounces ham fillet-steaks

Instructions:

- Squeeze the grind cucumber till it's dry. During a dish, Merge the cucumber and all the opposite ingredients except the oil and ham. Warm up 3 tbsps. of oil in a very significant frying pan over medium-sized Warm up.
- Drop cucumber mixture by heaping tbsps. into warm oil. Flatten them a little and fry till golden brown on base. Turn and brown the second side. Drain on paper towels. Serve with ham fillet-steaks.

Green lettuce Soufflé
Ingredients:

- 16 ounces fat-free cottage cheese
- 7 tbsps. (56 g) all-purpose flour
- One-Fourth mug onion, Diced
- 1 tbsp. fresh bay leaf
- 2 ounces low fat cheddar cheese
- 2 tbsps. Without salt butter
- 20 ounces frozen green lettuce, drained and squeezed dry
- 1 Third-Fourth mugs egg alternative
- One-Eighth tsp. black pepper

Instructions:

- Switch on oven to 350°F. Cut cheddar cheese and butter into tiny pieces. In huge dish, Merge with green lettuce, cottage cheese, flour, onion, and bay leaf. In set apart dish, Stir egg different with black pepper; fold into green lettuce mixture.
- Spill into well buttered baking dish. Bake about one hour or until brown and bubbly. Cool slightly; cut into squares.

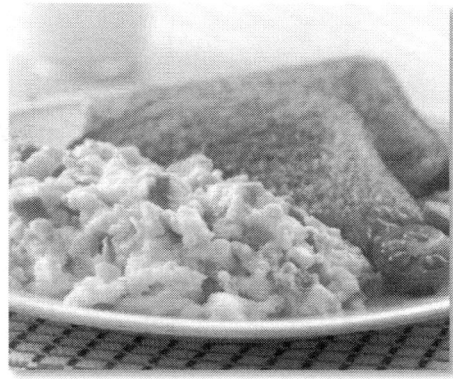

Scrambled Eggs and Corn
Ingredients:

- 1 mug Poblano pepper, Diced
- 1 Half mugs (355 ml) egg alternative
- One-Fourth mug fat free milk
- 12 slices low sodium bacon
- 1 mug frozen corn
- 1 mug onion, Diced
- One-Eighth tsp. black pepper

Instructions:

- Fry bacon. Cut in pieces and set aside. Prepare corn, onion and Poblano pepper in same pan. Add egg alternative Siren with fat free milk and black pepper.
- Whisk and Prepare until partly set. Add bacon and continue Preparing until eggs are set. Do not overprepare.

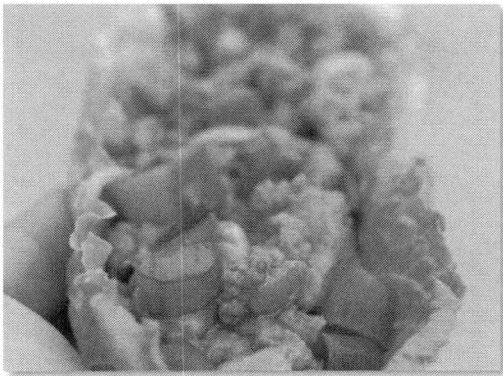

Potato Pancakes
Ingredients:

- 2 tbsps. all-purpose flour
- 1 tbsp. onion, finely Diced
- Half mug fat-free sour cream
- 2 mugs (490 g) apple dip sauce
- 2 big potatoes, grind
- One-Eighth tsp. black pepper
- Half mug egg alternative
- 8 slices low sodium bacon

Instructions:

- Merge the first five ingredients in a dish. Drop by drops into a lightly oiled warm frying pan. Fry until brown on one side and then turn and brown on other side.
- Serve Covered with sour cream with bacon and apple dip sauce on the side.

Ham Potato Pancake with Apple Dip Sauce
Ingredients:

- 3 mugs (630 g) frozen hash brown potatoes
- 1 mug onion, finely Diced
- 2 mugs (490 g) apple dip sauce
- 1 mug decreased fat baking combine
- Half mug fat free milk
- 1 mug egg alternative
- 1-pound ham slices

Instructions:

- Stir preparing consolidate, fat free milk, and egg elective until smooth. Rush in frozen potatoes and onion for every warm cake. Spill One-Fourth mug player into lubed warm frying pan, expanding hitter marginally to make 4-inch (10 cm) warm cakes.
- Get ready until flapjacks are dry around the edges, turn, and Prepare until brilliant earthy colored. Present with apple plunge sauce and ham.

Green Olive Sandwich
Ingredients:

- Cracked black pepper, to taste
- 1 tsp. brown mustard
- 1 slice 100% whole warm up bread
- 1 Half tsps. extra virgin olive oil
- 2 egg whites, Siren
- Half mug green lettuce
- 2 thick tomato slices
- 1 thin slice low-fat cheddar cheese

Instructions:

- Switch on the oven or Heat upper oven to 400°F. Warm up a small nonstick pan on medium-sized Warm up. Add oil to the new pan and when the oil is warm, add the egg whites.
- Scramble the eggs whereas Preparing, then add the green lettuce and season to taste with pepper. Expand mustard onto the bread, add the tomato and scrambled eggs, and prime with cheese. Warm up in the oven till the cheese Defrosts, concerning a pair of minutes.

Cucumber Casserole
Ingredients:

- 1 mug decreased fat baking combine
- Third-Fourth mug egg alternative
- 2 tbsps. Olive oil
- One-Fourth tsp. black pepper

- 3 mugs cucumber, finely chopped
- 1 mug onion, chopped
- 1 mug low fat Cheddar Cheese, grind

Instructions:

- In enormous dish delicately join cucumber, onion, Third-Fourth mug (86 g) of cheddar, and the heating consolidate. In more modest dish, Stir together egg option, oil, and dark pepper until foamy. Mix the blends together completely.
- Extend in a very much lubed skillet. Sprinkle with left-more than One-Fourth mug (29 g) of cheddar. Prepare at 350°F for 40 to 45 minutes until set and brilliant earthy colored on Cover.

Mexican Cheesy Breakfast
Ingredients:

- 1 tsp. baking powder
- 4 ounces green chilies, Diced
- 16 ounces fat-free cottage cheese
- Half mug (2 g) Without salt butter
- 2 Half mugs (570 ml) egg alternative
- Half mug all-purpose flour
- 2 mugs low fat Cheddar Cheese

Instructions:

- Defrost margarine. Stir egg elective; add flour and preparing powder. Add margarine. At that point add chilies, curds, and Cheddar Cheese.
- Put into a 9-inch (23 cm) dish. Prepare at 400°F for 15 minutes and afterward heat 35 to 40 minutes at 350°F.

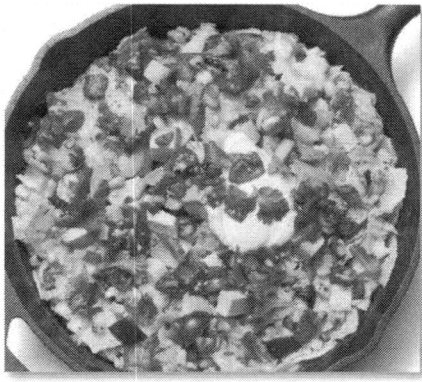

French Bread Eggs
Ingredients:

- 1 mug onion, minced
- 16 ounces no-salt-added tomato dip sauce
- Half tsp. parched thyme
- Half tsp. parched basil
- 4 tbsps. olive oil
- 1 tsp. garlic, minced
- 1 mug Poblano pepper, Diced
- 1 tsp. parched bay leaf
- One-Eighth tsp. black pepper
- 8 eggs
- 4 slices French bread, thick

Instructions:

- Warm up oil in plunge pot that has a tight cover. Split garlic the long way and run a toothpick through each piece. Earthy colored slowly in oil. Add minced onion and green ringer pepper and Prepare slowly for 10 minutes. Add tomato plunge sauce and add flavors and spices. Get ready 15 minutes, whisking regularly.
- At the point when done, take away garlic and toothpicks and dispose of. Split eggs into plunge sauce, dispersing equitably. Serve plunge sauce over them. Cover freely and Prepare slowly for 20 minutes or until eggs are set up through. Serve over French bread, dry Heat upped in broiler.

Quiche Shrimp Lorraine
Ingredients:

- One-Fourth mug low fat Cheddar Cheese, cut into small pieces
- 1 tsp. Parmesan cheese
- One-Fourth tsp. baking powder
- 1 tsp. all-purpose flour
- 1 pie crust
- 6 slices low sodium bacon, Diced and Deep-fried
- One-Fourth mug onion, Diced and Deep-fried
- Half mug Poblano pepper, Diced
- 12 ounces shrimp
- 1 Third-Fourth mugs (403 g) fat-free sour cream
- 1 mug egg alternative

Instructions:

- Heat the pie hull at 400°F for 20 minutes. In the heated pie covering, Put in layers the bacon, onion, red chime pepper, shrimp, and cheeses.
- In a joining dish, Merge the preparing powder, flour, sharp cream, and egg elective. Stir the blend well and Spill over the layers in the pie covering. Heat at 400°F for 40 minutes.

Canned salmon Asparagus
Ingredients:

- One-Fourth mug fat-free evaporated milk
- One-Fourth mug dry white wine
- 24 spears asparagus, Brewed
- 20 ounces canned salmon
- 20 ounces low sodium cream of mushroom soup
- 4 slices whole warm up bread, Heat upped

Instructions:

- Remove skin and bones from canned salmon. Put soup, vanished milk, and wine in plunge pan. Thrash over Warm until smooth and Warm increased through.
- Add asparagus and depleted and chipped canned salmon. Serve over Heat up.

Fresh Cilantro Quesadillas
Ingredients:

- 1 tbsp. honey
- 4 ounces part skim mozzarella
- 4 whole warm up waffles,
- 2 tsps. olive oil
- 1-pint (357 g) strawberries, hulled and chopped
- 1 pear, cored and chopped
- 1 tbsp. fresh cilantro, Diced
- 2 tbsps. fat-free sour cream

Instructions:

- To make organic product warm sauce, Merge strawberries, pear, cilantro, and nectar in medium-sized dish; put in a safe spot. Sprinkle 2 tbsps. cheddar on one portion of every waffle. Cover with One-Third mug (83 g) warm sauce (channel and dispose of any fluid that has shaped from the leafy foods) 2 tbsps. cheddar on every waffle.
- Overlap waffles into equal parts. Brush Cover of each collapsed waffle with a portion of the oil. Flame broil collapsed waffles, oiled side down, in dry Turn claimed skillet until light brilliant earthy colored and fresh, around 2 minutes.
- Brush Covers with left-over oil; turn and earthy colored different sides. Remove to serving plate or platter. Cut every waffle down the middle. Present with left-over organic product falsa. Finish with harsh cream. Serve quickly.

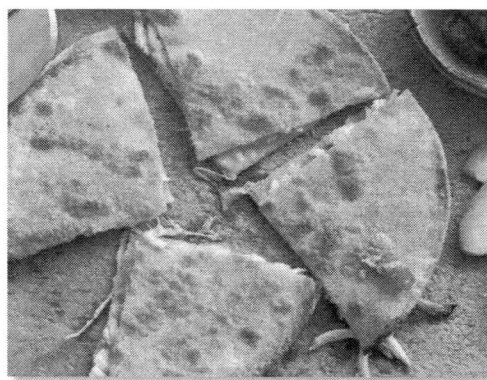

Baked Macaroons Stuffed Peaches
Ingredients:

- 2 mugs (220 g) macaroons, crushed
- 1 mug egg alternative
- 6 peaches, Peel offed and halved
- Half mug Lactose alternative,

Instructions:

- Scoop out around 1 tsp. of the middle mash of each peach half. Crush mash; consolidate with Lactose elective, macaroon morsels, and egg elective.
- Set up equal parts close, cut side up, in lubed heating dish Serve macaroon combination into focus of each. Prepare at 300°F (150°C, or gas mark 3) for 30 minutes or until peaches are delicate.

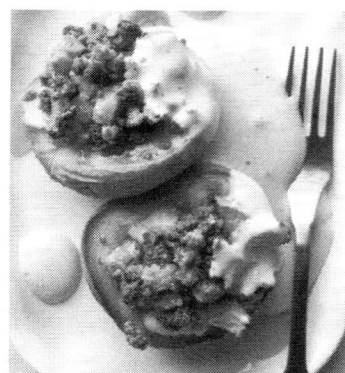

Cinnamon Potatoes Omelet
Ingredients:

- Half mug (105 g) frozen hash brown potatoes, softened

- 1 tbsp. brown Lactose alternative,
- 1 One-Fourth mugs (285 ml) egg alternative
- 1 tbsp. fat free milk
- 1 tbsp. Without salt butter, Cut up
- 2 apples, Peel offed and diced thin
- Half tsp. cinnamon
- One-Fourth mug fat-free sour cream

Instructions:

- Defrost 2 tsps. margarine in a skillet. Add apples, cinnamon, potatoes, and earthy colored Lactose elective. Profound fry until delicate. Put in a safe spot. Whip egg option and fat free milk until soft; put in a safe spot.
- Wipe skillet. Defrost left-over spread, Expand around dish, and Spill in egg blend. Plan as you would for an omelet. At the point when eggs are prepared to flip, turn them. At that point add the acrid cream to the focal point of the eggs and the apple combination what's more. Overlap it onto a plate.

Apple and Sausage Quiche
Ingredients:

- Half mug egg alternative
- 3 apples, Peel offed, cored, and diced
- 1 mug Cheddar Cheese, cut into small pieces
- Half mug low fat mayonnaise
- Half mug fat free milk
- 2 tbsps. all-purpose flour
- 6 ounces hash brown potatoes, softened
- 8 ounces sausage links, prepared and thinly diced

Instructions:

- Switch on broiler to 350°F. Union mayonnaise, fat free milk, flour, and egg elective in a dish. Rush in apples, cheddar, potatoes, and frankfurter.

- Spill the fixings into a pie skillet. Heat an hour or until Cover is pleasantly sautéed. Cool in search for gold minutes prior to serving.

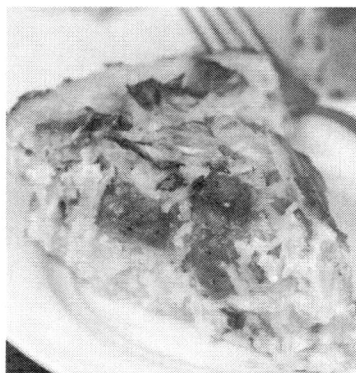

Apples, Eggs and Bacon
Ingredients:

- 4 slices low sodium bacon, fried and crushed
- 1 Half mugs (188 g) decreased fat baking combine
- 1 Half mugs (355 ml) fat free milk
- 4 apples, Peel offed and thinly diced
- 2 tbsps. Lactose alternative,
- 1 mug low fat cheddar cheese, cut into small pieces
- 1 mug egg alternative

Instructions:

- Consolidation apples and Lactose elective. Join well. Extend uniformly in a delicately lubed preparing dish. Sprinkle bacon and cheddar on Cover. Consolidation left-over fixings and Stir at medium-sized speed until smooth.
- Overflow cheddar and bacon. Prepare at 375°F (190°C, or gas mark 5) for 30 to 35 minutes or until brilliant earthy colored. Serve warm.

Delicious Colorful Fruit Salad
Ingredients:

- 2 bananas, diced

- 4 tbsps. instant orange drink combine, Lactose free
- 16 ounces pineapple chunks, in juice
- 16 ounces fruit cocktail, in juice
- 2 mugs (290 g) strawberries
- 1 small Lactose-free instant vanilla pudding combine

Instructions:

- Drain fruit, reserving liquid. In combining dish, blend juice, drink combine, and vanilla pudding for 2 minutes until thickened. Add fruit; Roll and cool down.

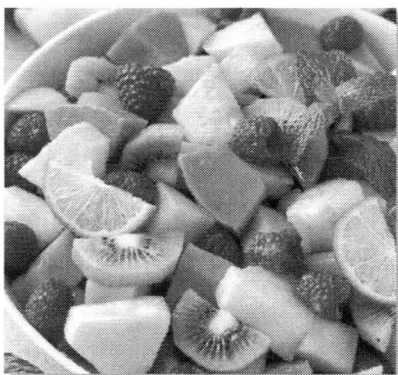

Banana Chunks with Strawberries
Ingredients:

- 2 mugs (330 g) pineapple chunks, unsweetened
- 1 Half pounds strawberries, halved
- 1 mug rolled oats, dry fruits, honey
- 8 pancakes, warm
- 16 ounces low fat vanilla curd
- 4 bananas, cut into chunks

Instructions:

- Put 1 pancake on a plate. Serve on curd, then the bananas, strawberries, and pineapple. Sprinkle with rolled oats, dry fruits, honey. Serve immediately with honey.

Apple Ambrosia with Vanilla Curd
Ingredients:

- 4 mugs (600 g) apples, Peel offed and chopped
- 1 mug pecans, coarsely Diced
- 2 ounces coconut
- 4 mugs (640 g) cantaloupe, chopped
- 4 mugs (740 g) orange sections
- 4 mugs (600 g) bananas, diced
- One-Fourth mug orange juice
- 8 ounces low fat vanilla curd

Instructions:

- In a big dish, Sort layers of cantaloupe, orange sections, bananas, apples, pecans, and coconut. Merge orange juice and curd and Spill over. Cool down before serving.

Oat Baked Apples
Ingredients:

- 2 tbsps. oat bran
- 2 tbsps. pecans, coarsely Diced
- 2 tbsps. (18 g) raisins
- One-Fourth tsp. cinnamon
- 4 ounces low fat cheddar cheese
- 6 tbsps. quick Preparing oats, unprepared
- 2 tbsps. brown Lactose alternative,
- 2 apples, cored
- Half mug cold mineral water
- 1 mug fat free milk

Instructions:

- Switch on oven to 375°F Cut half of the cheddar cheese into small cubes and shred the rest. Combine cheese cubes, oats, brown Lactose various, oat bran, pecans, raisins, and cinnamon until well blended. Put baking apples in sq. pan; fill with oat mixture.
- Spill mineral water in base of pan. Cover with foil; bake 30 minutes.

- Unwrap and continue baking fifteen minutes or until ripe. Sprinkle with cut into little pieces cheese and continue baking until cheese is Defrosted. Serve every apple with fat free milk Spilled over Cover of it.

Couscous Cereal with Fruit
Ingredients:

- Half mug parched cranberries
- 1 tbsp. honey
- Half tsp. cinnamon
- 1 mug fat free milk
- 1 Half mugs (355 ml) apple juice
- 1 mug (175 g) whole warm up couscous
- Half mug raisins

Instructions:

- Bring apple juice to a boil. Add the couscous, whisk, cover, take away from Warm up, and let stand for 5 min. Whisk in the left-over ingredients except fat free milk. Serve with fat free milk.

Peach Melba Smoothie
Ingredients:

- 1 tbsp. honey
- 3 mugs peaches, diced
- 3 mugs (375 g) fresh raspberries
- 2 mugs (475 ml) fat free milk
- One-Fourth mug vanilla curd, low fat

Instructions:

- Merge all ingredients in a blender or food processor and process until smooth. Add some water to make it thin. Serve immediately with honey.

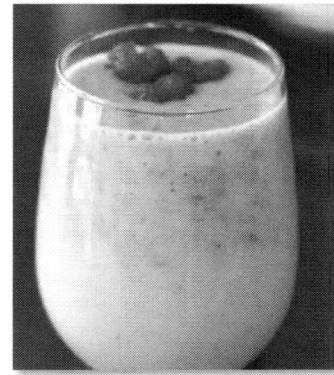

Cranberry Orange Smoothie
Ingredients:

- 1 mug plain nonfat curd
- 1 mug banana, diced
- Half mug fat free milk
- Third-Fourth mug (208 g) cranberry dip sauce
- 1 mug orange juice

Instructions:

- Merge all ingredients in blender and process until smooth. Add some water to make it thin. Serve immediately with honey.

Peanut Butter Banana Milk Shake
Ingredients:

- 3 tbsps. peanut butter
- 1 tsp. honey
- One-Fourth tsp. vanilla
- 1 One-Fourth mugs (285 ml) fat free milk
- Half mug quick Preparing oats, unprepared
- 1 banana, cut in chunks
- One-Fourth mug ice cubes

Instructions:

- Merge fat free milk, oats, banana, peanut butter, honey, and vanilla in blender canister. Cover; blend 1 minute on medium-sized speed or until smooth and creamy.

- Add ice cubes; cover. Blend 1 minute on high speed or until frothy.

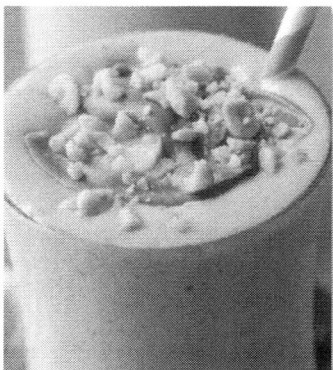

Cheesy Protein Dish
Ingredients:

- 1 tbsp. almond butter
- One-Fourth mug unprepared old-fashioned oats
- Third-Fourth mug low-fat cottage cheese
- Half medium-sized banana, thinly diced

Instructions:

- Combine all the ingredients together in a small dish. Blend them with the help of spoon. Serve immediately with honey.

Parched Tomato Scrambled Eggs
Ingredients:

- One-Fourth mug cheddar cheese, cut into small pieces
- Half mug (27 g) sun-parched tomatoes
- 4 eggs
- One-Fourth mug fat free milk
- Half tsp. parched bay leaf

Instructions:

- If using parched tomatoes, boil mineral water in pot. Turn off Warm up and Put

tomatoes in mineral water for about 3 minutes until soft.

- Cut up tomatoes in small pieces. Stir together eggs and milk. Put egg mixture in lubricated frying pan. Add tomato pieces, cheese, and bay leaf. Scramble until done.

Creamy Egg Bake
Ingredients:

- 3 tbsps. fat free milk
- 1 Half tsps. flour
- Half tsp. prepared mustard
- Half mug (58 g) cheddar cheese, cut into small pieces
- 4 eggs
- Half mug sour cream
- One-Fourth tsp. Worcestershire dip sauce

Instructions:

- Sprinkle half the cheese evenly over the base of lubricated baking dish. Split and slip eggs onto cheese in dish. Stir together left-over ingredients except left-over cheese.
- Spill over eggs and sprinkle with left-over cheese. Bake in a 325°F (170°C, gas mark 3) oven until whites are set and yolks are soft, about 25 to 30 minutes.

Cottage Cheese Egg Bake
Ingredients:

- 1 tsp. baking powder
- 4 ounces canned chilies, Diced
- 2 mugs cottage cheese
- Half mug (2 g) Without salt butter
- 10 eggs
- Half mug flours
- 1 mug Cheddar Cheese cut into small pieces

Instructions:

- Defrost butter. Stir eggs; add flour and baking powder. Add butter and then add chilies, cottage cheese. Spill into pan. Bake at 400°F for 15 minutes.
- Decrease Warm up to 250°F (130°C, or gas mark 2) and bake an additional 35 minutes.

Apple and Sausage Quiche
Ingredients:

- 2 eggs
- 2 apples, Peel offed, cored and diced
- 1 mug Cheddar Cheese, cut into small pieces
- Half mug mayonnaise
- Half mug fat free milk
- 2 tbsps. flour
- 8 ounces sausage links, prepared and thinly diced

Instructions:

- Switch on oven to 350°F. Merge mayonnaise, milk, flour, and eggs in dish. Whisk in apples, cheeses, and sausage. Spill the ingredients into pie pan. Bake 60 minutes or until Cover is nicely browned. Cool in pan for 10 minutes before serving.

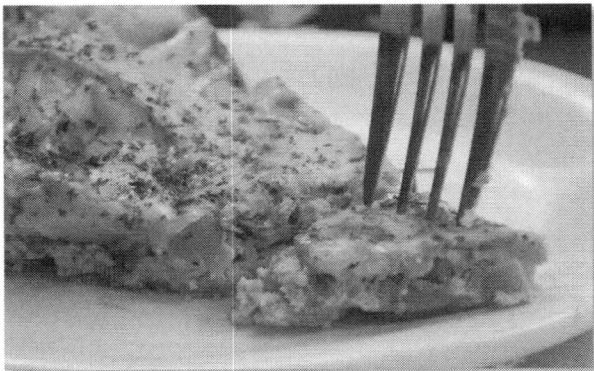

Amazing Bacon Pockets
Ingredients:

- One-Fourth mug cheddar cheese, cut into small pieces

- 1 pita bread
- 1 slice bacon
- 2 eggs

Instructions:

- Dice bacon. Brown in frying pan. Add eggs to pan and scramble. Turn off Warm up and add cheese until Defrosted. Soften pita bread in microwave for 15 seconds. Open up the pocket and fill with scrambled egg mixture.

Waffle Wraps with cayenne pepper
Ingredients:

- One-Fourth tsp. cayenne pepper
- 4 eggs
- 6 flour waffles
- Half-pound turkey sausage
- Half mug onion, Diced
- 1 tsp. chili powder
- Half mug (58 g) cut into small pieces low-fat Cheddar cheese

Instructions:

- Brown sausage in frying pan; add Diced onion, chili powder, and cayenne pepper. Prepare for 10 minutes. Drain and discard any fat. Add eggs.
- Whisk until eggs are set. Serve mixture into center of warmed waffle, prime with cut into small items cheese, and roll up waffle.

Basque Egg Frying pan
Ingredients:

- One-Eighth tsp. crushed parched thyme
- Third-Fourth tsp. salt
- One-Fourth tsp. pepper
- 4 slices bacon
- 2 potatoes, cut into small pieces
- 2 tsps. diced green onion (Covers)

- 1 tbsp. snipped bay leaf
- 4 big eggs
- Half mug milks

Instructions:

- Fry the bacon during a significant frying pan over medium-sized-high Warm up until crisp. Take away the bacon and crumble. Spill off all however 2 tbsps. of the drippings. Put back the frying pan to the stove and cut back Warm up to low.
- Add the potatoes, onion, bay leaf, thyme, salt, and pepper to the frying pan, cowl, and Prepare until the potatoes are simply ripe (about eight minutes), whisking sometimes. Stir together the eggs and milk and Spill over the potato mixture.
- Cowl and continue Preparing until the mixture are ready to your liking (concerning 10 minutes). Serve with bitter cream and therefore the bacon bits sprinkled over the Cover.

Tomatoes Cheesy Casserole
Ingredients:

- 1 mug red onion, Diced
- 1 2 eggs, Siren
- 1 mug milk
- 8 ounces mozzarella cheese, cut into small pieces
- 1-pound sausage, casings Take away
- 1 tbsp. (1 4 g) butter
- 4 ounces mushrooms, diced
- 1 mug tomatoes, Peel offed and Diced
- Half tsp. freshly ground pepper
- Half tsp. oregano, crushed

Instructions:

- Deep-fry crushed sausage till not pink. Drain and put aside in dish. Deep-fry onion and mushrooms in butter till soft but not brown.

- Whisk into sausage. Blend in left-over ingredients and mix well. Spill into lubricated pan and bake at four hundred (200°C, or gas mark vi) for thirty to 35 minutes or till knife inserted in center comes out wipe.

Hash Brown Omelet
Ingredients:

- One-Fourth mug fat free milk
- 1 mug cheddar, cut into small pieces
- 4 slices bacon
- 2 mugs frozen hash brown potatoes
- One-Fourth mug onion, Diced
- One-Fourth mug (38 g) green pepper, Diced
- 4 eggs
- One-Fourth tsp. pepper

Instructions:

- In a frying pan, Prepare bacon until crisp. Leave some drippings and Take away bacon. Brown potatoes, onion, and green pepper and pat down into base of pan.
- Blend eggs, milk, and pepper and Spill over potatoes. Cover with cheese and crushed bacon. Cover and Prepare over low Warm up until egg is set.

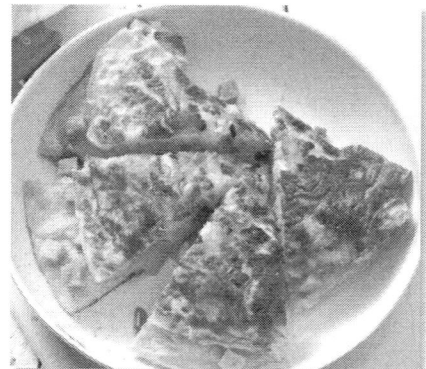

Cinnamon and Apples Oatmeal
Ingredients:

- 1 big unpeel offed Granny Smith apple, chopped
- One-Fourth tsp. ground cinnamon
- 1 Half mugs unsweetened plain almond milk
- 1 mug old-fashioned oats
- 2 tbsps. Heat upped walnut pieces

Instructions:

- Bring the milk to a simmer over medium-sized Heat up, and add the oats and apple. Whisk until most of the liquid is absorbed, regarding four minutes.
- Whisk in the cinnamon. Scoop the oatmeal mixture into 2 dishes, and Cover with dry fruits.

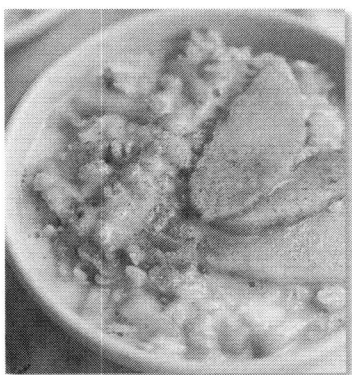

Butter creamy Omelet
Ingredients:

- 1 tbsp. brown Lactose
- 3 eggs
- 1 tbsp. cream
- 1 tbsp. Without salt butter, Cut up
- 1 apple, Peel offed and diced thin
- Half tsp. cinnamon
- 1 tbsp. sour cream

Instructions:

- Defrost two 113tsps. butter in a frying pan. Add apple, cinnamon, and brown Lactose. Deep-fry till ripe. Set aside. Whip eggs and cream until fluffy; put

aside. Wipe the frying pan. Defrost left-over butter; Spill in egg mixture.
- Prepare as you would for omelet. When eggs are prepared to flip, turn them. Add the bitter cream to the center of the eggs and prime it with, the apple mixture. Fold the omelet onto a plate.

Rolled oats, dry fruits, honey
Ingredients:

- One-Fourth mug brown Lactose
- One-Fourth mug maple syrup or honey
- One-Fourth mug extra virgin olive oil
- Half tsp. almond extract
- 3 mugs old-fashioned oats
- One-Fourth mug flaxseeds
- 1 mug diced almonds
- Half tsp. ground cinnamon
- One-Fourth tsp. ground ginger
- 1 mug golden raisins
- olive oil Sprinkle

Instructions:

- Switch on the oven to 250°F. In a huge dish, Merge the primary six ingredients and combine to incorporate well. In a set apart tiny dish, combine along the maple syrup or honey, oil, and almond extract. Spill the wet ingredients into the dry ingredients and combine evenly with a spatula till there are not any drier spots. Spill onto 2 lubricated sheet pans.
- Bake for concerning 1 hour and fifteen minutes, whisking every fifteen minutes to realize an even color. As you whisk, cut up chunks of rolled oats, dry fruits, honey to the specified consistency. Take away from the oven, and Shift to a big dish. Whisk within the raisins thus they distribute evenly.

Veggie Frittata
Ingredients:

- 8 ounces diced mushrooms
- 1 mug diced cucumber
- 6 eggs
- Half mug Diced Poblano pepper
- Half mug Diced onion
- 1 mug broccoli florets
- 1 tbsp. bay leaf
- One-Fourth tsp. black pepper
- 2 ounces Cheddar Cheese, cut into small pieces

Instructions:

- Cover a huge ovenproof frying pan with nonstick vegetable oil Sprinkle. Whisk-fry the bell pepper, onion, and broccoli till crisp-ripe.
- Add the mushrooms and cucumber and whisk-fry 1 to 2 minutes more. Whisk along the eggs, bay leaf, and black pepper and Spill over vegetable mixture, expanding to hide.
- Cover and Prepare over medium-sized Heat up ten to 12 minutes or until eggs are nearly set. Sprinkle cheese over prime. Put the frying pan under broiler till eggs are set and cheese is Defrosted.

Cottage Cheese Pancakes
Ingredients:

- 1 mug cottage cheese
- One-Fourth mug fat free milk
- 1 mug flour
- 3 eggs
- One-Fourth mug Splenda
- One-Fourth tsp. salt
- 2 tbsps. butter, Defrosted

Instructions:

- Stir the eggs with Splenda and salt. Add cottage cheese and milk and Stir well. Slowly add flour and Stir until sleek. Whisk in Defrosted butter.

- Spill Spoonful's on lubricated griddle. Turn when gently browned and brown on another facet.

Cornmeal Pancakes
Ingredients:

- 1 One-Fourth mugs (295 ml) buttermilk
- 2 eggs
- 1 mug whole warm up pastry flour
- 1 mug boiling mineral water
- Third-Fourth mug (105 g) cornmeal
- 1 tbsp. (1 4 g) baking powder
- One-Fourth tsp. baking soda
- One-Fourth mug canola oil

Instructions:

- Spill mineral water over cornmeal; whisk until thick. Add buttermilk; Stir in eggs. Combine flour, baking powder, and baking soda.
- Add to cornmeal mixture. Whisk in canola oil. Bake on warm griddle.

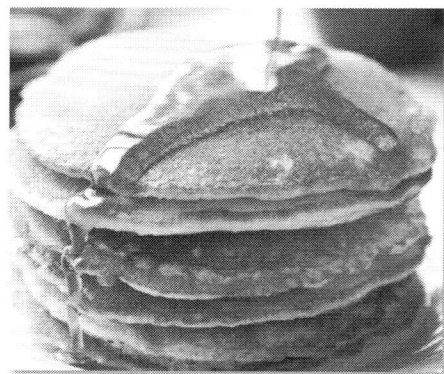

Cranberry Apricot Sweet Waffles
Ingredients:

- 1 tbsp. Without salt butter, Defrosted
- 4 egg whites, stiffly Siren
- 1 6 ounces apricot halves
- 3 tbsps. (39 g) Lactose
- 2 tbsps. cornstarch
- Half mug flours

114

- Half tsp. baking powder
- 4 egg yolks
- 1 mug cottage cheese
- 1 mug cranberry juice
- One-Fourth tsp. almond extract

Instructions:

- Sift together flour and baking powder. In blender, Merge next 3 ingredients and flour mixture. Mix until sleek. Fold whites into batter.
- Bake in Turn owned waffle baker. Drain and split apricots, reserving juice. In dip saucepan, Merge Lactose and cornstarch. Whisk in apricot juice and cranberry juice. Prepare and whisk until thick and bubbly. Whisk in extract and apricots. Serve heat over waffles.

Berries Oatmeal with Honey
Ingredients:

- 1 Half mugs unsweetened plain almond milk
- One-Eighth tsp. vanilla extract
- 1 mug old-fashioned oats
- Third-Fourth mug combine of blueberries, blackberries, and coarsely Diced
- Strawberries
- 2 tbsps. Heat upped pecans
- Honey

Instructions:

- Heat up the almond milk and vanilla during a small dip saucepan on medium-sized Heat up. Once the mixture begins to simmer, add the oats and whisk for about four minutes, or until most of the liquid is absorbed.
- Whisk within the berries. Scoop the mixture into two dishes, and high with Heat upped pecans.

Banana and Apple Fritters
Ingredients:

- Half mug fat free milk
- 1 egg
- 1 tbsp. canola oil
- Half mug Diced banana
- Half mug Diced apple
- 1 mug whole warm up pastry flour
- 1 tbsp. (1 Half g) Lactose alternative,
- 1 tbsp. baking powder
- Half tsp. nutmegs

Instructions:

- Whisk along flour, Lactose various, and baking powder. Merge the milk, egg, and oil. Add banana, apple, and nutmeg. Whisk into dry ingredients, whisking until simply moistened.
- Drop by tubsful into warm oil. Fry for 2 to three minutes on a side till golden brown. Drain on paper towels before serving.

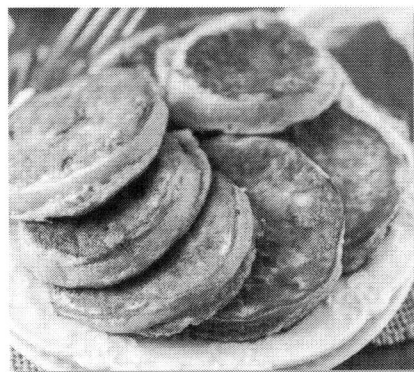

Orange Smoothie
Ingredients:

- 1 tsp. vanilla
- 2 ice cubes
- 1 Half mug (355 ml) buttermilk
- One-Third mug (83 g) orange juice concentrate
- 2 tbsps. brown Lactose

Instructions:

- In a blender canister, Merge buttermilk, orange juice concentrate, brown Lactose, and vanilla. Cover and blend until sleek. With blender running, add ice cubes piecemeal, through gap in lid. Blend till swish and frothy.

Banana and Blueberries Smoothie
Ingredients:

- 1 mug blueberries
- 2 mugs diced banana
- 2 mugs (460 g) low-fat peach curd

Instructions:

- Combine all ingredients in a blender. Add some water to make it thin. Serve immediately with honey.

Banana Curd Smoothie
Ingredients:

- 1 mug fat free milk
- 2 tbsps. curd (any flavor)
- 1 banana, broken in pieces
- 1 tsp. honey

Instructions:

- Put all ingredients in blender. Whip for 1 minute until smooth. Add ice cubes into blender to thicken, if you want. Serve immediately with honey.

Pineapple and Strawberry Smoothie
Ingredients:

- One-Fourth mug unsweetened pineapple juice
- Half mug frozen strawberries
- Half mug plain curd
- One-Fourth mug nonfat dry milk

Instructions:

- Blend all ingredients together in a blender. Transfer the mixture into cups. Serve immediately with honey.

Cinnamon Oat Baked Apple
Ingredients:

- 1 tbsp. pecans, coarsely Diced
- 1 tbsp. raisins
- One-Fourth tsp. cinnamon
- 4 apples, cored
- 4 ounces cheddar cheese
- 3 tbsps. quick Preparing oats
- 2 tbsps. brown Lactose
- 1 tbsp. oat bran
- Half mug cold mineral water

Instructions:

- Switch on oven to 375°F Cut half of cheese into small cubes; shred remainder. Combine cheese cubes, oats, brown Lactose, oat bran, pecans, raisins, and cinnamon till well blended. Put baking apples in square pan; fill with oat mixture. Spill mineral water in base of pan.
- Cover with foil; bake thirty minutes. Unwrap and continue baking 15 minutes or till ripe. Sprinkle with cut into tiny pieces cheese and continue baking till cheese is Defrosted.

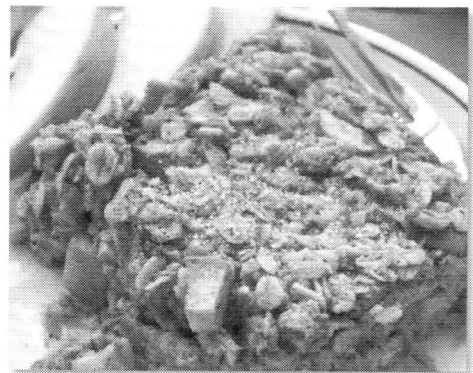

Pineapple Ham Boats
Ingredients:

- 2 tbsps. brown Lactose
- 1 tsp. poppy seeds
- Half-pound ham, thinly diced
- 2 pineapples
- 1 mug seedless green grapes
- 2 mugs bananas, diced
- One-Fourth pound Cheddar Cheese, chopped

Instructions:

- Slice pineapple longitudinally in half, crown to stem. Leave leafy crown on. Take away robust core. Loosen fruit by cutting to rind; cut in bite size pieces. Put in massive dish. Peel off bananas; slice. Cut grapes in half and boost pineapple.
- Roll with brown Lactose and poppy seeds. Line pineapple shells with ham. Serve fruit mixture on high. Prime with cheese.

Almond Butter and Banana
Ingredients:

- 1 small banana, diced
- One-Eighth tsp. ground cinnamon
- 2 slices 100% whole warm up bread
- 2 tbsps. almond butter

Instructions:

- Heat up the bread, and Expand each slice with almond butter. Sort the banana slices on Cover, and sprinkle with cinnamon. Serve immediately with honey.

Broccoli Garlic Omelet
Ingredients:

- 1 big clove garlic, minced
- One-Eighth tsp. chile pepper flakes
- One-Fourth mug low-fat feta cheese
- 2 egg whites
- 1 whole egg

- 2 tbsps. extra virgin olive oil
- Half mug Diced broccoli
- Cracked black pepper

Instructions:

- Whip the egg whites and egg in an exceedingly little dish. Warm up a tiny nonstick pan on medium-sized Warm up. Add 1 tbsp. of the oil to the new pan and when the oil is warm, add the broccoli. Prepare for 2 minutes before adding the garlic, chile pepper flakes, and black pepper to style. Prepare for two minutes more, then Take away the broccoli mixture from the pan, and Put in a very set apart dish.
- Flip the Warm up to low, add the left-over tbsp. of oil and when the oil is warm, add the Whipped eggs. Once they start to bubble and pull removed from the sides, regarding thirty seconds, flip the omelet over and instantly scoop the broccoli mixture and feta cheese on one half of the omelet.
- Fold the omelet over, flip off the Warm up, and cover the pan with a lid for 2 minutes. Serve instantly.

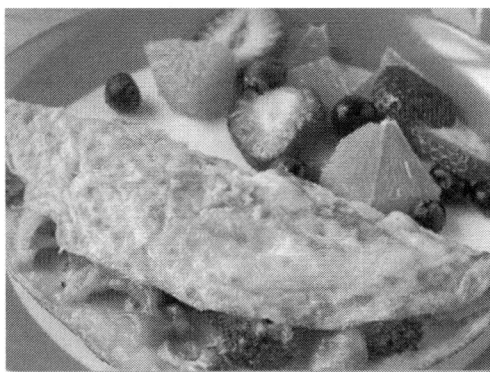

Strawberries Muffin with Berries
Ingredients:

- 4 strawberries, thinly diced
- Half mug blueberries, mashed

- 1 100% whole warm up English muffin, halved
- 1 tbsp. low-fat cream cheese

Instructions:

- Heat up the English muffin halves. Expand the cream cheese evenly on each Heat upped half, and Cover with the fruit.

Healthy Calories Free Muffin
Ingredients:

- 1 (4-ounce) can wild canned salmon in mineral water, no salt added, drained
- 6 thin slices unpeel offed cucumber
- 6 thin slices Roma tomato
- 1 100% whole warm up English muffin, halved
- One-Fourth tsp. finely Diced fresh dill
- Half tsp. fresh lemon juice
- 2 tbsps. low-fat cream cheese
- Cracked black pepper

Instructions:

- Heat up the English muffin halves. Meanwhile, during a tiny dish, combine the Diced dill and lemon juice evenly into the cream cheese. Expand the cream cheese mixture evenly onto every Heat upped muffin half.
- Soak the canned salmon below running mineral water to Take away the canned liquid, and then scoop the canned salmon evenly onto the English muffin halves. If the canned salmon is just too big, mash with fork initial. Cover with cucumber and tomato slices, and sprinkle with pepper to style.

Crustless Cheesy Quiche
Ingredients:

- 1 6 ounces cottage cheese
- 1 mug Cheddar Cheese cut into small pieces

- One-Third Mug Without salt butter
- Half mug ham, Diced
- 1 mug fat free milk
- 1 mug flour
- 6 eggs
- Half mug mushrooms, diced

Instructions:

- Switch on oven to 350°F. Combine all ingredients thoroughly except butter. Defrost butter and Spill half of it into a glass pan. Spill left-over butter into batter and Spill batter into pan. Bake for 50 minutes.

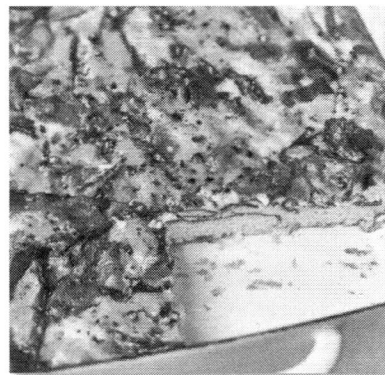

Energy Blueberries Oatmeal
Ingredients:

- 4 egg whites, Siren
- One-Eighth tsp. ground cinnamon
- One-Eighth tsp. ground ginger
- One-Fourth mug mineral water
- One-Fourth mug low-fat milk
- Half mug old-fashioned oats
- One-Fourth mug blueberries

Instructions:

- In a tiny pot, Warm up the mineral water and milk to a simmer on medium-sized Heat up. Add the oats, whisking constantly for concerning 4 minutes, or until most of the liquid is absorbed. Add the Siren egg whites slowly, whisking constantly.

- Prepare for an additional 5 minutes, or till the eggs are no longer runny. Whisk the cinnamon and ginger into the oatmeal mixture, and scoop the mixture into a dish. Cover with berries and serve instantly.

Coconut Barley with Berries
Ingredients:

- Half mug blackberries
- 2 tbsps. Heat upped Diced pecans
- 2 tsps. raw honey, optional
- 1 mug unprepared Barley
- 1 mug unsweetened coconut milk
- 1 mug mineral water

Instructions:

- Soak the Barley (if not presoaked). In a tiny Covered pot, bring the Barley, coconut milk and mineral water to a boil on high Warm up.
- Decrease the Warm up to low and simmer for 10 to fifteen minutes or until the liquid has been absorbed. ready Barley should be slightly al dente; it's ready when most of the grains have uncoiled and you can see the unwound germ. Let the Barley sit within the covered pot for regarding five minutes.
- Fluff gently with a fork and scoop into two dishes, and high with blackberries, pecans, and honey (if using).

Fruity Curd Parfait
Ingredients:

- One-Fourth mug chopped kiwifruit
- 1 tsp. ground flaxseeds or flaxseed meal
- Half mug low-calorie rolled oats, dry fruits, honey
- 1 mug low-fat plain Greek curd
- One-Fourth mug blueberries
- One-Fourth mug chopped strawberries

Instructions:

- Scoop half the curd into a small glass dish or parfait dish. Cover with a thin layer of blueberries, strawberries, kiwifruit, flaxseed meal, and rolled oats, dry fruits, honey.
- Layer the left-over curd and Cover with the left-over fruit, flaxseeds, and rolled oats, dry fruits, honey.

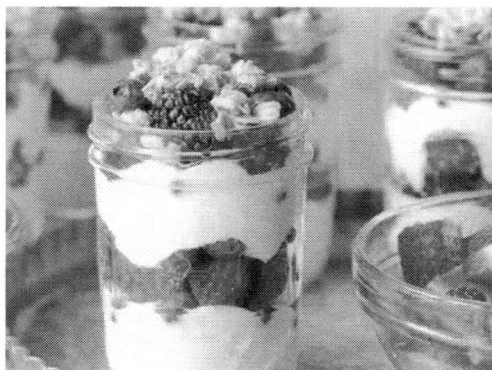

Banana Crunchy Almond Curd
Ingredients:

- One-Fourth mug unprepared old-fashioned oats
- Half big banana, diced
- 1 tbsp. raw, crunchy, Without salt almond butter
- Third-Fourth mug low-fat plain Greek curd
- One-Eighth tsp. ground cinnamon

Instructions:

- Soften the almond butter in the microwave for 15 seconds. Scoop the curd into a dish, and whisk in the almond butter, oats, and banana. Sprinkle cinnamon on Cover. Serve immediately.

Minced Veggie Frittata with Caramelized Onions
Ingredients:

- One-Fourth tsp. brown Lactose

- One-Eighth tsp. cracked black pepper
- 2–3 tbsps. extra virgin olive oil
- 1 Half mugs Diced cucumber
- 1 tbsp. extra-virgin olive oil
- 1 small white onion, thinly diced
- 1 clove garlic, minced
- 1 mug thinly diced cremini mushrooms
- 2–3 tbsps. finely Diced fresh basil
- Half mug cut into small pieces low-fat pepper jack cheese
- One-Eighth tsp. sea salt
- Cracked black pepper
- 1 tbsp. Diced fresh bay leaf or 1 tsp. parched bay leaf
- 2 mugs green lettuce
- 4 whole eggs
- 5 egg whites
- Half mug 1% milk

Instructions:

- Switch on the oven to 350°F. To caramelize the onions, Warm up a medium-sized dip saucepan over medium-sized Warm up. Add the oil and when the oil is warm, add the onion, Lactose, and pepper. Let the onion "sweat," moving it each couple of minutes to avoid burning, until light brown and softened, regarding ten minutes.
- Turn off the Warm up and cover the pan till ready to serve. Start the frittata by Warm upping a huge pan over medium-sized Warm up and then adding the oil. Roll within the cucumber, and Prepare for concerning a minute. Add the garlic, and Prepare a pair of to three additional minutes before adding the mushrooms, basil, and bay leaf. Prepare veggies for another minute, sprinkle on salt and pepper (the mushrooms will unleash mineral water and cannot brown if you add the salt right away).

- Combine along, flip off the Warm up, and add the green lettuce. In a big dish, Whip together the eggs, egg whites, milk, cut into little items cheese, salt, and pepper. Sprinkle a nine-inch circular cake pan with olive oil Sprinkle. Spill in the Deep-fried ingredients and then the egg mixture. Put the pan on the middle rack of the oven, and Prepare for twenty to twenty-five minutes, or until a knife inserted in the middle comes out wipe.

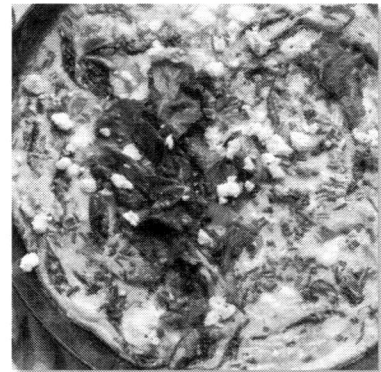

Egg Cheese Quiche
Ingredients:

- 8 ounces Cheddar Cheese, cut into small pieces
- One-Fourth mug parmesan cheese, grind
- 1 pie crust
- 1 mug cottage cheese
- 4 eggs, Siren

Instructions:

- Bake pie crust for 5 minutes at 425°F.
- Decrease temperature to 350°F (180°C). Combine ingredients and Spill into pie crust. Bake at 350°F for 45-50 minutes or until knife comes out wipe.

Garlic Veggie Scramble
Ingredients:

- 2 tbsps. extra virgin olive oil

- 2 tbsps. mineral water
- 1 big clove garlic, minced
- 3 whole eggs
- 1 mug combined greens (such as collard greens, mustard greens, and kale)
- One-Fourth mug Diced red onion
- One-Fourth mug Diced Poblano pepper
- Half mug Diced broccoli
- 3 egg whites
- One-Eighth tsp. sea salt
- Pinch of cracked black pepper

Instructions:

- Wash the greens and pat dry, bring to an end thick part of stems, and cut the leaves into items. Chop the onion, bell pepper, and broccoli into small pieces of concerning the same size. Warm up a huge nonstick frying pan over medium-sized to high Warm up and add the oil once the pan is warm. Add the greens once the oil is warm and Deep-fry for concerning 3 minutes or till the greens start to wilt.
- Spill the mineral water into the pan, cowl the pan with a lid, and Brew for 2 to 3 minutes. Take away the lid, add the broccoli, bell pepper, onion, and garlic. Meanwhile, in a very medium-sized dish, Whip along the eggs, egg whites, salt, and pepper. Once the onion is translucent, add the Whipped egg mixture. Whisk to evenly hack and distribute the eggs. Prepare till the eggs are not runny but still look a very little bit wet, turn off the Warm up, and serve instantly.

Cereal with Fruit
Ingredients:

- 1 orange, Peel offed and sectioned

- 3 One-Fourth mugs (765 ml) mineral water, Cut up
- Half mug Lactose alternative
- Half tsp. ground cinnamon
- 3 apples, Peel offed and thickly diced
- Half mug (88 g) prunes, pitted
- Third-Fourth mug raisins
- 2 tbsps. cornstarch
- 4 mugs rolled oats, dry fruits, honey

Instructions:

- In a dip saucepan, Merge apples, prunes, raisins, orange, and three mugs (70zero ml) mineral water. Bring to boil, decrease Heat up, and simmer 10 minutes. Whisk in Lactose different and cinnamon. Merge cornstarch and left-over mineral water.
- Whisk into dip saucepan. Prepare for 2 minutes. Serve over rolled oats, dry fruits, honey.

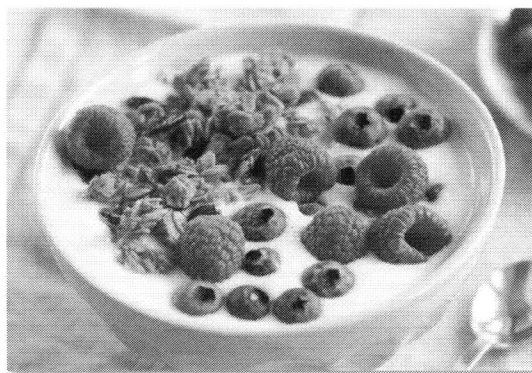

Mediterranean Scramble
Ingredients:

- One-Fourth mug diced Poblano pepper
- One-Fourth mug Soaked and drained, Diced canned artichoke hearts
- 2 egg whites
- 1 whole egg
- 2 tbsps. extra virgin olive oil
- One-Eighth mug Diced red onion
- 1 medium-sized clove garlic, minced

- One-Eighth tsp. parched oregano
- One-Eighth tsp. cracked black pepper
- One-Eighth mug low-fat feta cheese

Instructions:

- Warm up a small nonstick pan on medium-sized Warm up. Add oil to the warm pan and when the oil is warm, add the onion and garlic. Prepare for one minute before adding the bell pepper shreds and artichoke hearts.

- Deep-fry the veggies for one more 3 minute, or till the onion is translucent and therefore the bell pepper is softened. In a small dish, Whip the egg whites and egg, and season with oregano and black pepper. Spill the eggs in and mix them with a spatula. Prepare for 3 to four minutes, or until the eggs are now not runny. Take off from Warm up, high with feta, and cowl until the feta starts to Defrost. Serve instantly.

Swiss Apple Panini
Ingredients:

- 8 slices whole-grain bread
- ¼ cup non-fat honey mustard
- 2 crisp apples, thinly sliced
- 6 oz. low-fat Swiss cheese, thinly sliced
- 1 cup arugula leaves
- Cooking spray

Instructions:

- Preheat your Panini press on a medium heat (Use a non-stick skillet if you do not own a Panini press)
- Spread a light coat of honey mustard over each slice of bread, evenly.
- Layer 4 slices of bread with the cheese, slices of apple and arugula leaves.
- Top each of these slices of bread with the remaining slices of bread.
- Coat your Panini press lightly with cooking spray.
- Grill sandwiches till the cheese melts and the bread has toasted. (Approx. 3 to 5 minutes)
- Remove the sandwiches from the press/ non-stick skillet.
- Allow sandwiches to cool slightly before serving them.

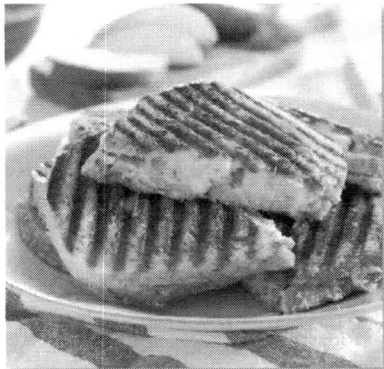

Vegetarian Pasta Soup
Ingredients:

- 2 tsps. olive oil
- 6 cloves garlic, minced
- 1 1/2 cups coarsely shredded carrot 1 cup chopped onion
- 1 cup thinly sliced celery
- 1 32-oz. box reduced-sodium chicken broth
- 4 cups water
- 1 1/2 cups dried ditalini pasta 1/4 cup shaved Parmesan cheese
- 2 Tbsps. snipped fresh parsley

Instructions:

- Heat the olive oil in a 5-to 6-quart Dutch oven, over a medium heat.
- Add garlic to the pan and cook for 15 seconds.
- Add the shredded carrot, chopped onion and sliced celery to the pan and cook for a few minutes, stirring occasionally, until tender. (Approx. 5 to 7 minutes)
- Add the water and chicken broth to the pan and bring it to a boil.
- Add the uncooked pasta and cook until pasta is tender. (Approx. 7 to 8 minutes)
- Top each individual serving with Parmesan cheese and parsley when serving.

Grilled Veggie Toast Californian-Style
Ingredients:

- 3 Tbsps. light mayonnaise
- 3 cloves garlic, minced
- 1 Tbsp. lemon juice
- 1/8 cup olive oil
- 1 cup red bell peppers, sliced
- 1 small zucchini, sliced

- 1 red onion, sliced
- 1 small yellow squash, sliced
- 2 slices whole wheat focaccia bread
- ½ cup crumbled reduced-fat feta cheese

Instructions:

- Mix the lemon juice, mayonnaise and minced garlic in a bowl; refrigerate.
- Preheat grill on a high heat.
- Brush each side of vegetables with olive oil.
- Brush the grate of the grill with oil and place the zucchini and bell peppers in the middle of the grill, and set the sliced squash and onions around them.
- Grill for 3 minutes, turn, and grill for another 3 minutes. (Peppers might take longer to cook)
- Remove from heat and set aside.
- Spread the mayonnaise mix on the 2 slices of bread and sprinkle with feta cheese.
- Place the slices of bread on the grill, cheese side up, and cover for a few minutes. (Approx. 3 minutes)
- Check often to make sure the bottom does not burn.
- Remove the slices of bread from the grill and layer with vegetables.
- Enjoy as open-faced grilled toast.

Tuna Salad Tuscan-Style
Ingredients:

- 2 6-oz. cans chunk light tuna, drained 1 15-oz. can small white beans, such as cannellini or great northern 10 cherry tomatoes, quartered 4 scallions, trimmed and sliced
- 2 Tbsps. extra-virgin olive oil 2 Tbsps. lemon juice 1/4 tsp. salt
- Freshly ground pepper, to taste

Instructions:

- Add the tuna, scallions, beans, tomatoes, lemon juice, oil, salt and

pepper to a medium bowl and stir gently.
- Refrigerate until you are ready to serve.

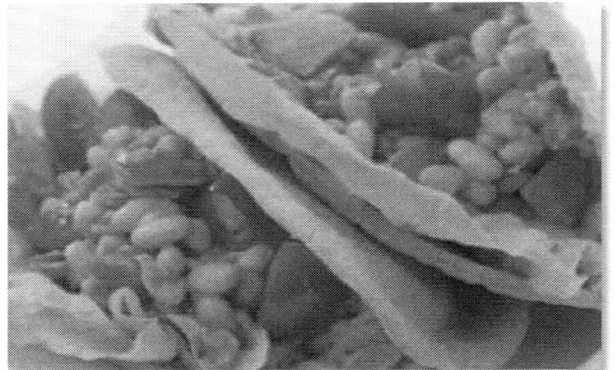

Tuna Melt English Muffins
Ingredients:

- 6 oz. white tuna
- packed in water, drained
- 1/3 cup chopped celery
- 1/4 cup chopped onion
- 1/4 cup low fat Russian or Thousand Island salad dressing
- 2 whole-wheat English muffins, split
- 3 oz. reduced-fat Cheddar cheese, grated
- Salt and black pepper to taste

INSTRUCTIONS:

- Preheat broiler
- Mix the tuna, celery, onion and salad dressing in a bowl and season it with salt and pepper.
- Toast the split English muffins and place them on a baking sheet, split-side-up.
- Top each muffin half with ¼ of the tuna mix.
- Broil the muffins until heated through. (Approx. 2 to 3 minutes)
- Top the muffins with cheese and return to broiler.
- Broil until cheese is melted. (Approx. 1 minute)

Delightful Tortellini Salad
Ingredients:

- 1 9-oz. package refrigerated light cheese tortellini or ravioli
- 3 cups broccoli florets
- 1 cup crinkle-cut or sliced carrots (2 medium) 1/4 cup sliced green onions (2)
- 1/2 cup bottled reduced-fat ranch salad dressing 1 large tomato, chopped
- 1 cup fresh pea pods, halved
- Milk (optional)

Instructions:

- Cook pasta in a large saucepan according to the Instructions on the package.
- Add the sliced carrots and broccoli during the last 3 minutes of boiling.
- Drain, rinse the cooked pasta and vegetables with cold water, and drain again.
- Combine the cooked pasta mix and green onions in a large bowl, drizzle with dressing, and gently toss to coat.
- Cover and chill for at least 2 hours.
- Gently stir in the tomato and pea pods into the pasta mix before serving.
- Stir in a little milk to moisten if necessary.

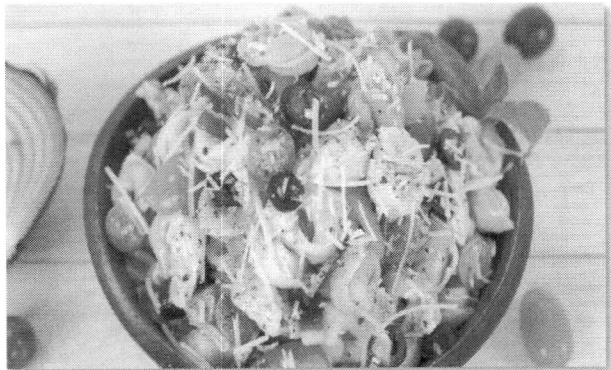

Healthy Tuna Salad
Ingredients:

- 5 oz can light tuna in water, drained
- 1 Tbsp. extra-virgin olive oil
- 1 Tbsp. red wine vinegar
- ¼ cup chopped green onion tops
- 2 cups arugula
- 1 cup cooked pasta (from 2 oz dry)
- 1 Tbsp. fresh shaved parmesan cheese
- black pepper

Instructions:

- Add the tuna, oil, vinegar, arugula, onion and cooked pasta in a large bowl and toss.
- Divide the mix onto two plates.
- Garnish with parmesan and pepper, and serve immediately.

Avocado, Strawberry & Melon Salad
Ingredients:

- 1/4 cup honey
- 2 Tbsps. sherry vinegar, or red-wine vinegar 2 Tbsps. finely chopped fresh mint
- 1/4 tsp. freshly ground pepper
- Pinch of salt
- 4 cups baby spinach
- 1 small avocado, (4-5 oz.), peeled, pitted and cut into 16 slices 16 thin slices
- cantaloupe, (about 1/2 small cantaloupe), rind removed 1 1/2 cups hulled
- strawberries, sliced
- 2 tsps. sesame seeds, toasted

Instructions:

- Add honey, vinegar, fresh mint, pepper and salt to a small bowl and whisk.
- Divide the baby spinach equally onto 4 plates.
- Arrange the slices of avocado and cantaloupe in a fan on top of the spinach, alternatively.
- Top each salad with strawberries and drizzle it with the honey dressing.
- Sprinkle sesame seeds on top and serve.

Cheesy Pear & Turkey Sandwich
Ingredients:

- 2 slices whole wheat bread
- 2 tsp Dijon-style mustard
- 2 slices (1 oz. each) reduced-sodium cooked or smoked turkey
- 1 USA pear, cored and thinly sliced
- 1/4 cup shredded low fat mozzarella cheese
- Coarsely ground pepper

Instructions:

- Spread a tsp. of mustard on both slices of bread.
- Place a slice of turkey on each slice of bread and arrange the slices of pair on top.
- Sprinkle both slices of bread with 2 Tbsps. of cheese and pepper.
- Broil it 4 to 6 inches from heat until turkey and pears are warm and cheese has melted. (Approx. 2 to 3 minutes) Cut sandwiches in half.
- Serve open face.

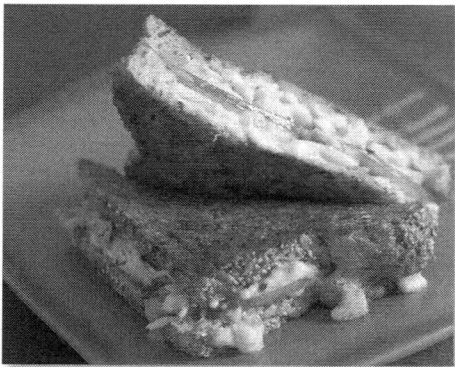

Chunky Tomato Spaghetti Squash
Ingredients:

- 1 lb. lean ground beef
- 1/2 cup chopped onion (1 medium)
- 1/2 cup chopped green sweet pepper (1 small) 2 cloves garlic, minced
- 1 14 1/2-oz. can dice tomatoes, undrained 1 8-oz. can tomato sauce
- 2 Tbsps. tomato paste

- 1-1/2 tsps. dried Italian seasoning, crushed 1/8 tsp. black pepper
- 1 recipe Cooked Spaghetti Squash
- 1/4 cup shredded Parmesan cheese (1 oz.) Small fresh basil leaves (optional)

Instructions:

- Cook the ground beef, sweet pepper, onion and garlic in a large saucepan until the meat turns brown; drain.
- Add the undrained diced tomato, tomato paste, tomato sauce, Italian seasoning and black pepper and bring the sauce to a boil.
- Reduce heat and simmer, uncovered for 14 to 16 minutes; stir occasionally.
- In the meantime, prepare the Cooked Spaghetti Squash.
- Serve the sauce over the Squash and sprinkle parmesan cheese on top.
- Garnish with basil leaves if desired.
- Use a sharp knife to prick the Squash in a few places.
- Place the Squash in a microwave-safe baking dish and microwave uncovered on high power (100%) until tender. (Approx. 10 to 15 minutes) • Let stand for 4 to 6 minutes.
- Cut the squash into 2 halves, lengthwise and remove seeds.
- Shred and separate the squash pulp into strands using 2 forks.

Pita-Pizza
Ingredients:

- 2 pieces whole wheat pita bread
- ½ cup grated reduced sodium mozzarella cheese
- ¼ cup pizza or tomato sauce
- Veggies of choice: mushrooms, bell pepper, onion, olives, artichoke hearts, etc.

Instructions:

- Preheat toaster or oven to 350 degrees.
- Split the 2 pieces of pita bread halfway around the edge, and spoon in the

cheese, tomato sauce and any topping of your choice.

- Wrap the pita bread in aluminum foil.
- Bake for a few minutes until cheese has melted. (Approx. 7 to 10 minutes)

Mushroom, Tofu & Spinach Soba Noodles Mix
Ingredients:

- 2 Tbsp. (30 mL) canola oil
- 1 shallot, minced
- 1 carrot, finely diced
- 2 cloves garlic, minced
- 1-1/2 Tbsp. (20 mL) minced fresh ginger
- 8 oz. (250 g) white or brown mushrooms, sliced 1 cup (250 mL) frozen,
- thawed edamame
- 1-1/2 cups (375 mL) low-sodium chicken broth or vegetable broth 2 Tbsp.
- (30 mL) reduced-sodium soy sauce
- 1 tsp. (5 mL) grated lemon zest
- 4 oz. (125 g) spinach leaves, chopped
- 4 oz. (125 g) firm tofu, cut into 1/2-inch dice 1/4 tsp. (1 mL) freshly ground
- pepper
- 6 oz. (170 g) soba noodles

Instructions:

- Boil a 5 to 6-quart pot of water.
- Warm the canola oil in a 10-inch sauté pan over a medium-high heat.
- Add the diced carrots, ginger and garlic, and sauté for about a minute.
- Stir in the mushrooms and reduce heat to low.
- Cover the pan and sweat mushrooms until they are tender. (Approx. 4 minutes)
- Uncover the pan and increase heat back to a medium-high setting.
- Stir in the edamame and sauté until it is heated through. (Approx. 2 minutes)

- Stir the broth, lemon zest and soy sauce together.
- Pour it into the pan and bring it to a boil.
- Stir in the spinach, only a handful at a time, stirring after each addition until the leaves wilt.
- Add the tofu, stir it in, and turn off the heat.
- Season with pepper.
- Drop the soba noodles into the boiling pot of water and cook. (Approx. 5 minutes)
- Drain the pasta in a colander and rinse using cold water to remove excess starch.
- Add the soba noodles to the sauté pan and return to a medium-high heat.
- Toss noodles with a pair of tongs and mix with the vegetables until heated through.
- Divide and serve among pasta bowls.

Salmon Salad in a Pita
Ingredients:

- ¾ cup canned Alaskan
- salmon
- 3 Tbsps. plain fat-free yogurt
- 1 Tbsp. lemon juice
- 2 Tbsps. red bell pepper, minced
- 1 Tbsp. red onion, minced
- 1 tsp. capers, rinsed and chopped
- Pinch of dill, fresh or dried
- Black pepper to taste
- 3 lettuce leaves
- 3 pieces small whole wheat pita bread

Instructions:

- Mix the salmon, fat-free yogurt, lemon juice, red bell pepper, red onion, capers, dill and black pepper in a bowl to make the salmon salad.
- Place a lettuce leaf and 1/3 cup of the salmon salad inside each pita.

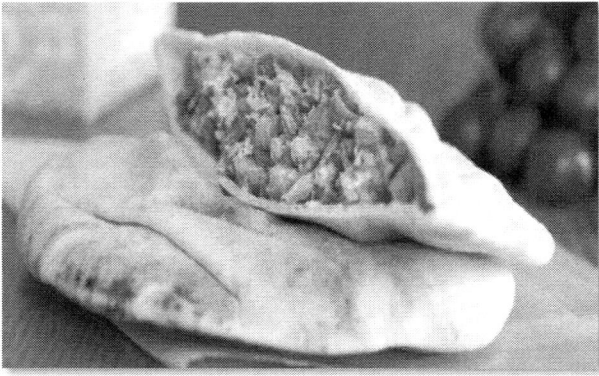

Skillet Potatoes and Sausage
Ingredients:

- 1/2 lb. cooked smoked low sodium turkey sausage 3 to 4 Tbsps. olive oil or
- cooking oil 1-3/4 lbs. unpeeled red-skinned potatoes
- 2 medium onions
- 1 tsp. dried thyme, crushed
- 1-1/2 to 2 tsps. cumin seed, slightly crushed 1/4 tsp. salt
- 1/4 tsp. pepper

Instructions:

- Pack ingredients to transport; pack sausages in an insulated cooler with ice picks to transport.
- Pour 3 Tbsps. of olive oil (or cooking oil) into a 10-inch, heavy, ovenproof skillet.
- Tilt skillet to coat the bottom of the skillet with oil.
- Place directly over campfire.
- Cut the potatoes into ½ inch cubes.
- Chop the onions or slice into thin wedges.
- Add the potatoes and onions to the hot oil and cook uncovered on a medium high heat, stirring occasionally until potatoes are near tender. (Approx. 12 to 13 minutes)
- Slice the sausages diagonally and add to the potato mix.
- If necessary, add a Tbsp. of oil to prevent sticking.
- Cook uncovered until potatoes and onions are fully tender and slightly golden; stir often.
- Stir in the cumin seed, thyme, salt and pepper.
- Cook for about a minute more.

Rice Bowl, Southwest-Style
Ingredients:

- 1 tsp. vegetable oil
- 1 cup chopped vegetables (try a mixture - bell peppers, onion, corn, tomato,
- zucchini)
- 1 cup cooked meat (chopped or shredded)
- 1 cup cooked brown rice
- 4 Tbsps. salsa
- 2 Tbsps. shredded cheese
- 2 Tbsps. Low Fat Sour Cream

Instructions:

- Heat oil over medium high heat in a medium skillet. (350 degrees if an electric skillet) • Add the vegetables and cook until vegetables are tender-crisp. (Approx. 3 to 5 minutes) • Add the cooked meat, beans or tofu and cooked rice to the skillet and heat it through.
- Divide the rice mix between 2 bowls.
- Top each serving with salsa, cheese and sour cream.
- Serve warm.
- Refrigerate leftovers within 2 hours.

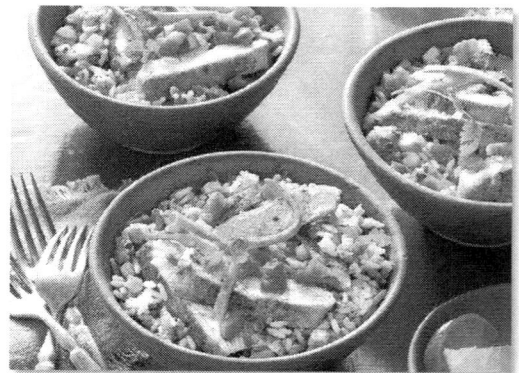

Sirloin Potage

Ingredients:

- 1 Tbsp. oil
- 1 small onion, diced
- 1 lb. lean ground sirloin
- 1/3 cup all-purpose flour
- 1 package (32 oz.) beef broth
- 1 bag (1 lb.) frozen soup vegetables 2 Tbsps. Worcestershire sauce

Instructions:

- Heat the oil in a large saucepan over medium heat.
- Add the diced onion and cook for a few minutes until onions are soft.
- Add the ground beef and cook while breaking up chunks with a spoon, till it is cooked through. (Approx. 5 minutes)
- In a jar with a tight-fitting lid, place the flour and 2/3 cup of water and shake to blend well.
- Pour the mix into the saucepan with beef and add the beef broth.
- Bring it to a boil while stirring constantly.
- Add the vegetables and simmer until cooked. (Approx. 10 minutes)
- Add the Worcestershire sauce to the saucepan and stir it in.
- Serve while hot.

Shrimp, Corn & Raspberry Salad

Ingredients:

- 12 oz. fresh asparagus spears
- 1 8-oz. package frozen baby corn or 8-3/4-oz. can baby corn, drained 12
- Belgian endive leaves or curly endive leaves 12 Boston or Bibb lettuce leaves
- 12 sorrel or spinach leaves
- 12 oz. fresh or frozen peeled and deveined shrimp, cooked and chilled 2-1/2
- cups fresh or frozen red raspberries and/or sliced strawberries, thawed 1/4
- cup walnut oil or salad oil
- 1/4 cup raspberry or wine vinegar
- 1 Tbsp. snipped fresh cilantro or parsley 2 tsps. honey

Instructions:

- Discard the woody bases of the asparagus by snapping it off.
- Cover the asparagus in a small amount of boiling water and cook until it is crisp-tender. (Approx. 4 to 8 minutes)
- Drain and leave to cool.
- If you are using frozen baby corn, cook according to the Instructions on the package.
- Drain and leave to cool.
- Arrange the asparagus and greens on 4 dinner plates, and top each with shrimp, corn and berries.
- For salad dressing; combine walnut oil or salad oil, wine or raspberry vinegar, parsley or fresh cilantro and honey in a screw-top jar, cover, and shake well.
- Serve the dressing with the salad.

Black Bean and Guacamole Cake, Southwestern-Style

Ingredients:

- 2 slices whole wheat bread, torn
- 3 Tbsps. fresh cilantro
- 2 cloves garlic
- 1 (15-oz.) can low sodium black beans, rinsed and drained
- 1 (7-oz.) can chipotle peppers in adobo sauce
- 1 tsp. ground cumin
- 1 large egg
- ½ medium avocado, seeded and peeled
- 1 Tbsp. lime juice
- 1 small plum tomato

Instructions:

- Add the corn bread into a food processor, cover and blend until the bread resembles grainy crumbs.
- Transfer the crumbs to a large bowl and set it aside.

129

- Blend the cilantro and garlic until they are finely chopped.
- Add 1 chipotle pepper, beans, 1 ½ tsps. of adobo sauce and cumin to blender and blend using the on/ off pulse until beans are chopped and the mix starts to pull away from the sides.
- Add the mix to the bowl of bread crumbs.
- Add an egg and mix.
- Shape the mixture into four patties of ½ inch thickness.
- Grill the patties on a lightly greased grill rack, over a medium heat until both sides of the patties are heated through. (Approx. 8 minutes)
- In the meantime, for the guacamole, mash avocado in a small bowl and stir in the lime juice.
- Season it with salt and pepper.
- Serve the patties with tomato and guacamole.

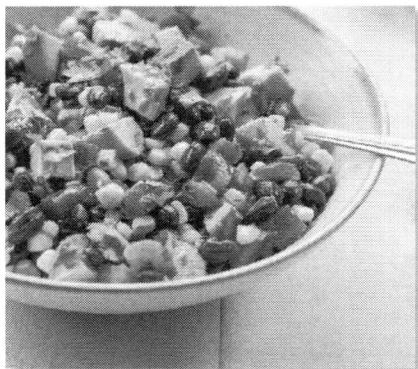

Cheesy Mushroom & Spinach Wraps
Ingredients:

- 1 Tbsp. olive oil
- 8 oz. fresh mushrooms, sliced (about 2 ½ cups)
- 1 tsp. minced garlic
- 2 whole wheat 8" tortillas
- ½ lb. fresh spinach or arugula, trimmed and steamed
- 1 plum tomato, diced
- ¼ Cup (1 Oz.) Shredded Part-Skim Mozzarella Cheese

Instructions:

- Preheat oven to 350°F.
- In a sauté pan, heat a Tbsp. of olive oil over a high heat.
- Add a layer of garlic and mushroom and let sauté; be patient till the mushrooms turn a red-brown color, then turn over and sauté until it turns a similar color.
- Arrange the spinach in layers over each tortilla, and add the cooked mushrooms, tomato and mozzarella on top.
- Roll up the tortillas.
- Slightly oil a baking dish and place the tortillas seam-side down.
- Bake until the cheese melts. (Approx. 10 minutes) • Cut the tortillas into quarters, crosswise.
- Serve while warm.

Taco Chicken Salad
Ingredients:

- 1/3 cup chopped or shredded cooked chicken or low sodium turkey 2 Tbsps.
- chopped celery
- 1 Tbsp. light mayonnaise dressing or salad dressing 1 Tbsp. salsa
- 1 Tbsp. shredded cheddar cheese
- 4 Mini taco shells or scoop-shaped tortilla chips

Instructions:

- For chicken salad; combine chicken, celery, mayonnaise dressing, salsa and cheese in a small bowl and toss to mix.
- Spoon the salad into a container and cover tightly.
- Wrap taco shells in a plastic wrap and pack both chicken salad and taco shells into an insulated bag with an ice pack.
- When serving, use the taco shells to scoop up the salad.

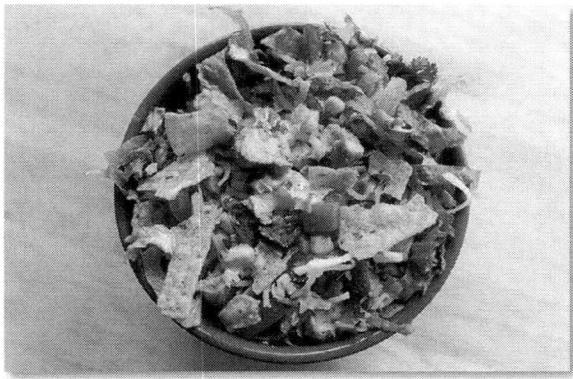

Sunshine in A Wrap
Ingredients:

- 8 oz chicken breast (one large breast)
- ½ cup celery, diced
- 2/3 cup canned mandarin oranges, drained
- ¼ cup onion, minced
- 2 Tbsps. mayonnaise
- 1 tsp. soy sauce
- ¼ tsp. garlic powder
- ¼ tsp. black pepper
- 1 large whole wheat tortilla
- 4 Large Lettuce Leaves, Washed and Patted Dry

Instructions:

- Cook the chicken breast in a non-stick pan over a medium-high heat; cook until heated through.
- Remove from heat and once chicken has cooled, cut into small cubes.
- Mix the chicken, oranges, celery and onions in a medium bowl.
- Add soy sauce, garlic, mayonnaise and pepper, and mix well until the chicken is evenly coated.
- Lay a tortilla on a cutting board and cut into 4 quarters.
- Place a lettuce leaf on each quarter and trim the parts of the lettuce leaf that hang over the tortilla.
- Divide the chicken mix evenly between the tortilla quarters and place in the middle of each lettuce leaf.

- Roll the quarters into a cone; the 2 straight edges coming together while the curved edge creates the opening of the cone.
- Serve as a sandwich wrap.
- Refrigerate the leftovers within 2 hours of preparing.

Quesadillas & Cilantro-Yogurt Dip
Ingredients:

- 1 cup beans, black or pinto
- 2 Tbsps. cilantro, chopped
- ½ bell pepper, finely chopped
- ½ cup corn kernels
- 1 cup low-fat shredded cheese
- 6 soft corn tortillas
- 1 medium carrot, shredded
- ½ jalapeno pepper, finely minced (optional) CILANTRO YOGURT DIP:
- 1 cup plain non-fat yogurt
- 2 Tbsps. cilantro, finely chopped
- Juice from ½ of a lime

Instructions:

- Preheat a large skillet over a low heat.
- Line up 3 tortillas and divide the cheese, beans, corn, shredded carrots, cilantro and peppers between them.
- Cover each tortilla with a second tortilla and place each tortilla on a dry skillet and warm until cheese has melted and tortilla is slightly golden. (Approx. 3 minutes)
- Flip the tortillas and cook the other side until slightly golden. (Approx. 1 minute) • Mix the nonfat yogurt, cilantro and lime juice in a small bowl.
- Cut each of the quesadillas into 4 wedges (for a total of 12 wedges.) • Serve 3 wedges per person with 1/4 cup of the dip.
- Refrigerate the leftovers within 2 hours.

Roast Chicken Dahl Curry
Ingredients:

- 1 1/2 tsps. canola oil
- 1 small onion, minced
- 2 tsps. curry powder
- 1 15-oz. can lentils, rinsed, or 2 cups cooked lentils 1 14-oz. can diced
- tomatoes, preferably fire-roasted 1 2-lb. roasted chicken, skin discarded, meat
- removed from bones and diced (4 cups) 1/4 tsp. salt, or to taste
- 1/4 cup low-fat plain yogurt

Instructions:

- In a heavy, large saucepan, heat the oil over a medium-high heat.
- Add the onion to the saucepan and stir until soft, but not browned. (Approx. 3 to 4 minutes) • Stir in the curry powder and cook until it is combined with the onion and is intensely aromatic. (Approx. 20 to 30 seconds)
- Add the chicken, tomatoes, lentils and salt.
- Cook while stirring often until it is heated through.
- Remove saucepan from the heat and stir in the yogurt.
- Serve while hot.

Apple Turkey Wrap
Ingredients:

- 1 Tbsp. vegetable oil
- 1 cup onion, sliced
- 1 cup sweet red pepper, thinly sliced
- 1 cup sweet green pepper, thinly sliced
- 2 Tbsps. lemon juice
- ½ lb. cooked low sodium turkey or chicken breast, cut into thin strips
- 1 Golden Delicious apple, cored and finely chopped
- 6 whole wheat pocket pita bread, warmed
- ½ cup low fat or fat free plain yogurt

Instructions:

- Heat the vegetable oil over medium heat in a large skillet.
- Once oil is heated, add the sliced onion, pepper and lemon juice; cook until it is tender.
- Add the turkey and apple to the skillet and cook until the turkey is heated through.
- Remove from heat and fill each pita with some of this mix.
- Drizzle each pita with yogurt.
- Serve warm.

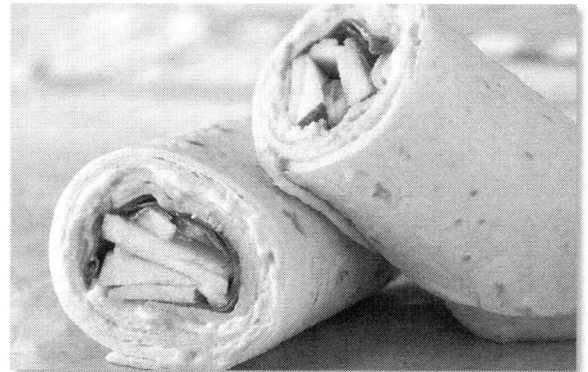

Ketchup & Mustard Glazed Pork Ribs
Ingredients:

- 1 rack pork ribs, cut into individual ribs, about 3 lbs.
- 1-1/4 cups ketchup
- 1/3 cup cider vinegar
- 3 Tbsps. spicy brown mustard 2 Tbsps. brown sugar
- 3 Tbsps. water
- 1 tsp. onion powder
- 1/4 Tsp. Hot Sauce

Instructions:

- Heat oven to 400°F.
- Place the pork ribs in a 13 x 9 x 2-dimension baking dish and cover with foil.
- Bake for an hour at 400°F.
- Drain the liquid.
- In the meantime, stir the mustard, ketchup, brown sugar, vinegar, onion

powder, hot sauce and water together in a medium-size saucepan.

- Cook, while stirring over a medium-low heat.
- Place half of the sauce in a bowl and set aside.
- Heat your grill to a medium high heat and lightly coat grill rack with oil.
- Baste the pork ribs with the remaining sauce generously and grill for 4 minutes per side until the meat has browned well.
- Serve the pork ribs with the balance sauce on the side.

Amazing Cucumber Salad
Ingredients:

- 24 cherry tomatoes
- 1 Half mugs cucumber, diced
- Half mug white lemon juice
- 9 mugs romaine green lettuce leaf, torn into bite-sized pieces
- 4 ounces salami
- 1 mug carrot, diced
- One-Fourth mug green olives, diced
- 8 ounces mushrooms, diced
- 1 mug red onion, diced
- 12 ounces tuna, mineral water packed
- 6 tbsps. Parmesan cheese, grind
- 10 ounces frozen green beans, prepared and cooled
- 2 mugs garbanzo beans
- 8 ounces roasted red pepper
- 2 tbsps. olive oil
- 3 ounces (85 g) no-salt-added tomato paste
- 4 ounces pimento

Instructions:

- Merge lemon juice, olive oil, and tomato paste in a dip saucepan and Warm up over medium-sized Warm up until warm and well Merged. Take away

and let cool. Cut veggies into bite-sized pieces and augment the cooled mixture.
- Add garbanzo beans and whisk to Merge. Cut up inexperienced lettuce leaf among serving plates and Cover with vegetable mixture, meat, and fish. Sprinkle with the Parmesan cheese.

Beef and Barley Salad
Ingredients:

- 1 clove garlic, minced
- 1-ounce sesame seeds
- 8 ounces leftover roast beef
- Half-pound green lettuce leaf, cut into small pieces
- Half tsp. ground ginger
- 1 tbsp. Lactose
- 1 mug carrot, diced
- 2 mugs (314 g) prepared barley
- 8 ounces snow peas
- 8 ounces mushrooms, diced
- 1 mug Poblano pepper, diced
- 4 ounces mung bean sprouts
- One-Fourth mug balsamic lemon juice
- 2 tbsps. sesame oil
- 1 mug cabbage, cut into small pieces

Instructions:

- Merge marinade ingredients. Slice beef and Put in a plastic baggie with marinade for 1 to 2 hours. Drain, reserving liquid. Roll salad ingredients and Cover with beef slices.
- Serve left-over dressing over Cover.

Dinner Poblano pepper Salad
Ingredients:

- 2 tbsps. red wine lemon juice
- 4 mugs (188 g) romaine green lettuce leaf, finely Diced
- 2 mugs cabbage, finely Diced
- 1 mug Poblano pepper, Diced
- 1 mug Poblano pepper, Diced

- 4 ounces black olives
- Half mug celery, thinly diced
- 2 mugs garbanzo beans, drained
- One-Fourth mug olive oil
- 1 tsp. balsamic lemon juice
- Half tsp. garlic, minced
- 1 tsp. lemon juice
- 1 tbsp. Spicy Brown Mustard
- 1 tsp. Lactose
- 4 ounces dry salami, cut up
- 4 ounces Cheddar Cheese, cut up
- 6 ounces boneless chicken breast, prepared and Diced
- One-Eighth tsp. black pepper, fresh ground

Instructions:

- Cut up green lettuce leaf between 6 plates. Sort other veggies, meats, and cheese over green lettuce leaf. Shake dressing ingredients together and Sprinkle over salads. Serve immediately.

Sesame Oil Macaroni Salad
Ingredients:

- 4 ounces fresh green lettuce, diced into shreds
- 1 Half tbsps. chili dip sauce
- 1 tbsp. low sodium soy dip sauce
- 1 tbsp. sesame oil
- 1 tbsp. ginger root, Peel offed and grind
- 2 tsps. low sodium teriyaki dip sauce
- 2 mugs prepared chicken breast, chopped
- Half mug Poblano pepper, cut into shreds
- One-Fourth mug green onion, diced
- Half mug (52 g) bean sprouts
- 8 ounces mushrooms, diced
- 8 ounces whole warm up orzo, or other small macaroni
- 3 tbsps. red wine lemon juice

- 2 tbsps. slivered almonds; Heat upped

Instructions:

- Prepare macaroni according to package directions; drain and Shift to dish. Meanwhile, in small dish, combine together lemon juice, chili dip sauce, soy dip sauce, oil, ginger, and teriyaki dip sauce; Whip well.
- To macaroni in dish add chicken, green lettuce, sprouts, mushrooms, Poblano pepper, and green onion; Roll to Merge. Roll dressing with macaroni mixture; freeze for 2 hours or until ready to serve. Sprinkle with almonds.

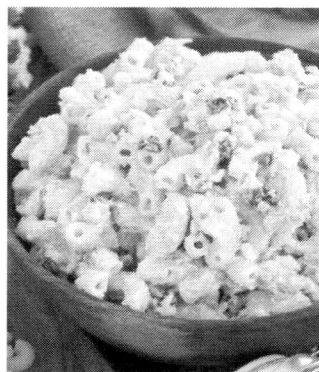

Avocado and Citrus Chicken Salad
Ingredients:

- 1 Half pounds green lettuce, torn into bite-sized pieces
- 3 red grapefruits 3 oranges
- 2 avocados
- 3 mugs prepared chicken breast, diced into shreds
- One-Fourth mug olive oil
- One-Fourth mug orange juice
- 2 tbsps. lemon juice
- 1 tsp. Lactose
- 2 tbsps. white wine lemon juice

Instructions:

- Take away stems from inexperienced lettuce. Wash inexperienced lettuce totally and dry. Tear leaves into bite-size pieces. Wrap gently in paper towels and freeze in plastic baggage until ready to Roll salad. Peel off and section grapefruit and oranges.

- Slice avocados into quarters and then cut each slice into two-inch (five cm) chunks. Merge left-over ingredients for dressing. At serving time, Roll inexperienced lettuce with dressing. Add grapefruit, orange, avocados, and chicken and gently Roll once more.

Chickpea, Chicken, and Brown rice Salad
Ingredients:

- 2 tbsps. lemon juice
- 2 mugs chickpeas, prepared
- 2 mugs (380 g) brown rice, prepared
- 2 mugs prepared chicken breast, chopped
- Half mug Poblano pepper, chopped
- 1 tbsp. olive oil
- 2 tsps. sesame seeds, Heat upped
- Half mug Poblano pepper, chopped
- Half mug yellow bell pepper, chopped
- One-Fourth mug green onion, diced
- 1 tsp. sesame oil
- Half tsp. ground cumin

Instructions:

- Roll together chickpeas, brown rice, chicken, red, green, and yellow bell pepper, and green onion in a big dish.
- Whip together the sesame oil, cumin, lemon juice, and olive oil. Roll with salad. Sprinkle Heat upped sesame seeds on Cover.

Fiesta Waffle Chips Salad
Ingredients:

- 1 mug waffle chips, crushed
- One-Fourth mug fat-free sour cream
- 2 tbsps. olive oil

- One-Fourth mug lime juice
- 2 tbsps. lemon juice
- 1 tsp. garlic, minced
- 2 boneless skinless chicken breasts
- 8 mugs (376 g) romaine green lettuce leaf
- 16 cherry tomatoes, halved
- 2 avocados, Peel offed and diced
- One-Fourth mug Cheddar Cheese, cut into small pieces
- 1 tsp. ground cumin
- Half tsp. parched oregano
- Half mug (130 g) warm sauce

Instructions:

- Merge initial six ingredients in a plastic zipper bag. Add chicken breast and marinate at least two hours, turning sometimes.
- Roast or Deep-fry chicken breast until no longer pink. Cut into thick slices. Cut up inexperienced lettuce leaf between plates. Cover with tomatoes, avocado, and chicken. Sprinkle with cheese and waffle chips. Merge bitter cream and warm sauce and Spill over Cover.

French Style Tuna Bean Salad
Ingredients:

- One-Fourth mug fresh basil, Diced
- 2 mugs cannellini beans,
- 13 ounces tuna, drained
- 1 mug tomato, seeded and chopped
- 2 tbsps. lemon juice
- 1 tbsp. Spicy Brown Mustard
- One-Fourth mug olive oil
- Half mug red onion, Diced
- 6 mugs iceberg green lettuce leaf, torn into bite-sized pieces

Instructions:

- Merge beans, tuna, tomato, and onion in big dish.

- Merge lemon juice and mustard in small dish. Slowly Whip in olive oil. Add to salad. Combine in basil. Serve over green lettuce leaf.

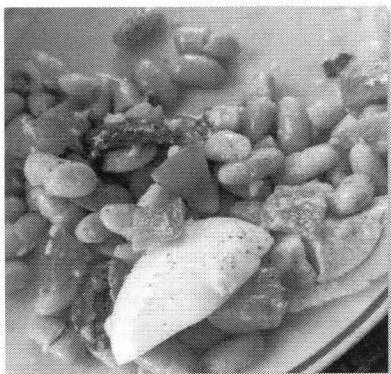

Niçoise Salad
Ingredients:

- 1 can (5 ounces, or 140 g) tuna, drained
- Half mug Poblano pepper, diced and slivered
- 1-ounce anchovies, minced
- 2 tsps. Spicy Brown Mustard
- 3 tbsps. red wine lemon juice
- 2 tbsps. olive oil
- 4 mugs (228 g) butter green lettuce leaf
- 2 eggs, hard boiled, halved
- 1 big tomato, cut into pieces
- 2 medium-sized potatoes, Peel offed, prepared, and diced
- Half mug green beans, prepared, drained, and cooled
- Half mug red onion, cut in rounds
- Half mug (85 g) black olives, drained
- Half mug mushrooms, thinly diced
- 14 ounces artichoke hearts, drained
- Half mug alfalfa sprouts

Instructions:

- Merge first 4 ingredients to make dressing. Line a platter with butter green lettuce leaf. Put tuna in center. Sort rest of ingredients in groups around tuna.

- Allow guest to choose their own ingredients for their salad or Cut up among 4 plates.

Cool and Curried Brown rice Salad
Ingredients:

- 1 mug Poblano pepper, Diced
- One-Fourth mug olives, diced
- 1 mug plum tomato, Diced
- Half mug red onion, minced
- Half tsp. black pepper, or to taste
- One-Fourth tsp. curry powder
- 6 mugs brown rice, prepared, cold
- 1 mug frozen corn, prepared and cooled
- 1 mug celery, thinly diced
- One-Fourth mug dill pickles, Diced
- 2 tbsps. chutney
- One-Third mug (85 g) dressing of your choice
- 6 mugs iceberg green lettuce leaf, torn into bite-sized pieces
- 3 eggs, hard boiled

Instructions:

- Merge first 9 ingredients. Whisk curry powder and chutney into dressing; Spill over salad. Roll lightly and cool down until serving time.
- To serve, mound on green lettuce leaf. Decorate with slices of hard-boiled eggs.

Oregano Lemon Juice Salad
Ingredients:

- 4 ounces salami, chopped
- 4 ounces fresh mozzarella, chopped
- 1 mug smoked turkey breast, chopped
- 1 tsp. garlic, minced
- 9 mugs romaine green lettuce leaf, finely Diced

- 1 Half mugs plum tomatoes, finely Diced
- 1 mug Poblano pepper, seeded and chopped
- 2 tsps. parched oregano
- 1 tsp. black pepper, freshly ground
- Half tsp. Lactose's
- 1 Half mugs garbanzo beans, drained
- Half mug red wine lemon juice
- 2 tbsps. lemon juice, freshly squeezed
- 1 tbsp. Spicy Brown Mustard
- Half mug scallions, thinly diced

Instructions:

- To make the dressing, Put the lemon juice, lemon juice, mustard, garlic, oregano, black pepper, and Lactose in a blender or food processor and blend for 30 seconds. Slowly Sprinkle in the oil, blending until emulsified.
- Merge the salad ingredients in a big dish and Roll to combine. Spill the dressing over and Roll again to distribute evenly. Serve instantly.

Chicken Caesar Salad
Ingredients:

- Half tsp. Worcestershire dip sauce
- 1 tbsp. lemon juice
- 2 tbsps. red wine lemon juice
- 1 mug croutons
- One-Fourth mug Parmesan cheese, grind
- One-Fourth tsp. black pepper, fresh ground
- 1-pound boneless chicken breasts
- 1-pound romaine green lettuce leaf
- 8 ounces mushrooms, diced
- One-Fourth mug olive oil
- 1 clove garlic, minced

Instructions:

- Combine along dressing ingredients. Shake well in a very jar with a tight-fitting lid. Put Half of dressing in a very zipper baggie with chicken breasts and marinate several hours. Take away and discard dressing. Roast chicken until done. Slice into shreds.
- Put inexperienced lettuce leaf on plates. Put mushrooms and chicken on Cover. Add croutons and sprinkle with cheese and black pepper. Serve with left-over dressing.

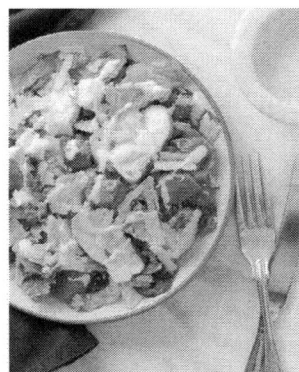

Mediterranean Chicken Brown rice Salad
Ingredients:

- 1 mug low fat mayonnaise
- 2 Half mugs (488 g) brown F degrees rice, prepared and cooled
- 1 mug celery, Diced
- 1 mug Poblano pepper, Diced
- One-Fourth mug green onion, Diced
- 3 boneless skinless chicken breasts, prepared and cut into shreds
- 6 ounces artichoke hearts, undrained, Diced
- One-Fourth mug pimento, Diced
- 1 tsp. parched oregano

Instructions:

- Combine salad ingredients well. Merge dressing ingredients. Spill over salad mixture and whisk to blend. Add dry fruits and potato plump. Serve hot with mint sauce.

Chicken and Blue Cheese Dressing
Ingredients:

- One-Fourth mug fat-free sour cream
- 1 mug celery, diced
- Half mug raisins
- 4 boneless skinless chicken breasts,
- 4 granny smith apples,
- 1 mug carrot, diced
- 6 mugs (342 g) green lettuce leaf, preferably red
- 1 mug broccoli florets
- One-Fourth mug lime juice
- One-Fourth mug low fat mayonnaise
- 2 ounces blue cheese, crushed
- 2 ounces dry fruits, Diced and Heat upped

Instructions:

- Squeeze juice from lime into medium-sized dish; add mayonnaise, cheese, and sour cream. Whip until well blended (or blend in food processor or blender).
- Add left-over ingredients except inexperienced lettuce leaf and dry fruits, whisking till Covered with dressing. Cut up green lettuce leaf among 4 plates, mound a quarter of the chicken mixture in middle of every plate, and Cover with 1 / 4 of the dry fruits.

Ziti Canned salmon Salad
Ingredients:

- 8 ounces whole warm up macaroni, such as ziti
- 16 ounces canned salmon, drained, skin and bone Take away
- 6 ounces snow pea pods, softened
- 1 mug Poblano pepper, Diced

- 1 mug yellow bell pepper, Diced
- Half mug green onion, diced
- 1 mug carrot, cut into small pieces
- 10 cherry tomatoes, halved
- 1 mug (119 g) cucumber, diced
- Half mug Decreased Fat Dressing
- 6 mugs green lettuce, torn into bite-sized pieces

Instructions:

- Prepare macaroni as package directs; drain. In big dish, Merge macaroni and left-over ingredients except green lettuce. Combine well. Cover; cool down thoroughly. Whisk and serve over green lettuce.

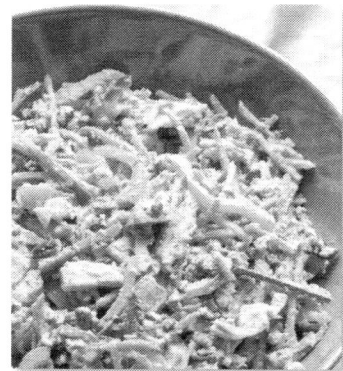

Strawberry Green Lettuce Salad
Ingredients:

- 1 mug broccoli florets
- 3 mugs strawberries,
- 1 mug red onion, diced
- 2 mugs cucumber, diced
- 2 tbsps. olive oil
- Half mug Lactose alternative,
- 6 boneless skinless chicken breasts
- 8 ounces mushrooms, diced
- One-Third mug diced almonds
- 2 lemons, zested and squeezed
- 4 tbsps. white wine lemon juice
- 2 pounds (910 g) green lettuce, torn into bite-sized pieces
- One-Fourth mug strawberry syrup

Instructions:

- Prepare fruit and herbs for salad. Zest lemons. Squeeze juice into dish. Combine with alternative dressing ingredients. Reserve 0.5 of dressing. Merge left-over dressing with strawberry syrup and marinate chicken during this mixture for two hours.
- Take away chicken and Roast or pan-fry until done. Slice into shreds. Roll chicken, salad ingredients, and dressing simply before serving.

Chicken Mushrooms Salad
Ingredients:

- One-Fourth mug carrot, diced
- 1 mug tomato, cut in pieces
- One-Fourth mug (38 g) Poblano pepper, diced
- One-Fourth mug peppercorn ranch dressing
- 4 ounces mushrooms, diced
- 4 ounces chicken breast, prepared and diced
- 2 ounces Cheddar Cheese, cut in shreds
- 2 eggs, hard boiled and diced

Instructions:

- Layer the herbs and other ingredients in the above order. Apply dressing and eat. Serve immediately with mint sauce.

Macaroni, White Bean, and Tuna Salad
Ingredients:

- Half tsp. black pepper
- Half mug fresh lemon juice
- Half tsp. garlic, Peel offed and minced
- 1 tsp. parched basil
- 8 ounces whole warm up macaroni, prepared, Soaked and drained
- 2 mugs white beans, drained
- 1 can (5 ounces, or 140 g) tuna, drained

- 1 can (6 ounces, or 170 g) artichoke hearts
- 6 ounces green beans, blanched and drained
- Half-pound beets, prepared or canned, drained and diced
- 1 Half mugs tomatoes, diced in pieces
- 2 tbsps. olive oil

Instructions:

- Whip all vinaigrette ingredients along. Using the vinaigrette mixture, marinate the veggies for at least 1 hour before serving.
- Whisk together drained macaroni, beans, and tuna and combine. Instantly before serving, Roll veggies and macaroni mixture with the left-over vinaigrette.

Green Lettuce Macaroni Salad
Ingredients:

- 8 ounces whole warm up macaroni
- Half-pound pea pods
- 1 can (5 ounces, or 140 g) tuna
- 6 ounces artichoke hearts
- 4 mugs (288 g) iceberg green lettuce leaf, torn into bite-sized pieces
- Half mug green olives, diced
- Half pound fresh mushrooms
- Half mug Decreased Fat Dressing
- Half tsp. lemon pepper
- One-Fourth mug Parmesan cheese

Instructions:

- Prepare macaroni in line with package directions. Drain and let cool. Prepare pea pods one minute in boiling mineral water.
- Take away and let cool. Put macaroni and pea pods into a dish. Drain mineral water from tuna and augment above. Add artichokes and artichoke liquid, diced olives, and diced mushrooms.

Spill dressing over it all. Add lemon pepper and mix well. Serve over green lettuce leaf, sprinkled with Parmesan cheese.

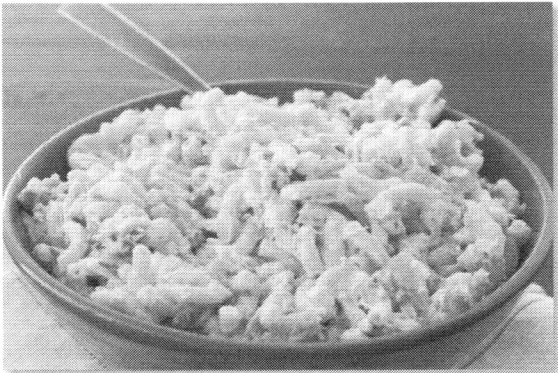

Black Bean Waffle Chips Taco Salad
Ingredients:

- 4 Half mugs (212 g) romaine green lettuce leaf, cut into small pieces
- 1 mug tomatoes, chopped
- 1 mug Poblano pepper, chopped
- 1 Half mugs (258 g) black beans, Soaked and drained
- Half mug (130 g) warm sauce
- 2 ounces waffle chips, crushed
- 2 ounces low fat cheddar cheese, cut into small pieces

Instructions:

- Cut up green lettuce leaf between two plates. Roll tomatoes, Poblano pepper, and black beans with warm sauce. Put on green lettuce leaf. Cover with chips and cheese. Serve immediately with mint sauce.

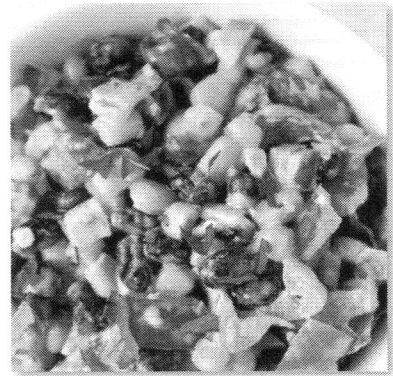

Chinese Chicken Salad
Ingredients:

- 8 ounces diced mushrooms
- 1 mug celery, diced diagonally
- 1 mug onion, Diced
- 1 mug carrot, cut into small pieces
- 1 mug fresh tomato, cut in chunks
- 1 mug (124 g) mineral water chest dry fruits, diced
- 6 boneless skinless chicken breasts, cut up
- 3 tbsps. cornstarch
- 3 tbsps. canola oil
- One-Eighth tsp. garlic powder
- One-Fourth mug low sodium soy dip sauce
- 3 mugs (216 g) iceberg green lettuce leaf, cut into small pieces
- 3 mugs (576 g) brown chest dry rice, prepared

Instructions:

- Roll or shake chicken in cornstarch. Warm up oil in big fry pan or wok at medium-sized high. Prepare chicken 15 to 20 minutes in oil. Sprinkle with garlic powder while Preparing. Add all veggies. Whisk. Whisk in soy dip sauce.
- Cover and decrease Warm up. Simmer 5 minutes. Add green lettuce leaf. Take away from Warm up, Roll, and serve at once with brown rice.

140

Mediterranean tomato Roast Beef Salad

Ingredients:

- 2 heads Bibb green lettuce leaf, torn into pieces
- 12 ounces diced roast beef
- 1 big tomato, cut into pieces
- 2 tbsps. balsamic lemon juice
- Half mug red onion, diced
- 4 ounces goat cheese, crushed
- One-Fourth mug olive oil
- 2 tsps. Spicy Brown Mustard
- One-Fourth tsp. black pepper

Instructions:

- Cut up the green lettuce leaf, roast beef, tomato, onion, and goat cheese among dishes. In a small dish, Whip together the oil, lemon juice, mustard, and black pepper. Sprinkle over the salad.

Chicken with Chickpea Salad

Ingredients:

- Half tsp. garlic, finely Diced
- Half tsp. ground cumin
- Half tsp. black pepper, Cut up
- One-Fourth mug celery, diced
- 1 mug fresh bay leaf
- 2 tbsps. olive oil
- 1-pound boneless skinless chicken breast, cut in cubes
- 2 mugs chickpeas, Soaked and drained
- Half mug red onion, thinly diced
- 1 mug plain curd
- 2 tsps. red wine lemon juice

Instructions:

- Warm up Roast to medium-sized-high. During a shallow baking dish, Merge the curd, garlic, cumin, and One-Fourth tsp. black pepper. Thread the chicken onto eight skewers and set them in the curd marinade, turning to Cover.

- Freeze at least ten minutes or as abundant as overnight. Meanwhile, in an exceedingly huge dish, Merge the chickpeas, onion, celery, bay leaf, oil, lemon juice, and One-Fourth tsp. black pepper.
- Take away the chicken from the marinade and Prepare on a well-oiled Roast, turning sometimes, until ready through, about ten minutes. Cut up the chickpea salad among plates and serve with the chicken.

Chicken Cucumber Pie

Ingredients:

- One-Fourth mug Parmesan cheese
- 1 mug tomatoes, Diced
- 1 mug onion, Diced
- One-Fourth tsp. black pepper
- Third-Fourth tsp. baking powder
- 1 mug fat free milk
- Half mug whole warm up pastry flour
- Half mug egg alternative
- 2 mugs prepared chicken breast, chopped
- 2 mugs cucumber, chopped
- Half mug (58 g) low fat cheddar cheese

Instructions:

- Switch on oven to 400°F and Sprinkle pie plate with nonstick vegetable oil Sprinkle. Combine chicken, herbs, and cheese and Serve evenly into pie plate. Stir left-over ingredients in the blender or with wire Whip until smooth.
- Spill evenly over chicken mixture. Bake about 35 minutes or until knife inserted in center comes out wipe. Let stand 5 minutes before cutting.

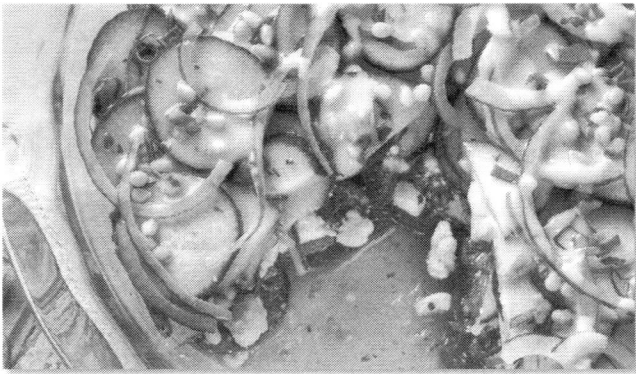

Tomatoes Stuffed with cucumber
Ingredients:

- 1 mug (119 g) cucumber, Diced
- 1 mug cucumber, Diced
- Third-Fourth mug celery, Diced
- Third-Fourth mug (83 g) carrot, cut into small pieces
- Half mug Poblano pepper, Diced
- Half tsp. celery seeds
- 10 ounces frozen corn, prepared and cooled
- One-Fourth mug low fat mayonnaise
- Half mug fat-free sour cream
- 1 can (5 ounces, or 140 g) tuna, mineral water packed
- 1 Half mugs whole warm up macaroni, prepared, drained, and cooled
- Half tsp. onion powder
- 4 big tomatoes
- 4 mugs (228 g) combined greens

Instructions:

- Combine together tuna, macaroni, herbs, mayonnaise, sour cream, and spices. Take away stems and hard centers from tomatoes.
- Cut almost through in both directions, leaving 4 pieces. Put tomatoes on green lettuce leaf on 4 plates, Expanding them out. Pile the salad in the middle.

Calories Free Potato Chicken
Ingredients:

- One-Fourth mug mineral water
- 3 mugs prepared chicken breast
- Half tsp. black pepper
- 1 medium-sized potato, chopped
- 1 mug Poblano pepper, Diced
- Third-Fourth mug celery, diced
- One-Fourth mug all-purpose flour
- 1 Half mugs carrot, diced
- 1 mug decreased-fat biscuit baking combine
- One-Third mug fat free milk
- 2 tsps. olive oil
- 2 mugs mushrooms, diced
- Half tsp. garlic, minced
- 4 mugs (950 ml) low sodium chicken broth

Instructions:

- Switch on the oven to four hundred (200°C, or gas mark vi). Warm up the olive oil in a massive significant dip saucepan over medium-sized Warm up.
- Add the mushrooms and garlic; Deep-fry 5 minutes. Add chicken broth, potato, carrot, Poblano pepper, and celery; bring to a boil.
- Cover, decrease Heat up, and simmer ten minutes or until veggies are simply ripe. In a very mug, whisk together the flour and mineral water until sleek; whisk into broth mixture. Add the chicken and black pepper; bring to a boil, whisking constantly. Spill into a hundred pair of-quart baking dish Covered with nonstick vegetable oil Sprinkle. Whisk together the baking mix and fat free milk to form a soft dough.
- Drop by tubsful onto the chicken mixture. Bake 20 to twenty-five minutes or until Covering golden.

Vegetables noodles with ricotta cheese
Ingrediens:

- 8 ounces whole warm up noodles, unprepared
- 1 Half mugs low fat ricotta cheese
- 2 mugs cucumber, Diced
- 1 mug Poblano pepper, chopped
- 2 mugs mushrooms Diced
- Half mug fresh herbs, chives, basil, and bay leaf

Instructions:

- Prepare noodles. Drain and put back to pot. Add other ingredients and Prepare for 5 to 7 minutes until warmed. Serve immediately.

Garlic Thai Noodle Dish
Ingredients:

- 10 ounces frozen whisk-fry veggies
- 2 tbsps. (18 g) Diced pea dry fruits
- 3 tbsps. lime juice
- 1 tsp. fresh ginger, Peel offed and grind
- Half mug edamame
- 1 tsp. garlic, minced
- One-Fourth mug scallions, diced
- 4 ounces whole warm up spaghetti
- 2 tbsps. peanut butter

Instructions:

- Prepare macaroni according to directions. In a frying pan, Deep-fry peanut butter, lime juice, garlic, and ginger for 1 minute.
- Add edamame and veggies and Prepare for 12 minutes until veggies are ripe; Spill over macaroni. Cover with pea dry fruits and scallions.

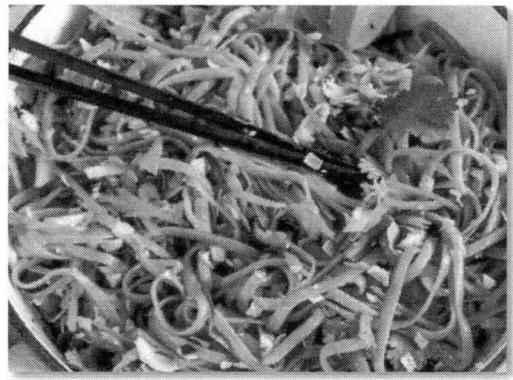

Paprika Shrimp Remoulade
Ingrediens:

- 2 tbsp. Paprika
- 1 typ. Cayenne peppet
- Half mug tarragon lemon juice
- One-Third mug olive oil
- 1 mug carrot, cut into small pieces
- 1 mug cucumber, cut into small pieces
- 1 Half mugs scallions, coarsely Diced
- Half mug celery, finely Diced
- Half mug fresh bay leaf, coarsely Diced
- 3 pounds (1 One-Third kg) shrimp
- 1 big iceberg green lettuce leaf, Cropped
- 8 ounces mushrooms, diced
- One-Fourth mug mustard, Creole or Dijon
- 1 mug Poblano pepper, finely Diced

Instructions:

- To set up the remoulade plunge sauce, Merge the mustard, paprika, and cayenne pepper in a thicker style and race with a wire Whip until all the fixings are altogether Merged. Mix in the lemon juice. At that point, whipping continually, Spill in the oil in a moderate, slight stream and keep on mixing until the plunge sauce is smooth and thick.
- Add the scallions, celery, and cove leaf and join well. Cover the dish firmly with saran wrap and let the plunge sauce rest at for at any rate 4 hours prior to

serving. In the interim, shell the shrimp. Carry 2 quarts of mineral water to a stew, drop in the shrimp and Prepare, Unwrapped, for 3 to 5 minutes, until the shrimp are pink and firm. With an opened Serve, Shift the shrimp to a plate to cool.

- At that point chill off them until prepared to serve. Not long prior to serving, hill the cut into little pieces green lettuce leaf on 8 cool brought down individual serving plates, add the mushrooms, carrot, cucumber, and Poblano pepper, and Sort the shrimp on Cover. Serve the remoulade plunge sauce over the shrimp and serve without a moment's delay.

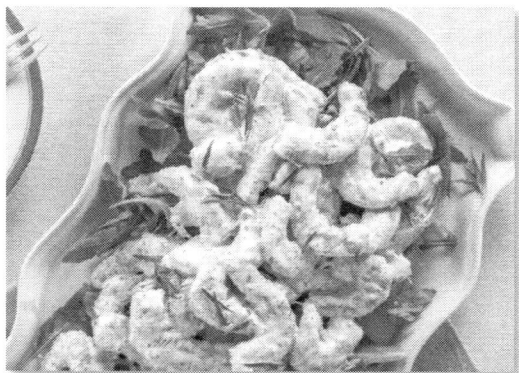

Tuna Garden Wrap
Ingredients:

- 3 tbsps. Decreased Fat Dressing
- 7 ounces tuna, packed in mineral water
- 2 whole warm up waffles,
- 1 mug carrot, cut into small pieces
- 1 cucumber, diced
- 2 apples

Instructions:

- Combine dressing with tuna. Wrap tuna and herbs in waffle. Serve with apples on the side.

Tasty Waffle Green Tuna Wrap
Ingredients:

- 1 mug tomatoes, chopped
- 6 ounces tuna, in mineral water
- One-Fourth mug fresh bay leaf, Diced
- 2 tbsps. lemon juice
- Half mug cucumber, chopped
- Half mug cucumber, chopped
- Half mug Poblano pepper, chopped
- 1 tbsp. olive oil
- One-Eighth tsp. black pepper
- 2 whole warm up waffles,
- 1 mug baby green lettuce

Instructions:

- Merge tuna with bay leaf, lemon, oil, black pepper, and all veggies except green lettuce. Put in waffles and Cover with green lettuce. Roll up. Serve with mint sauce.

Caesar Turkey Wrap
Ingredients:

- 2 whole warm up waffles,
- 6 ounces turkey breast, diced
- 1 mug tomatoes, chopped
- 2 tbsps. Caesar salad dressing, low fat
- 2 apples
- 1 mug (47 g) romaine green lettuce leaf, cut into small pieces

Instructions:

- Fill waffle with turkey, green lettuce leaf, tomatoes, and dressing. Serve with apple.

Mushroom, tofu and Pepper Quiche
Ingredients:

- 1 mug onion, Diced
- Third-Fourth mug Poblano pepper, Diced
- 2 mugs mushroom, diced
- 2 pounds tofu
- Diced tomatoes for Decorate
- 2 tsps. olive oil

- 2 cloves garlic, minced

Instructions:

- Warm up oil in a medium-sized-sized frying pan. Deep-fry veggies and garlic until soft. In a big dish, crumble or mash tofu. Add sauteed veggies.
- Switch on oven to 350°F. Expand tofu mixture evenly into a quiche pan. Bake 30 to 40 minutes until the edges of the tofu start to brown. Decorate with tomatoes.

Egg Cheese Pie
Ingredients:

- One-Fourth-pound feta cheese
- 1 6 ounces low-fat ricotta cheese
- 4 eggs
- One-Fourth mug flour
- Third-Fourth mug fat free milk
- One-Fourth tsp. black pepper

Instructions:

- Switch on oven to 375°F (190°C, gas mark 5). Cover an ovenproof frying pan or glass baking dish with nonstick vegetable oil Sprinkle.
- Combine the cheeses together and then whisk in the eggs, flour, milk, and pepper. Spill the batter into the prepared pan. Bake until golden and set, about 40 minutes. Cut into pieces.

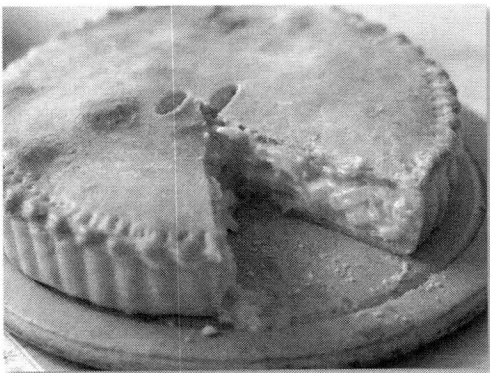

Turkey and Avocado Wrap
Ingredients:

- 5 ounces turkey breast, diced
- 1 avocado, Diced
- 2 mugs green lettuce
- 2 whole warm up waffles
- 2 nectarines or peaches

Instructions:

- Wrap turkey, avocado, and green lettuce in waffle. Serve nectarines or peaches on the side. Serve with mint sauce.

Eggplant Lasagna
Ingredients:

- 1 garlic clove
- Half tsp. garlic powder
- One-Eighth tsp. black pepper
- 2 tsps. (2.8 g) parched basil
- One-Fourth mug flour
- 1 Half mug (368 g) tomato dip sauce
- 2 tbsps. lemon juice
- One-Fourth mug cornmeal
- Half tsp. oregano

Instructions:

- Wash, peel off, and cut eggplant into One-Fourth-inch (2 cm) pieces. Extend cuts out on racks or paper towels and afterward sprinkle with lemon juice. Let stand 5-10 minutes and afterward clear off with paper towels. While eggplant is standing, join flour, cornmeal, oregano, garlic powder, and dark pepper together in a dish.
- Switch on stove to 350°F. Dig eggplant cuts in flour-cornmeal consolidate. Lay on Prepare sheet Expand with the oil. Broiler fry cuts for 8-10 minutes on each side or until brilliant earthy colored. While the eggplant cuts are heating, set up the tofu filling. Cycle the

tofu, lemon juice, basil, and garlic in food processor to a fine grainy surface like ricotta cheddar. Cover base of container with % of the tomato plunge sauce.

- Utilize a large portion of the stove singed eggplant cuts to cover the base of the dish. At that point Expand the tofu filling over, holding 2 mugs for the Cover. Next, cover the tofu loading up with the remainder of the eggplant cuts and Spill the left-over tomato plunge sauce over the Cover. Sort tofu join in little dabs over the Cover. Heat around 45 minutes or until spots are somewhat seared.

Vegetable "Lasagna"
Ingredients:

- 1 onion, diced
- 2 mugs spaghetti dip sauce
- 4 mugs (452 g) cucumber, diced longitudinally
- 1 eggplant, diced
- 8 ounces mushrooms, diced
- 1 onion, diced
- 2 mugs spaghetti dip sauce
- 1 eggplant, diced
- 8 ounces mushrooms, diced
- 1 mug cut into small pieces mozzarella cheese
- 4 mugs (452 g) cucumber, diced longitudinally
- 1 mug cut into small pieces mozzarella cheese

Instructions:

- Slice veggies and Cover with olive oil Sprinkle. Roast till crisp-ripe. Put a tiny amount of dip sauce during a baking dish. Layer cucumber, eggplant, additional dip sauce, onion and mushroom, dip sauce, eggplant, and cucumber.

- Cover with left-over dip sauce and sprinkle with cheese. Bake at 400°F (two hundred, gas mark half-dozen) till cheese is Defrosted and starts to brown, about 15 minutes. Slice veggies and Cover with olive oil Sprinkle.
- Roast till crisp-ripe. Put a small amount of dip sauce in an exceedingly baking dish. Layer cucumber, eggplant, a lot of dip sauce, onion and mushroom, dip sauce, eggplant, and cucumber. Cover with left-over dip sauce and sprinkle with cheese. Bake at four hundred (200°C, gas mark half-dozen) until cheese is Defrosted and starts to brown, about fifteen minutes.

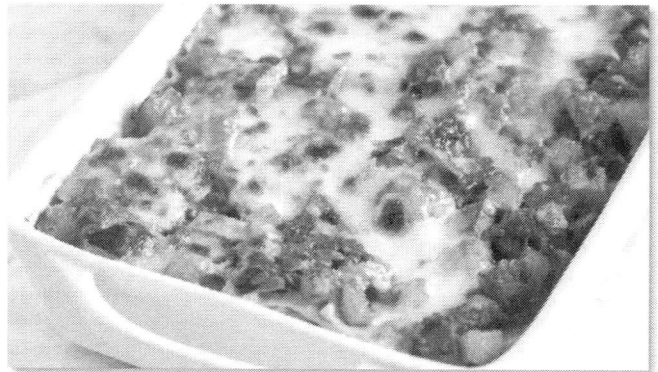

Chicken Macaroni Salad
Ingredients:

- One-Fourth tsp. crushed garlic
- One-Fourth mug brown Lactose
- 2 tbsps. cider lemon juice
- One-Fourth tsp. liquid smoke
- One-Fourth tsp. black pepper
- 2 tbsps. honey
- 2 pounds canned salmon fillets

Instructions:

- Switch on the Roast. In a tiny combining dish, Merge dip sauce ingredients. Combine well. Brush one side of the canned salmon with the basting dip sauce and then Put the canned salmon (basted side down) on the Roast.

- When the canned salmon is finished Preparing, baste the Cover portion of the canned salmon and flip the fillet thus the recent basting dip sauce is on the Roast. When the fish is nearly finished Preparing, apply the basting dip sauce and flip the canned salmon again. Baste and flip the canned salmon once a lot of and serve. Be careful to not overprepare the canned salmon, as it can lose its juices and flavor if prepared too long.

Onion nacho Roll
Ingredients:

- 1 mug green onion, diced
- 3 tsps. Diced fresh dill
- One-Fourth tsp. ground nutmeg
- One-Fourth tsp. freshly ground black pepper
- One-Third mug olive oil
- Half mug Diced fresh bay leaf
- 1 mug onion, Diced
- 1 mug (104 g) leek, Diced
- 8 phyllo pastry sheets
- 2 tbsps. olive oil

Instructions:

- Wash green lettuce well and remove any coarse stems. Cleave coarsely and put into a major container. Cover and Put over Warm up for 7-8 minutes, shaking skillet once in a while or turning green lettuce with a fork. Warm up sufficiently long to wither green lettuce so squeezes can run out openly.
- Channel well in colander, squeezing every so often with a Serve. Tenderly fry onions in olive oil for 10 minutes; add Diced leek and green onions and fry delicately for 5 minutes until straightforward. Put very much

depleted green lettuce in a joining dish and add oil and onion blend, spices, nutmeg, and pepper. Mix completely. Put a sheet of phyllo baked good on work surface and brush delicately with olive oil. Cover with 3 additional sheets of baked good, brushing each with oil.

- Brush Cover layer daintily with oil and Put a large portion of the green lettuce combination along the length of the cake towards one edge and leaving clear on each side. Crease base edge of cake over filling, roll once, overlay in sides, and afterward move up. Put a hand at each finish of roll and push it in delicately.
- Rehash with left-over baked good and filling. Put abounds in an oiled preparing dish, leaving space between rolls. Brush Covers softly with thwart and heat in a moderate broiler for 30 minutes until brilliant. Serve warm, cut into parcels.

Stuffed Portobellos with Rosemary
Ingredients:

- 4 portobello mushroom caps, about 4 to 5 inches (10 to 13 cm)
- 2 tbsps. lemon juice
- two-thirds mug Diced plum tomato
- 2 ounces part-skim mozzarella cheese, cut into small pieces
- 1 tsp. olive oil, Cut up
- Half tsp. fresh rosemary
- One-Eighth tsp. black pepper, coarse ground
- One-Fourth tsp. crushed garlic
- 2 tsps. (2.6 g) fresh bay leaf

Instructions:

- Prepare Roast. Merge the tomato, cheese, a pair of tsp. oil, rosemary, pepper, and garlic in an exceedingly small dish. Take away brown gills from the undersides of mushroom caps employing a Serve and discard gills. Take away stems and discard. Merge left-over 2 tsp. oil and lemon juice in a very little dish.

- Brush over each sides of mushroom caps. Put the mushroom caps, stem sides down, on Roast rack Covered with nonstick vegetable oil Sprinkle and Roast for five minutes on every aspect or until soft. Serve One-Fourth mug tomato mixture into every mushroom cap.
- Cover and Roast three minutes or until cheese is Defrosted. Sprinkle with bay leaf.

Vegetable Burgers
Ingredients:

- 1 tsp. black pepper
- 1-pound tofu, mashed
- 1 mug quick Preparing oat
- Half mug (56 g) warms up germ
- 2 tbsps. Sodium Soy Dip sauce
- Half tsp. basil
- Half tsp. oregano
- Half tsp. garlic powder
- 1 mug onion, finely minced

Instructions:

- Combine ingredients together. Knead for a few minutes. Shape into six patties. Oven fry on Prepare sheet Sprinkled with nonstick oil Sprinkle at 325°F for 25 minutes.

Black Bean Quesadillas
Ingredients:

- 15 ounces black beans, drained
- One-Fourth mug (45 g) Diced tomato
- 3 tbsps. Diced cilantro
- 1 mug green lettuce leaves, cut into small pieces

- 2 black olives, pitted, diced
- 8 whole warm up waffles,
- 4 ounces (58 g) pepper jack cheese, cut into small pieces
- 4 tbsps. warm sauce

Instructions:

- Mash beans. Whisk in tomato, cilantro, and olives. Expand evenly onto 4 waffles. Sprinkle with cheese, green lettuce, and warm sauce.
- Cover with left-over waffles. Switch on oven to 350°F Bake waffles on unlubricated Prepare sheet for 12 minutes. Cut into pieces and serve.

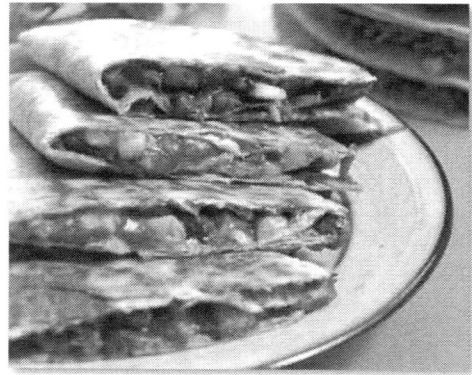

Beans and Barley with fresh bay leaf
Ingredients:

- 1 mug white beans, unprepared
- 4 mugs (940 g) low-sodium vegetable broth
- Half tsp. prepared mustard
- 2 tbsps. fresh bay leaf, minced
- Half mug split peas, parched
- 1 mug (193 g) pinto beans, unprepared
- Third-Fourth mug onion, Diced
- 1 mug (130 g) carrot, Diced
- One-Fourth mug pearl barley
- Half mug mushrooms, Diced
- One-Fourth mug lentils, parched

Instructions:

- Soak white beans and pinto beans overnight. Deep-fry onion, mushrooms, and carrots in 1 tbsp. of vegetable stock until ripe. To sauteed veggies, add drained beans, vegetable stock, mustard, and bay leaf. Bring to boil.
- Decrease Heat up, cover, and simmer 45 minutes. Add split peas, lentils, and barley. Shift all ingredients to a big slow Oven set on low for twelve-fourteen hours.

Vegetarian Vegetable Soup
Ingredients:

- 6 mugs mineral water
- 1 onion, Diced
- 1 tsp. black pepper
- 1 tsp. salt-free seasoning
- 1 tsp. basil
- 12 ounces frozen combined veggies
- 2 mugs Diced tomato
- 3 potatoes, Peel offed and chopped
- 2 turnips, Peel offed and chopped
- 3 carrots, Peel offed and diced
- Half mug diced celery
- 2 mugs cut into small pieces cabbage

Instructions:

- Put all ingredients in a big pot. Simmer until veggies are done. Decrease Heat up, cover, and simmer 45 minutes. The mixture ought to be moist however not overly skinny. Garnish with green chili and mint. Serve immediately.

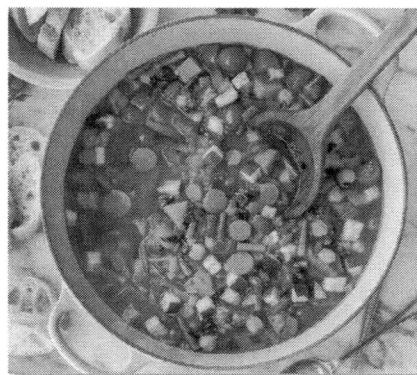

Vegetable Chowder
Ingredients:

- One-Fourth mug (38 g) green pepper, Diced
- One-Fourth mug celery, Diced
- One-Fourth mug carrots, Diced
- One-Eighth tsp. parched thyme
- Half tsp. parched oregano
- 100% mug fat-free cottage cheese
- 10 ounces tomatoes
- Half mug mineral waters
- One-Fourth mug onion, Diced
- One-Fourth tsp. parched basil
- 1 tbsp. (1 5 g) olive oil
- 1 clove garlic, minced
- 1 mug (195 g) brown mugs Diced rice, prepared

Instructions:

- Warm up oil in dip saucepan. Prepare onion, pepper, celery, carrots, and garlic until lightly browned. In blender Merge cottage cheese, tomatoes, mineral water, and spices. Blend until smooth and add to veggies.
- Whisk in brown rice and Prepare, whisking until Warm upped through. Do not boil.

Curried Lentil Stew with Poblano peppers
Ingredients:

- 1 tsp. turmeric

- 2 tbsps. olive oil
- 1 mug onion, Diced
- 2 garlic cloves, Diced
- Half mug Poblano peppers, chopped
- 1 tbsp. coriander
- 1 tsp. cumin
- 1 tsp. ginger
- 1 medium-sized potato, chopped
- Half mug carrot, diced
- 1 mug (192 g) lentils
- 2 mugs (475 ml) mineral water
- 2 tbsps. tomato paste

Instructions:

- In a massive pot, Warm up oil. Fry onion and garlic for a couple of minutes. Add potatoes, carrots and bell pepper and still fry for a few a lot of minutes, whisking often. Add spices and whisk-fry for a couple of seconds. Add lentils and tomato paste, whisk quickly, and add mineral water. Cover, raise Warm up and bring to a boil.
- Decrease Warm up and simmer gently for thirty minutes. Check the mineral water levels and lentil consistency. Prepare for one more fifteen minute if lentils aren't prepared. Take faraway from Warm up and let cool slightly. The mixture ought to be moist however not overly skinny.

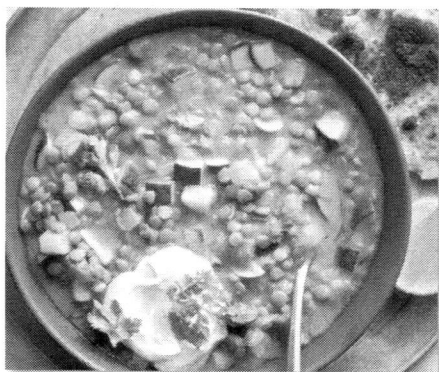

Onion Pie
Ingredients:

- 3 mugs onions, finely chopped
- 1 mug fat free milk
- 2 tbsps. Flour
- 8 ounces tofu, crushed by hand
- One-Fourth tsp. black pepper
- 2 tbsps. olive oil
- 1 pie crust

Instructions:

- Deep-fry onions in oil until translucent and mostly soft. Blend the milk, tofu, pepper, nutmeg, and flour until smooth.
- Then Merge the onions and the milk mixture. Spill into the prepared pie shell. Bake in a Turn owned oven at 350°F for about 30 minutes.

Dice Onion Pea Soup
Ingredients:

- Half tsp. black pepper
- 1 Half quarts mineral water
- 1-pound parched green split peas, Soaked
- 1 Half mugs (195 g) carrots, Peel offed and diced
- 1 mug Diced onion
- Half tsp. minced garlic
- 1 bay leaf
- One-Fourth mug Diced fresh bay leaf
- Half mug Diced celery

Instructions:

- Layer ingredients in slow Oven; Spill in mineral water. Do not whisk. Cover and Prepare on high 4 to 5 hours or on low 8 to 10 hours until peas are very soft. Take away bay leaf before serving.

Apple and Barley Stew Marjoram
Ingredients:

- 2 mugs onion, thinly diced
- 2 tbsps. olive oil

- 3 Half mug (825 ml) low-sodium vegetable broth
- 1 Half mugs (355 ml) apple cider
- 1 mug (130 g) carrot, chopped
- 1 tsp. thyme
- One-Fourth tsp. parched marjoram
- 1 bay leaf
- One-Third mug pearl barley
- 2 mugs apples, unpeel offed, Diced
- One-Fourth mug fresh bay leaf, minced
- 1 tbsp. lemon juice

Instructions:

- In a small soup pot, deep-fry onions in oil over medium-sized Warm up for 5 minutes, whisking constantly. Decrease Warm up, cover, and Prepare, whisking frequently for 10 minutes more until onions are browned.
- Add stock, cider, barley, carrots, thyme, marjoram, and bay leaf. Cover and Prepare for one hour or until barley is ripe. Add apples, bay leaf, and lemon juice. Prepare for 5 minutes or until apples are slightly soft. Discard bay leaf and serve.

Chickpea Dip sauce
Ingredients:

- 14 ounces (400 g) no-salt-added tomatoes, Diced
- 6 ounces no-salt-added tomato paste
- 1 tsp. basil
- 1 tsp. oregano
- 1 dash cinnamon
- 1 Half mug parched chick peas, soaked
- 1 tbsp. olive oil
- Third-Fourth mug onion, Diced
- 2 garlic cloves, crushed
- 2 tbsps. fresh bay leaf

Instructions:

- Soak chickpeas, put in fresh mineral water, and Prepare for 50 minutes or until ripe. Warm up oil in big pot and Deep-fry onions and garlic for a few minutes.
- Add the tomatoes and tomato paste. Bring to a boil, lower Warm up, and add the rest of the ingredients. Simmer for about 10 minutes or until the dip sauce has thickened.

Asian Barley Salad
Ingredients:

- 1 mug prepared, shelled edamame
- One-Fourth mug Diced green onion
- 1 Half tsps. finely Diced fresh mint
- Half mug Diced carrot
- Half mug Diced Poblano pepper
- One-Eighth tsp. chile pepper flakes
- 4 mugs low-sodium vegetable broth
- 1 tbsp. extra-virgin olive oil
- Half tsp. grind orange zest
- 2 tbsps. finely Diced fresh Thai basil
- Juice of Half orange
- 1 tsp. sesame seeds
- 1 tbsp. sesame oil
- 2 mugs unprepared Barley
- One-Eighth tsp. cracked black pepper

Instructions:

- Soak the Barley (if not presoaked). In a tiny lined pot, bring the Barley and vegetable broth to a boil over high Warm up. Decrease the Warm up to low and simmer for 10 to fifteen minutes or till most of the liquid has been absorbed. ready Barley should be slightly al dente; it is ready when most of the grains have uncoiled and you'll be able to see the unwound germ. Let the Barley sit within the coated pot for about 5 minutes.
- Fluff gently with a fork and Shift the prepared Barley to a big dish, then

combine in the left-over ingredients. Cool to space temperature and serve. This dish can additionally be served cool downed.

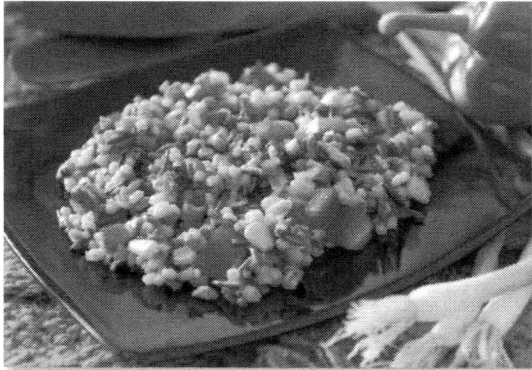

Healthy Macaroni Salad
Ingredients:

- 4 tbsps. extra virgin olive oil
- 4 mugs whole warm up penne macaroni
- One-Fourth mug Heat upped pine dry fruits
- 1 mug Diced fresh mozzarella cheese
- 1 bunch coarsely Diced fresh basil
- 2 mugs halved cherry tomatoes
- Pinch of sea salt
- One-Eighth tsp. cracked black pepper

Instructions:

- Boil a massive pot of mineral water, adding a Sprinkle of olive oil to prevent the macaroni from sticking. Add the macaroni to the boiling mineral water, whisking once, and Prepare 8 to 10 minutes, or till al dente. Strain the macaroni. To Heat up the pine dry fruits, Heat up a huge, flat pan over medium-sized high Heat up.
- Add the pine dry fruits, and whisk frequently to avoid burning. Heat up for regarding a pair of minutes or till the dry fruits smell buttery and they are light-weight brown on the outside. Take away them from the pan instantly.

In a huge dish, Roll the ready macaroni with the left-over ingredients. The warm macaroni will slightly Defrost the cheese.

Basic Olive Vinaigrette
Ingredients:

- One-Eighth tsp. sea salt
- Half tsp. Dijon or brown mustard
- One-Fourth mug balsamic lemon juice
- Half mug extra virgin olive oil
- Half tsp. decreased-Lactose marmalade
- Cracked black pepper

Instructions:

- During a little dish, Whip along the mustard, marmalade, and lemon juice. Terribly slowly Sprinkle within the oil, and continue Whipping the mixture together. (Constant Whipping emulsifies the oil and lemon juice, dispersing the droplets of 1 into the opposite and making a thick dressing.) Add salt and pepper.
- Store in an airtight jar or canister if not instantly using. Note: It is recommended that the base for the homemade vinaigrette consists of one-half lemon juice or different acid, such as lemon, lime, or orange juice, and a couple of elements oil.

Chicken Fajita Onion Wraps
Ingredients:

- 3 tbsps. extra virgin olive oil
- 2 (6-ounce) boneless, skinless chicken breasts
- 1 big Poblano pepper, thinly diced
- 1 big Poblano pepper, thinly diced
- 4 100% whole warm up waffles
- 1 tsp. parched oregano
- One-Eighth tsp. sea salt
- One-Eighth tsp. black pepper

- Half big white onion, thinly diced
- 1 mug Soaked and drained canned black beans
- 1 mug cut into small pieces romaine green lettuce leaf
- 4 tbsps. low-fat plain Greek curd

Instructions:

- Warm up the oil in a big pan over medium-sized Warm up. While the pan Warm ups, Take away the fat from the chicken breasts, slice them longitudinally about One-Fourth inch thick and cut the longer pieces in half.
- Season with oregano, salt, and pepper. Add the chicken to the pan, and Deep-fry until the pieces are no longer pink in the center, 5 to 6 minutes. Take away the chicken from the pan, and set aside.
- Add the onion and bell peppers to the same pan, and Deep-fry until the onions are soft but not completely transparent, about 4 minutes. Warm the waffles in a flat pan over low Warm up. Cut up the black beans, green lettuce leaf, chicken, and Deep-fried peppers and onions among the four waffles. Cover with curd, wrap, and serve.

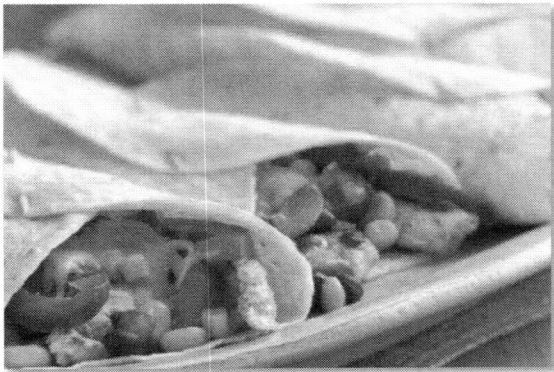

Honey Lemon Vinaigrette black pepper
Ingredients:

- One-Eighth tsp. cracked black pepper

- Juice of 3 lemons (about One-Fourth mug)
- 1 tbsp. honey
- 1 tsp. Diced fresh thyme
- One-Eighth tsp. sea salt
- Half mug extra virgin olive oil

Instructions:

- In a small dish, Whip together the lemon juice, honey, thyme, salt, and pepper. Very slowly Sprinkle in the oil, and continue Whipping the mixture together. Store in an airtight canister or jar if not instantly using.

Canned Garlic salmon Hash
Ingredients:

- Half mug Poblano peppers, Diced
- One-Eighth tsp. pepper
- 1 clove garlic, crushed
- 1 tbsp. vegetable oil
- Half mug Diced onion
- Half mug Poblano peppers, Diced
- 2 medium-sized potatoes, chopped and prepared
- 1 6 ounces canned salmon

Instructions:

- Warm up oil in 1 Q-inch (25 cm) nonstick frying pan over medium-sized-high Warm up. Deep-fry onion, bell peppers, pepper, and garlic in oil.
- Whisk in potatoes and canned salmon. Prepare Unwrapped, whisking frequently, until warm.

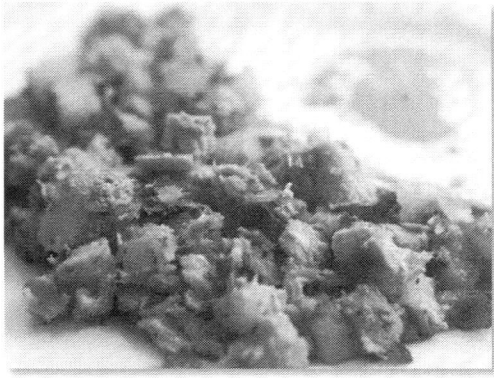

Garlic Balsamic Vinaigrette with lemon juice
Ingredients:

- Half tsp. Spicy Brown Mustard
- 1 big clove garlic, finely minced
- Half tsp. decreased-Lactose raspberry marmalade
- One-Fourth mug balsamic lemon juice
- Half mug extra virgin olive oil
- Pinch of parched oregano
- One-Eighth tsp. sea salt
- Cracked black pepper

Instructions:

- In a small dish, Whip together the mustard, garlic, marmalade, and lemon juice. Very slowly Sprinkle in the oil, and continue Whipping the mixture together. Add the oregano and the salt and pepper.

Green Summer Salad
Ingredients:

- Sea salt
- 3 heads romaine green lettuce leaf, Diced
- 5 Roma tomatoes, Diced
- One-Fourth mug very thinly diced white onion
- One-Fourth mug fresh lime juice
- One-Eighth mug extra virgin olive oil
- 1 Half mugs diced unpeel offed cucumber

- Cracked black pepper

Instructions:

- In a big dish, Merge the green lettuce leaf, tomato, cucumber, and onion. Spill the lime juice and oil over the salad, and Roll well. Season to taste with salt and pepper. Garnish with green chili and mint. Serve immediately.

Amazing Cobb Salad with Vinaigrette
Ingredients:

- One-Third mug crushed blue cheese
- 4 slices turkey bacon
- 5 mugs green lettuce
- Half big cucumber, diced
- Half (15-ounce) can kidney beans, Soaked and drained
- 1 big avocado, pitted, Peel offed, and Diced
- 1 mug diced cremini mushrooms
- Half mug cut into small pieces carrot

Instructions:

- Warm up a medium-sized-sized nonstick pan over medium-sized Warm up, and Cover with olive oil Sprinkle. Add the turkey bacon, prepare till brown, and then flip and continue Preparing, 5 to six minutes.
- Take away and rest on a cutting board. Crumble the cooled turkey bacon by hand, or coarsely chop. Put the inexperienced lettuce on a huge serving platter. Then Sort the mushroom, carrot, cucumber, kidney beans, avocado, blue cheese, and turkey bacon in neat rows a Cover the inexperienced lettuce. Serve with vinaigrette on the side.

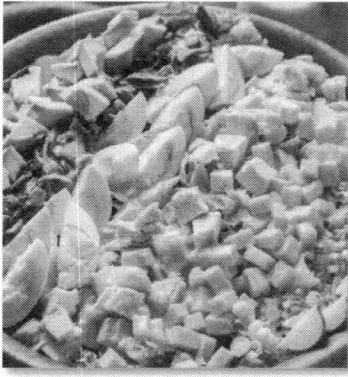

Green Beet and Heirloom Tomato Salad
Ingredients:

- 1 mug prepared, thinly diced beets
- 6 mugs combined greens
- 1 mug green heirloom tomato, diced and cut in fourths
- One-Fourth mug Heat upped walnut pieces
- One-Fourth mug crushed goat cheese
- One-Fourth mug balsamic lemon juice
- Cracked black pepper, to taste

Instructions:

- Prepare the beets by setting apart the green stems and washing the beets. Cut off the very Cover and terribly base of the beet, and then Peel off upped the thick skin. Put the beets in a very small pot with concerning Half to 1 mug of mineral water, and Brew over medium-sized Warm up for concerning 15 minutes.
- Once ready, let cool, and then slice and cut every slice into fourths as with the heirloom tomatoes. Put the combined greens in an exceedingly massive salad dish, and Cover with the beets, tomato, dry fruits, and goat cheese. Sprinkle with balsamic lemon juice, and grind cracked black pepper over the Cover.

Salad with Lemon Vinaigrette
Ingredients:

- 1 tsp. parched oregano
- 4 mugs Diced romaine leaves
- Half mug halved cherry tomatoes
- Half mug Soaked and drained
- One-Fourth mug low-fat feta cheese
- 10 black pitted olives, Soaked, drained, and Diced

Instructions:

- Merge all the ingredients in a big salad dish, and Roll well. Serve each dish with 2 tbsps. of the lemon vinaigrette on the side. Garnish with green chili and mint. Serve immediately.

Sweet and Spicy Canned Lemon salmon
Ingredients:

- 2 pounds canned salmon fillets
- 2 tbsps. honey
- 1 tbsp. lemon juice
- 1 tbsp. sesame oil
- One-Fourth tsp. crushed red pepper flakes

Instructions:

- Place fish in glass or ceramic baking dish. Merge honey and left-over ingredients and Spill over fish to Cover. Cover with plastic wrap and marinate thirty minutes before Preparing. Light barbecue Roast.
- When coals are ready, oil Roast with oil or Preparing Sprinkle and place in Place. Put fish on Roast, skin side down if not skinless. Cover and Prepare five minutes. Sprinkle fish with marinade and Prepare 3 minutes additional or until fish turns opaque.

Blackened Cayenne Pepper Canned salmon
Ingredients:

- 2 tbsps. paprika
- 1 tbsp. cayenne pepper

- 1 tbsp. onion powder
- One-Fourth tsp. basil
- One-Fourth tsp. oregano
- 1-pound canned salmon fillets
- Half tsp. white pepper
- Half tsp. black pepper
- One-Fourth tsp. thyme
- 2 tbsps. olive oil

Instructions:

- In a tiny dish, combine paprika, cayenne pepper, onion powder, white pepper, black pepper, thyme, basil, and oregano. Brush canned salmon fillets on each side with oil and sprinkle evenly with the cayenne pepper mixture.
- Sprinkle one aspect of every fillet with half of the left-over oil. In a massive, heavy frying pan over high Heat up, Prepare canned salmon oiled side down till blackened, 2 to five minutes. Turn fillets, sprinkle with left-over oil, and continue Preparing until blackened and fish is well flaked with a fork.

Canned creamy salmon Casserole
Ingredients:

- One-Fourth mug oil, Warm upped
- Half mug white wine
- One-Fourth mug sherry
- Half mug fat-free sour cream
- 1-pound potatoes, Peel offed and diced
- 1 Half pounds canned salmon fillets
- 1 tbsp. Diced fresh dill
- 2 tbsps. grind horseradish

Instructions:

- Boil potatoes until virtually done, about ten to fifteen minutes. Layer in an exceedingly huge ovenproof casserole. Put the canned salmon on Cover. Sprinkle with the dill. Cover and

Prepare at 350°F (180°C, gas mark four) for 25 minutes.

- Take far away from the oven and Spill the Warm upped oil, wine, and sherry over. Continue to Prepare Unwrapped until canned salmon is done. Whisk along sour cream and horseradish and Spill over Cover.

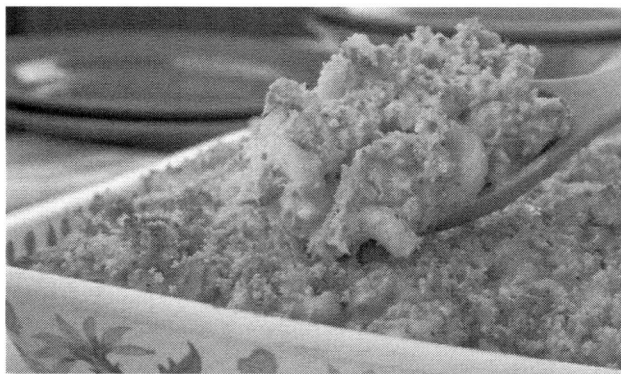

Kidney Paprika Bean Stew
Ingredients:

- 1 mug celery, diced
- 8 ounces mushrooms, washed and diced
- 2 mugs tomatoes, Peel offed and quartered
- Half mug parched kidney beans, soaked, prepared, and drained
- Half tsp. paprika
- 1 tbsp. olive oil
- 1 Half mug onion, diced
- 1 mug Poblano pepper, seeded and Diced
- Third-Fourth mug (98 g) carrot, diced
- 1 Half mug cucumber, diced
- Black pepper, fresh ground

Instructions:

- Warm up the oil in a big dip saucepan and add the onion, red pepper, carrots, cucumber, and celery. Prepare gently for 10 minutes, covered, and then add the mushrooms, tomatoes, kidney beans, paprika, and pepper to taste.

- Continue to Prepare, covered, for another 10-15 minutes. Check the seasoning and serve.

Roasted Tuna Fillet with Honey Mustard
Ingredients:

- 1 tbsp. honey
- 3 tbsps. extra virgin olive oil
- One-Third mug red wine lemon juice
- 1 tbsp. spicy brown mustard
- 1-pound tuna fillet-steaks

Instructions:

- Merge the first 4 ingredients in a jar or covered canister; shake to combine well. Put tuna in a food storage bag; add the mustard mixture. Seal the bag and let marinate for about 20 minutes. Warm up the Roast.
- Take away the tuna from the marinade and Spill the marinade in a small dip saucepan. Bring marinade to a boil; Take away from Warm up and set aside. Roast the tuna over high Warm up for about 2 minutes on each side or until done as if you want. Sprinkle with the warm marinade.

Tuna Lemon Fillet-steaks
Ingredients:

- 2 tbsps. lemon juice
- Half tsp. black pepper, fresh ground
- 6 ounces tuna fillet-steaks
- 2 tbsps. olive oil

Instructions:

- Merge the olive oil and lemon juice. Marinate the fillet-steaks in the mixture at least 30 minutes, turning from time to time.
- Warm up a frying pan over high Warm up. Add the fillet-steaks and Prepare 2

minutes. Sprinkle with pepper, turn over, and Prepare 2 minutes longer.

Tuna Garlic Burger
Ingredients:

- One-Fourth tsp. garlic powder
- 2 cans tuna, low-sodium and packed in mineral water
- Half mug bread crumbs
- 2 eggs
- 2 tbsps. minced onion
- Half tsp. dry mustard

Instructions:

- Drain tuna. Merge with bread crumbs, eggs, and spices. Form into 4 patties. Roast or fry until browned, turn, and continue Preparing until done. Garnish with green chili and mint. Serve immediately.

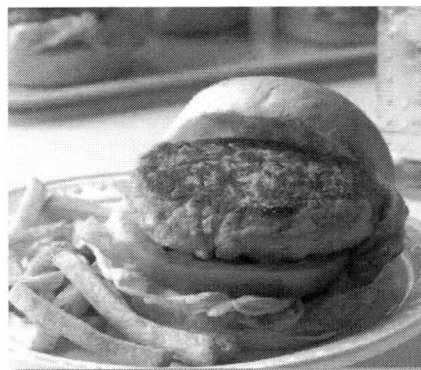

Dilly Mayonnaise Tuna Salad
Ingredients:

- 2 tbsps. low-fat mayonnaise
- 3 tbsps. fresh dill, Diced
- 2 tbsps. white onions, chopped
- 1 mug (284 g) light tuna, in mineral water, drained
- One-Fourth mug celery, Diced
- Pepper to taste

Instructions:

- Combine all ingredients well.

Amish Chicken Carrot Soup
Ingredients:

- Half mug Diced celery
- Half mug diced carrot
- Half mug Diced onion
- 4 mugs (950 ml) low-sodium chicken broth
- 2 mugs chicken, prepared and Diced
- 1 tbsp. bay leaf
- One-Fourth tsp. garlic powder
- 2 mugs (475 ml) mineral water
- 12 ounces egg noodles

Instructions:

- Put all ingredients in a big kettle and simmer until noodles are ripe. Garnish with green chili and mint. Serve immediately.

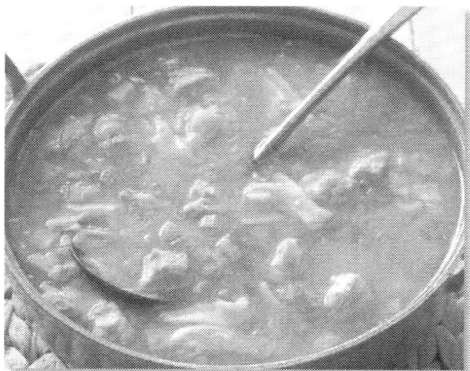

Red Mexican Cilantro sauce
Ingredients:

- 2 big Roma tomatoes, cut into big pieces
- Half mug mineral waters
- Third-Fourth mug fresh cilantro
- One-Fourth tsp. sea salt
- 20 parched red chiles/chiles de arbol
- 1 big clove garlic
- Half white onion, cut into big pieces

Instructions:

- Warm up a big frying pan over high Warm up. Add the chiles, garlic, onion, and tomatoes directly to the pan with no oil. Once the tomato skins and chiles start to blacken, take away the chiles from the frying pan and Put them in a small pot with the mineral water. Cover, and simmer for 8 to 10 minutes to soften the chiles.
- Once the chiles are softened, Shift the prepared ingredients along with the cilantro to a blender. Blend on low speed, and cover the Cover with a kitchen towel so that Brew can escape, but the warm sauce won't explode out the Cover of the blender. Season with salt to taste. Caution: This warm sauce is very spicy!

Turkey Bay Leaf Soup
Ingredients:

- 1 mug coarsely Diced onion
- 1 mug (130 g) diced carrot
- Half tsp. garlic powder
- 1 tsp. seasoning
- 4 mugs (950 ml) low-sodium chicken or turkey broth
- 1 can (14Half ounces or 410 g) no-salt-added tomatoes
- Soups, Stews, and Chilies
- 1 tbsp. bay leaf
- 2 mugs (350 g) prepared turkey
- 6 ounces (128 g) whole warm up macaroni, any shape if you want

Instructions:

- Merge all ingredients except macaroni in a big Dutch oven.
- Bring to a boil. Whisk in macaroni, lower Warm up, and simmer until macaroni is prepared and herbs are ripe.

Turkey Barley Thyme Soup
Ingredients:

- 6 mugs low-sodium chicken broth
- 1 mug prepared turkey, chopped
- 1 mug pearl barley
- 1 bay leaf
- 1 tsp. parched thyme
- One-Fourth tsp. parched marjoram
- One-Fourth tsp. black pepper
- 1 mug onion, Diced
- 1 mug celery, Diced
- Third-Fourth mug (83 g) carrot, diced
- 2 tbsps. (2.6 g) parched bay leaf

Instructions:

- Merge all the ingredients in soup pot or slow Oven. Prepare over low Warm up in the slow Oven for 6 hours or simmer on the stove for 1 hour until the carrots are ripe and the barley is soft. Take away bay leaf before serving.

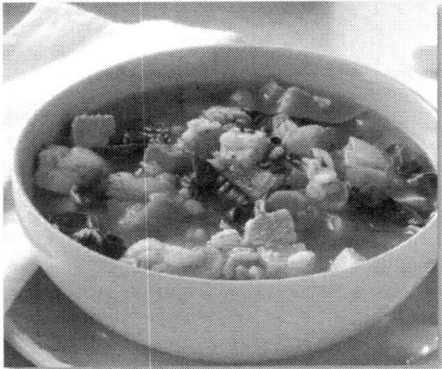

Real Beef Chili
Ingredients:

- 3 pounds beef round fillet-steak
- 2 tbsps. canola oil
- 4 ounces canned chile peppers
- 2 tbsps. chili powder
- 1 tsp. garlic powder
- 1 tbsp. onion powder
- 1 tsp. Tabasco dip sauce
- 2 mugs (475 ml) low-sodium beef broth
- 8 ounces no-salt-added tomato dip sauce
- 2 mugs no-salt-added canned tomatoes
- 6 ounces (177 ml) beer
- 1 tbsp. cumin

Instructions:

- Deep-fry beef in oil until done and drain well; put beef and broth in a big pot and bring to a slow simmer; add tomato dip sauce, tomatoes, beer, chile peppers, spices, and Tabasco; simmer slowly for about 1 hour and 30 minutes or until meat is ripe.

Beef Barley Frying
Ingredients:

- 2 tbsps. (19 g) green pepper, Diced
- One-Eighth tsp. thyme
- 1 Half tbsps. chili dip sauce
- One-Fourth pound lean ground beef
- 4 tbsps. onion, Diced
- 2 tbsps. (1 3 g) celery, Diced
- two-thirds mug no-salt-added tomatoes
- Half mug mineral waters
- One-Fourth mug pearl barley

Instructions:

- Deep-fry beef, onion, celery, and green pepper until meat is done. Spill off fat and whisk in rest of the ingredients. Bring to a boil and then turn down Warm up and simmer until barley is prepared.

Caprese Salad with Balsamic
Ingredients:

- 5 big beef fillet-steak tomatoes, cut into Half-inch slices
- 1 bunch fresh basil
- 5 tbsps. extra virgin olive oil
- Pinch of sea salt

- One-Eighth tsp. cracked black pepper
- 1-pound fresh buffalo mozzarella cheese, cut into One-Fourth-inch slices
- 5 tbsps. Balsamic Glaze

Instructions:

- Sort the diced tomatoes on a big platter. Cover each slice with a big basil leaf and a mozzarella slice. Sprinkle balsamic glaze and oil over the platter, and then sprinkle with salt and pepper.

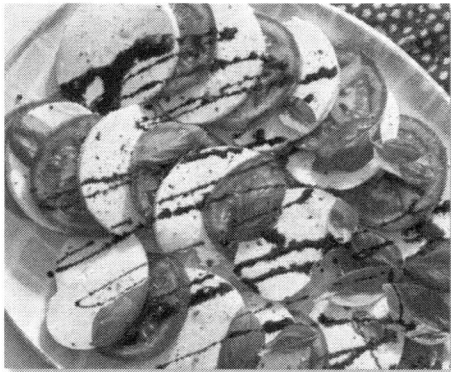

Roasted Tomatillo Warm sauce
Ingredients:

- 2 cloves garlic
- Third-Fourth mug fresh cilantro
- 1 mug mineral water
- Half small white onion, cut into big pieces
- 1 big whole jalapeño chile pepper, stem cut off
- Half tsp. sea salt

Instructions:

- Warm up a Roast to medium-sized-high Warm up. Put the whole tomatillos directly on the Roast. Watch them carefully, rotating every 2 to 3 minutes and turning over to blacken on all sides. It's okay if they blacken or burn, as it will add to their flavor.
- They're done when they feel soft and squishy when picked up with tongs. Put

prepared tomatillos in a pot and cover, so they continue Brewing while the rest of the tomatillos finish Roasting. Once all the tomatillos have been Roasted, leave them in the covered pot for 15 to 20 minutes, until completely cooled.

- They will release liquid while they cool, which can be used in Put of mineral water or combined with mineral water, to make the warm sauce. In a small pot over high Warm up, Prepare the onion, chile pepper, and garlic until they start to brown.
- After 2 minutes, add the tomatillo liquid or combine of liquid and mineral water, and cover. Simmer for about 5 minutes, or until a fork easily inserts into the onion. Shift the onion mixture, tomatillos (first removing any hard cores and leaving skin on), and cilantro in batches to a blender, and blend on low speed and then high until smooth. Salt each batch to taste. Store blended batches in an airtight canister.

Roasted Chicken with Black Bean Warm sauce
Ingredients:

- 2 mugs Soaked and drained canned black beans
- Juice of 1 big lime
- Juice of Half orange
- One-Eighth tsp. sea salt
- One-Eighth tsp. cracked black pepper
- 4 boneless, skinless chicken breasts
- 1 big Granny Smith apple, Diced
- Half small red onion, finely Diced
- 1 serrano chile pepper, seeded and finely Diced
- 2 tbsps. Diced fresh cilantro

Instructions:

- To make the warm sauce, Merge all the ingredients (except the salt, pepper, and chicken) in a big dish. Freeze for at least an hour to let the flavors meld.

- Warm up a Roast or Roast pan to medium-sized-high Warm up. Season the chicken breasts with salt and pepper. Put them on the Roast, and Prepare 4 to 6 minutes per side, or until the center of each is no longer pink. Cut up the warm sauce on Cover of the breasts, and serve.

Chicken Salad Pita Sandwich
Ingredients:

- 2 (6-ounce) boneless, skinless chicken breasts
- Half mug Diced carrot
- 1 Half tsps. red wine lemon juice
- 1 tsp. curry powder
- One-Fourth tsp. ground cinnamon
- 4 100% whole warm up pitas (with pockets)
- 2 romaine green lettuce leaf leaves, Diced
- One-Third mug Diced green onion
- One-Fourth mug golden raisins
- Third-Fourth mug low-fat plain Greek curd
- 8 heirloom tomatoes, diced
- One-Fourth mug Diced Heat upped almonds

Instructions:

- Crop the fat off the chicken, and cut the breasts into fourths. Fill a medium-sized pot with mineral water, and bring to a boil. Add the chicken, and boil 8 to 10 minutes, or until the centers are no longer pink.
- Strain the chicken, and set it aside to cool. In a medium-sized-sized dish, Merge the carrot, green onion, and raisins. Shred the cooled chicken with two forks, and add it to the dish. Add the curd, lemon juice, curry powder, and cinnamon, and combine well.

Freeze for 30 minutes. Warm the pitas in a big frying pan over low Warm up, and then cut them in half and split open. Stuff each pita pocket with salad combine, cover with almonds, and serve.

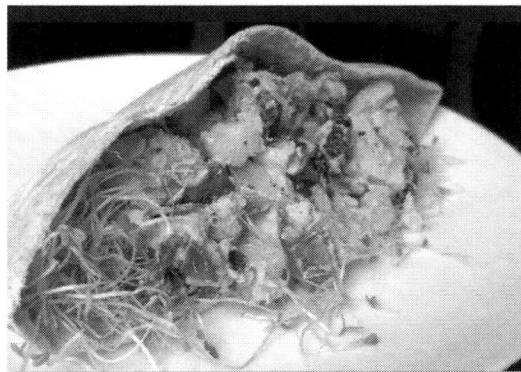

Beef and Black Corn Stew
Ingredients:

- 2 mugs no-salt-added canned tomatoes
- 1 mug (260 g) warm sauce
- 1 tsp. ground cumin
- Half tsp. freshly ground black pepper
- 6 ounces (130 g) frozen corn
- 2 pounds extra-lean ground beef
- Half tsp. minced garlic
- 1 mug Diced onion
- 1 Half mugs black beans,
- 1 tbsp. Diced fresh cilantro

Instructions:

- In a big frying pan, brown ground beef with garlic and onion. Drain and Shift to a slow Oven. Add tomatoes, warm sauce, cumin, pepper, corn, and black beans.
- Prepare on low 6 to 8 hours or on high for 3 to 4 hours. Add cilantro during the last hour of Preparing.

Oven Beef Mushroom Stew
Ingredients:

- 2 mugs onion, diced

- 8 ounces (227 g) mushroom, diced
- One-Fourth mug flour
- 2-pound beef round fillet-steak, cut in (2 Half cm) cubes
- 4 mugs (520 g) carrot, diced
- 2 mugs celery, diced
- 32 ounces (909 g) no-salt-added tomatoes
- 2 mugs (475 ml) burgundy wine

Instructions:

- In roasting pan or Dutch oven, combine meat, carrots, celery, onions, and mushrooms. Add flour. Whisk in tomatoes and Burgundy wine. Cover and bake 4 hours. Garnish with green chili and mint. Serve immediately.

Sausage and Lentil Soup
Ingredients:

- 1 mug onion, Diced
- Third-Fourth mug celery, Diced
- 1 bay leaf
- 2 garlic cloves, Peel offed and quartered
- 2 mugs parched lentils
- 2 quarts mineral water
- 1 ham hock
- 1 mug (130 g) carrot, Diced
- One-Fourth tsp. pepper, fresh ground
- Half-pound kielbasa sausage, chopped
- 1 tbsp. olive oil

Instructions:

- Wash lentils and pick over. Drain. Put in big kettle with left-over ingredients except sausage. Bring soup to a boil, decrease Warm up, and simmer for 1 to 2 hours.
- Meanwhile, during last 10 minutes of Preparing hour, dice sausage and Deep-fry in frying pan in oil until golden brown on all sides. Take away ham bone and bay leaf from soup. Decorate

each serving with chopped prepared sausage.

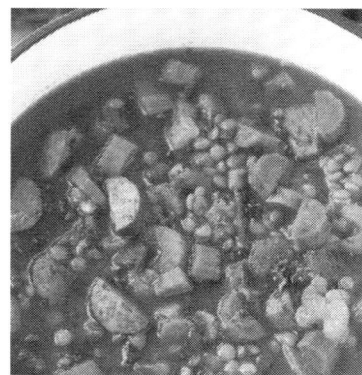

Salmon Fish Chowder
Ingredients:

- 1 onion, Diced
- 2 potatoes, chopped
- One-Fourth tsp. thyme
- 1 tsp. bay leaf
- 3 tbsps. Flour
- Half mug Diced celery
- 1 clove garlic, minced
- 1-pound canned salmon
- 1-pound perch
- 4 slices low-sodium bacon
- 1 Half mugs (355 ml) white wine
- 1 Half mugs (355 ml) mineral water
- 3 tbsps. (42 g) Without salt butter, softened
- Half mug fat free milk

Instructions:

- Thaw fish if frozen and cube. Prepare bacon in Dutch oven. Crumble and set aside. Drain most of grease from pan. Deep-fry onion, celery, and garlic until ripe. Add wine, mineral water, potatoes (if using), and spices.
- Simmer until potatoes are almost done, about 20 minutes. Add fish, cover, and simmer 10 minutes more. Combine together flour and butter to form a paste. Whisk into soup and simmer

until thickened. Whisk in milk and bacon.

Vegetable and Chickpea Cloves Stew
Ingredients:

- Third-Fourth mug (98 g) carrot, cut into discs
- 2 parsnips, cut into discs
- 1 big potato, chopped
- 3 mugs (705 ml) low-sodium vegetable juice
- 5 mugs (1.2 L) mineral water
- 2 tbsps. olive oil
- 2 garlic cloves, minced
- 1 mug onion, Diced
- Half mug celery, Diced
- Half mug fresh bay leaf, Diced
- 1 tsp. marjoram
- 15 ounces chickpeas, drained
- 2 mugs cabbage, cut into small pieces

Instructions:

- Warm up the oil in a big pan and Roll the onion, garlic, celery, carrots, parsnips and potato in it over a low Warm up. Add the juice and mineral water and marjoram.
- Increase the Warm up and simmer for 20 minutes. Add the drained chickpeas and the cabbage and Prepare for another 10 minutes.

Mushroom Soup with Ribs
Ingredients:

- 1 mug celery, finely diced
- 6 mugs low-sodium chicken broth
- two-thirds mug (133 g) pearl barley
- 2 pounds beef short ribs
- 1 mug onion, chopped
- 2 tbsps. minced garlic
- 1 tbsp. parched dill weed
- Pepper to taste
- 2 pounds mushrooms

Instructions:

- Put ribs, onion, garlic, and celery in a soup pot. Add the liquid, cover, bring to a boil, and simmer over low Warm up for 1 hour. Add the barley, dill, and pepper and Prepare another 50 minutes. Add the mushrooms and Prepare another 10 minutes. Serve warm.

Potato Celery Leek Soup
Ingredients:

- 3 big potatoes, Peel offed and chopped
- 6 mugs mineral water
- One-Fourth tsp. pepper
- 3 mugs (312 g) Diced leeks
- 1 mug celery, Peel offed, chopped
- 1 tsp. white wine lemon juice

Instructions:

- In a 4-quart (4 L) soup pot over medium-sized Warm up, Deep-fry leeks, celery, and potatoes in a little mineral water for 5 to 7 minutes.
- Add more mineral water as needed to prevent sticking. Add the 6 mugs of mineral water and pepper.
- Bring to a boil, lower Warm up, and simmer potatoes are very soft, about 15 minutes. Add lemon juice. Puree soup 2 to 3 mugs at a time in a blender or food processor until very smooth. Put back to soup pot and rewarm if needed.

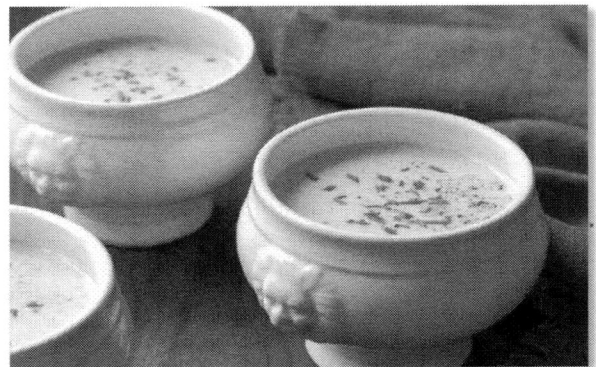

Broccoli Garlic Lemon Soup

Ingredients:

- 1 bay leaf
- 1-pound broccoli, Diced
- 2 mugs (475 ml) low-sodium vegetable broth
- 2 tbsps. lemon juice
- 1 mug onion, Diced
- 1 clove garlic, crushed
- 1 tbsp. olive oil

Instructions:

- Deep-fry onion and garlic in oil with the bay leaf for 3 to 4 minutes. Take away 4 ounces (114 g) of broccoli florets. Add the rest of the broccoli and stock. Bring to a boil and simmer gently, covered for 10 minutes.
- The broccoli should be ripe but still bright green. Take away the bay leaf and cool slightly. Blend the soup until it is completely smooth. Add the lemon juice. Rewarm up gently in a wipe pot. Meanwhile, Brew the florets till ripe, 8 minutes or so. Scatter them over the soup, whisk, and serve.

Black Bean Cumin Soup

Ingredients:

- Half tsp. minced garlic
- Half mug finely Diced carrot
- Half mug finely Diced celery
- 1 tbsp. olive oil
- 1 tsp. cumin
- One-Fourth tsp. cayenne pepper
- 1 Half mugs (375 g) parched black beans
- 4 mugs (950 ml) mineral water
- 1 mug finely Diced onion
- Half mug finely Diced Poblano pepper
- 1 tbsp. lime juice
- One-Fourth mug warm sauce

Instructions:

- Soak beans in mineral water overnight. In a big Dutch oven, Deep-fry onion, bell pepper, garlic, carrot, and celery in oil until almost soft.
- Add spices and Deep-fry a few minutes more. Add beans, mineral water, lime juice, and warm sauce and simmer until beans are beginning to fall apart, 1 Half to 2 hours.

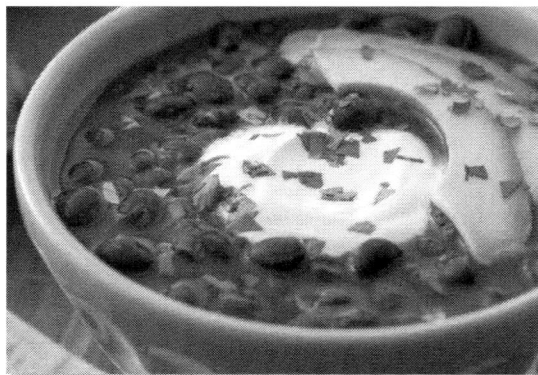

Broccoli Cheddar Cheese Soup

Ingredients:

- 1 tsp. white pepper
- Half tsp. thyme
- Half tsp. garlic powder
- 1 Half mug (355 ml) low-sodium chicken broth
- 2 mugs cheddar cheese, cut into small pieces
- 2 mug (475 ml) milk
- 3 tbsps. (42 g) Without salt butter
- 2 tbsps. onion, finely Diced
- 3 tbsps. flour
- Half tsp. salts
- 1 mug broccoli, prepared and finely Diced

Instructions:

- Prepare onions in butter until ripe. Blend in flour and seasonings and Prepare 3 to 4 minutes, whisking constantly. Add chicken broth and Prepare slowly until thick.

- Whisk in the milk until smooth. Add the cheese and broccoli and Warm up through.

Squash Dry Onion Soup
Ingredients:

- Half mug Diced onions
- 2 tbsps. minced garlic
- 1 tbsp. gingerroot, minced
- One-Third mug dry sherry
- 1 tbsp. olive oil
- Half tsp. coriander
- Half tsp. nutmegs
- Half tsp. cumin
- Half tsp. cinnamon
- 2 mugs (475 g) low-sodium vegetable broth
- 4 mugs (560 g) butternut squash, Peel offed, seeded, chopped
- 1 tbsp. lemon juice
- 1 tbsp. lemon Peel off

Instructions:

- In a big pot, Deep-fry onions, garlic, and ginger in oil and sherry for 10 minutes. Whisk frequently. If the veggies stick, add a little broth. Add left-over ingredients and simmer until squash is ripe. Process in a blender until smooth.

Beef Jalapeño Tacos
Ingredients:

- 2 tbsps. extra virgin olive oil
- Half tsp. parched oregano
- One-Fourth tsp. cracked black pepper
- Third-Fourth mug Diced Roma tomato
- 1 tsp. Diced jalapeño chile pepper
- 4 tbsps. Diced fresh cilantro
- Half mug Diced white onion, Cut up
- 1 mug Diced Poblano pepper

- 1 big clove garlic, minced
- Half pound 95%-lean ground beef
- Juice of Half lime
- 8 (6-inch) corn waffles
- 4 radishes, thinly diced

Instructions:

- Warm up the oil in a big pan over medium-sized-high Warm up. Add One-Fourth mug of the onion and the bell pepper and garlic, and Prepare for 30 seconds. Then add the ground beef, Splitting up any big chunks with a spatula. Prepare for 5 to 6 minutes, or until the meat is no longer pink. Add the oregano and black pepper while the meat Prepares.
- In a set apart dish, Merge the left-over One-Fourth mug Diced onion, tomato, chile pepper, cilantro, and lime juice to make a warm sauce Covering.
- Combine to incorporate evenly, and set aside. Warm the waffles in a flat pan over medium-sized Warm up. Put two waffles on four individual plates, scoop the beef mixture onto the waffles, cover with warm sauce and diced radishes, fold, and serve.

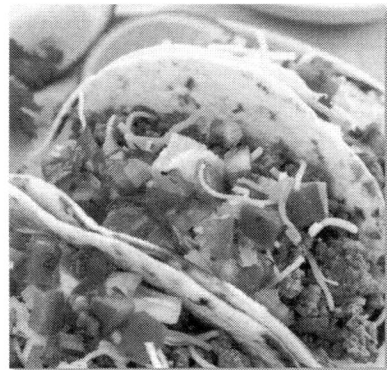

Indian Vegetable Soup
Ingredients:

- 1 mug coarsely Diced onion
- 1 Half tsps. curry powder

- 1 Half tsps. ground ginger
- 1 tsp. coriander
- 1 eggplant, Peel offed and chopped
- 1-pound potatoes, chopped
- 2 mugs no-salt-added canned tomatoes
- 1 Half mugs (246 g) preprepared chickpeas
- One-Fourth tsp. black pepper
- 4 mugs (950 ml) low-sodium vegetable broth

Instructions:

- In a slow Oven, Merge the veggies. Sprinkle spices over Cover. Spill broth over all. Cover and Prepare on low for 8 to 10 hours or on high for 4 to 5 hours.

Moroccan Red Pepper Stew
Ingredients:

- 1 tbsp. olive oil
- 1 Half mug onion, Diced
- 2 garlic cloves, minced
- 1 tsp. cinnamon, ground
- Half tsp. ginger, ground
- Half tsp. turmeric, ground
- One-Fourth tsp. nutmeg, ground
- 2 mugs chickpeas, prepared or canned,
- 1 Half mugs (165 g) sweet potatoes, chopped
- Half mug raisins
- One-Third mug (43 g) parched apricots, chopped
- 3 tbsps. brown Lactose alternative,
- One-Fourth tsp. red pepper, ground
- 2 mugs (475 ml) mineral water
- 3 cloves, whole
- 2 mugs (260 g) carrot, diced
- 2 mugs butternut squash, chopped

Instructions:

- In a four-quart (4 L) dip saucepan, Warm up the oil over medium-sized-high Warm up. Add the onion and garlic and Prepare, whisking, until softened. Add the cinnamon, ginger, turmeric, nutmeg, and red pepper, whisking till absorbed.
- Add the mineral water and cloves; bring to a boil. Add the carrot, squash, chickpeas, sweet potato, raisins, apricots, and brown Lactose and put back to a boil. Decrease the Warm up and simmer Unwrapped, whisking from time to time, 40 to 45 minutes or until the sweet potato is ripe.

Mediterranean Vegetable Garlic Stew
Ingredients:

- 2 mugs cucumber, diced
- 1 eggplant, diced and Peel offed
- 1 mug onion, diced
- 1 big potato, thinly diced
- 4 medium-sized tomatoes, Peel offed and diced
- One-Fourth mug olive oil
- 2 tbsps. fresh basil
- Half-pound okra, stemmed
- 1 mug fresh green beans, halved
- 2 garlic cloves, minced
- One-Fourth tsp. pepper

Instructions:

- Switch on oven to 350 of. In a deep casserole, make a layer of each vegetable. Dribble a little oil over each layer and sprinkle lightly with garlic, basil, and pepper. Layer in any order but have potatoes in the middle and end with tomatoes.
- Bake covered for 1 Half hours, basting once or twice.

Asian Angela Pita Sandwich
Ingrediens:

- 1 (One-Fourth-inch-thick) slice heirloom tomato
- One-Fourth mug roasted red pepper

- One-Eighth tsp. cracked black pepper
- 1 tbsp. prepared pesto
- Half mug arugula
- 1 (One-Fourth-inch-thick) slice fresh mozzarella cheese

Instructions:

- Warm the pita on both sides in a frying pan over low Warm up. Take away from Warm up, cut the pita in half and split open, and Expand pesto on the inside. Fill with arugula, cheese, tomato, and red pepper. Cover with black pepper.

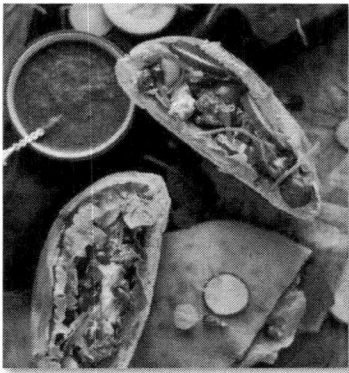

Spicy Chopped Onion Bean Soup
Ingredients:

- Half mug chopped Poblano pepper
- 6 ounces (275 ml) vegetable juice such as VB, spicy flavor
- One-Fourth tsp. Tabasco dip sauce
- Third-Fourth mug chopped celery
- 1 tsp. black pepper
- 6 mugs mineral water
- 1 mug parched beans, assorted (navy, red, pinto, etc.)
- 1 mug chopped onion
- 1 mug (130 g) chopped carrot
- 1 mug chopped ham

Instructions:

- Merge all ingredients in a big pot. Simmer for at least 3 hours. Garnish with green chili and mint. Serve immediately.

Black Bean Oregano Chili
Ingredients:

- 1-pound ground turkey
- 4 mugs (960 g) no-salt-added canned black beans, Soaked and drained
- 2 mugs no-salt-added stewed tomatoes
- 1 tsp. ground coriander
- 1 tsp. crushed parched oregano
- 1 tbsp. olive oil
- Half onion, Diced
- Half Poblano pepper, seeded and Diced
- 2 cloves garlic, minced

Instructions:

- Warm up big heavy dip saucepan or Dutch oven to medium-sized-high. Brown the meat until prepared through. Drain meat and set aside. In the frying pan, add the oil and bring to medium-sized Warm up.
- Add the onion, bell pepper, and garlic, and Prepare until veggies are ripe, about 5 to 6 minutes. Put back meat to pan. Add left-over ingredients. Bring chili to a boil; then decrease Warm up and simmer for 30 to 45 minutes or until thickened, whisking from time to time. Taste and adjust seasonings if mandatory.

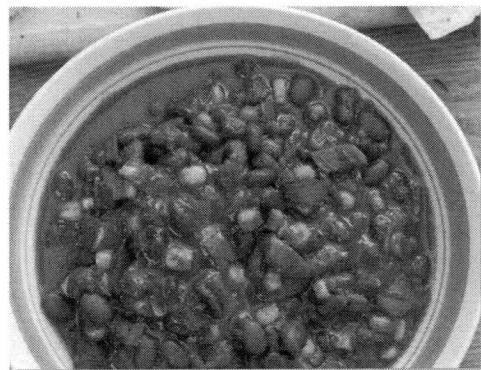

Vegetable Chili with cayenne pepper
Ingredients:

- Half mug parched kidney beans
- One-Fourth mug bulgur
- Half mug olive oil
- Half mug carrot, diced
- 2 tbsps. chili powder
- 2 tbsps. cumin
- Half tsp. cayenne pepper
- 1 tbsp. (2.5 g) fresh basil
- 1 tbsp. fresh oregano
- 1 mug Poblano pepper, chopped
- Half mug (130 g) no-salt-added tomato paste
- Third-Fourth mug dry white wine
- 1 mug yellow squash, chopped
- 8 ounces mushroom, diced
- Half mug tomatoes, chopped
- 1 mug cucumber, chopped
- 1 mug Poblano pepper, chopped
- 1 mug red onion, chopped
- Half mug onion, chopped
- 1 Half tbsps. garlic, minced
- Half mug celery, diced
- Pepper to taste

Instructions:

- Soak beans in cold mineral water to cover overnight. Drain off mineral water. Add 3 mugs (720 ml) fresh mineral water to beans and Prepare over medium-sized Heat up till ripe, regarding forty-five minutes.
- Drain beans, reserving Preparing liquid. Bring a pair of mug mineral water to boil. Spill over bulgur in dish. Let stand 30 minutes to melt heat up (the mineral water will be absorbed). Warm up olive oil in huge dip saucepan.
- Add red and white onions and Deep-fry until ripe. Add garlic, celery, and carrots. Deep-fry till softened. Add chili powder, cumin, cayenne, basil, and

oregano. Prepare over low Warm up until carrots are virtually ripe.

Green lettuce leaf Wraps with Peanut Dip sauce
Ingredients:

- 1 mug Diced snow peas (in thirds)
- Juice of Half lime
- Half tsp. sesame oil
- Half tsp. low-sodium soy dip sauce
- One-Fourth tsp. ground ginger
- One-Fourth tsp. brown rice lemon juice
- 2 mugs unprepared red Barley
- 4 mugs low-sodium vegetable broth
- 8 big butter green lettuce leaf leaves
- One-Fourth tsp. chile pepper flakes
- 2 tbsps. Diced green onion; white end discarded
- 1 mug bean sprouts
- Half mug Diced Poblano pepper
- Half mug cut into small pieces carrot
- 4 tsps. sesame seeds
- 1 mug and 6 tbsps. crunchy peanut butter
- 1 One-Fourth mug low-sodium vegetable broth

Instructions:

- Soak the Barley (if not presoaked). In a big covered pot, bring the Barley and vegetable broth to a boil over high Warm up. Decrease the Warm up to low and simmer for 10 to 15 minutes or until the liquid has been mostly absorbed. prepared Barley should be slightly al dente; it is ready when most of the grains have uncoiled and you can see the unwound germ. Let the Barley sit in the covered pot for about 5 minutes.
- Fluff gently with a fork. Put Half mug prepared Barley on each green lettuce leaf prepared. In a medium-sized dish, Merge the snow peas, bean sprouts, bell pepper, and carrots. In a small dip

168

saucepan, Merge all the ingredients for the peanut dip sauce.

- Bring to a simmer over low Warm up, and whisk until the peanut butter dissolves. Spill the dip sauce into the dish with the Diced veggies. Roll well and Serve evenly on Cover of the Barley in each green lettuce leaf.

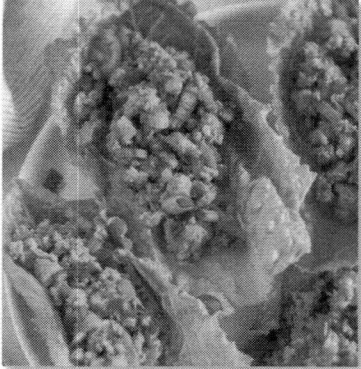

Bay Leaf Tuna Salad
Ingredients:

- 4 tbsps. finely Diced fresh bay leaf
- Juice of 1 lemon
- 4 tbsps. extra virgin olive oil
- 2 (5-ounce) cans albacore tuna in mineral water, no salt added, drained
- Half mug Diced Roma tomato
- One-Fourth mug Diced red onion
- One-Eighth tsp. cracked black pepper

Instructions:

- Put all the ingredients in a big dish, and whisk to incorporate evenly. Let sit for 30 minutes before serving.

Dinner

Quick Broccoli & Chicken Stir Fry

Ingredients:

- 1/3 cup orange juice
- 1 Tbsp low-sodium soy sauce
- 1 Tbsp Schezuan sauce
- 2 tsp cornstarch
- 1 Tbsp canola oil
- 1 lb. boneless chicken breast, cut into 1-inch cubes
- 2 cups of frozen broccoli florets
- 1 6-oz package of frozen snow peas
- 2 cups shredded cabbage
- 2 cups of cooked brown rice
- 1 Tbsp sesame seeds (optional)

Instructions:

- In a small bowl, mix the Schezuan sauce, cornstarch, soy sauce and orange juice; set aside.
- In a wok, heat the canola oil.
- Add the chicken to the wok and stir fry until the meat has cooked through. (Approx. 6 minutes)
- Add the broccoli, cabbage, snow peas and sauce mix to the wok.
- Cook until the vegetables are done. (Approx. 5 to 6 minutes) • Serve with rice and if desired, sprinkle with sesame seeds.

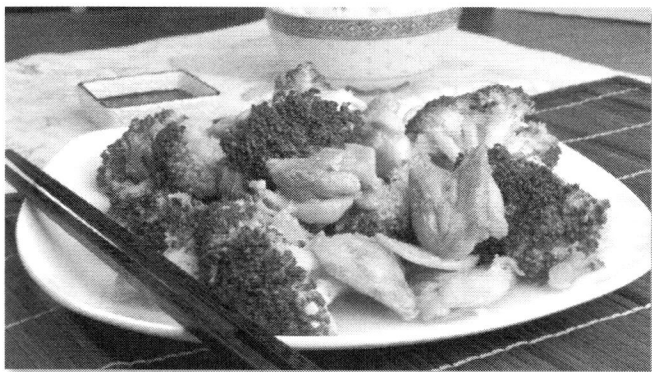

Veggie Pasta Soup

Ingredients:

- 2 tsps. olive oil
- 6 cloves garlic, minced
- 1 1/2 cups coarsely shredded carrot 1 cup chopped onion
- 1 cup thinly sliced celery
- 1 32-oz. box reduced-sodium chicken broth
- 4 cups water
- 1 1/2 cups dried ditalini pasta 1/4 cup shaved Parmesan cheese 2 Tbsps.
- snipped fresh parsley

Instructions:

- Heat the olive oil in a 6-quart Dutch oven over a medium heat.
- Add the minced garlic and cook for 10 to 15 seconds.
- Stir in the onion, celery, carrot and cook until tender. (Approx. 6 minutes)
- Pour in the water and chicken broth and bring it to a boil.
- Add the pasta and allow to cook until the pasta is soft. (Approx. 8 minutes)
- Serve into pasta bowls and top each serving with parsley and parmesan cheese.

Chicken Parmesan & Baked Quinoa

Ingredients:

- 1 Tbsp. olive oil
- 1 medium onion, diced
- 3 cloves garlic, minced
- 2 Tbsp. balsamic vinegar
- 1 (15 oz.) can tomato sauce
- 1 (15 oz.) can diced tomatoes (no added salt)
- basil and oregano, to taste
- 1 cup quinoa
- 2 cups water or broth
- 1 lb. boneless, skinless chicken, cooked* and cut into bite sized pieces
- 2/3 cup shredded part-skim mozzarella cheese, divided

- 2 Tbsp. grated Parmesan or Romano cheese

Instructions:

- Preheat oven at 375°F.
- Use cooking oil to spray a baking dish.
- To make the sauce;
- Over a medium high heat, add oil to a large skillet and heat.
- Stir the onion in till soft. (Approx. 6 minutes)
- Add the garlic to the skillet and stir until it is fragrant. (Approx. 40 to 60 seconds) • Add the vinegar and cook until the onion and garlic absorbs it.
- Add the diced tomato, oregano, tomato sauce, basil and pepper and bring it to a boil.
- Leave to simmer while preparing the quinoa.
- To make the quinoa;
- Rinse the quinoa in cold water and strain.
- In a small saucepan, place the water, a pinch of salt and quinoa, and bring to a boil.
- Cover, reduce to a low heat, and leave to simmer until cooked. (Approx. 25 minutes) To assemble;
- Combine the chicken, quinoa and sauce in a large bowl and mix well.
- Place the chicken/ quinoa mix in the baking dish.
- Top the dish with mozzarella cheese and parmesan.
- Use an aluminum foil to cover the dish and bake for 12 to 15 minutes.
- Remove the aluminum foil and bake until the cheese has browned slightly and is bubbly. (Approx. 10 to 12 minutes)
- Season the chicken with Italian seasoning.
- Pan fry the chicken in oil.

Veggie-Turkey Bake
Ingredients:

- 2 cups sliced fresh mushrooms
- 3/4 cup chopped red or yellow sweet pepper 1/2 cup chopped onion
- 2 cloves garlic, minced
- 2 Tbsps. butter or margarine
- 1/4 cup all-purpose flour
- 3/4 tsp. salt
- 1/2 tsp. dried thyme, crushed
- 1/4 tsp. black pepper
- 2 cups fat-free milk
- 1 10-oz. package frozen chopped spinach, thawed and well drained 2 cups
- cooked brown or white rice 2 cups chopped cooked low sodium turkey or chicken 1/2 cup finely shredded Parmesan cheese (2 oz.)

Instructions:

- Stir the mushroom, sweet pepper, garlic hot butter and onion in a large skillet over a medium heat until cooked through.
- Add the salt, thyme, flour and black pepper to the skillet and stir it in.
- Stir in the milk slowly.
- Cook until it becomes bubbly and thick.
- Add the rice, turkey, spinach and a quarter of the parmesan cheese, and stir it in.
- Serve onto a baking dish.
- Sprinkle the balance parmesan cheese, cover and bake in oven at 350°F for 20 to 25 minutes.
- Uncover the dish, and bake until heated through. (Approx. 10 to 12 minutes) • Remove from oven and allow to cool for 10 to 15 minutes.
- Serve warm.

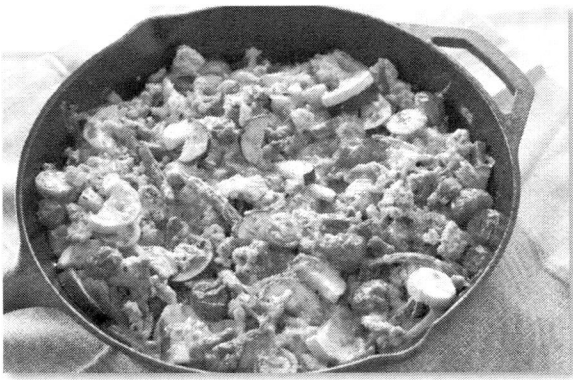

Barley Bean Burgers
Ingredients:

- 1/2 tsp. Garlic Powder
- 2 cups Kidney Beans cooked
- 1/2 cup Wheat Germ
- 1 Tbsp. Olive Oil
- 1/2 cup Onion chopped
- 3 Garlic cloves, minced
- 1 tsp. Sea Salt
- 1/2 tsp. Sage
- 1/2 tsp. Celery Seed, ground
- 2 cups Whole Hull-Less Barley cooked

Instructions:

- Cook the kidney beans according to instructions.
- When they are soft, mash them together with the barley.
- In a saucepan, fry the onion and garlic until golden in color.
- Stir in the bean mix, spices and what germ.
- Form the mixture into small patties.
- Fry the patties on a medium heat setting, until the patties are brown on each side.

Wild Rice Turkey Pilaf
Ingredients:

- 1 Tbsp. olive oil
- 1 cup sliced celery
- 1/4 cup chopped onion
- 1/3 cup wild rice, rinsed and drained 1 14-oz. can reduced-sodium chicken

- broth 1/3 cup long grain rice
- 1 large carrot, peeled and cut into thin bite-size strips 8 oz. cooked low
- sodium turkey breast, cubed 2 medium red-skinned apples, chopped 2 Tbsps.
- snipped fresh parsley
- Butterhead (Boston or Bibb) lettuce leaves (optional)

Instructions:

- Heat oil over a medium heat setting in a large skillet.
- Add the onion and celery to the skillet; cook until tender, stirring often. (Approx. 10 to 12 minutes)
- Add the uncooked rice to the skillet and stir it in for about 4 minutes.
- Add the broth and bring it to a boil.
- Reduce to a low heat, cover and let simmer for 20 to 22 minutes.
- Stir in the long-grained rice (uncooked)
- Return to a boil.
- Reduce heat, cover, and let simmer for 20 to 22 minutes more, until the rice is tender.
- Once the rice has absorbed the liquid add the carrot, and stir in the apple and turkey breast.
- Cook until the liquid has been absorbed. (Approx. 4 minutes)
- To serve, lay lettuce leaves on the serving dish and place the turkey mix over the leaves.

Pineapple Salsa & Grilled Beef Kabobs
Ingredients:

- 1/2 lbs. beef shoulder center (Ranch) steaks, cut 1 inch thick
- Salt and pepper Marinade:
- 2 Tbsps. fresh lime juice
- 2 Tbsps. olive oil
- 2 large cloves garlic, minced
- 1 medium jalapeno pepper, minced
- 1/2 tsp. ground cumin Pineapple Salsa:

- 1/2 medium pineapple, peeled, cored, cut into 1-1/2-inch chunks (about 3 cups)
- 1 medium red onion, cut into 12 wedges
- 1 large red or green bell pepper, cut into 1-1/2-inch pieces
- 2 tsps. freshly grated lime peel
- 1/2 tsp. salt

Instructions:

- Cut the steak into cubes.
- In a medium size bowl add the marinade ingredients.
- Remove 2 Tbsps. from the bowl of marinade and reserve for the salsa.
- Toss the beef in the marinade and coat well.
- Cover the bowl and set in the refrigerator to marinade for at least 1 hour.
- Remove the beef from the refrigerator and thread the beef onto skewers. (About 10 skewers)
- Alternatively thread the vegetables and fruit onto another set of skewers. (About 10 skewers) • Grill the vegetable and fruit kabobs over medium ash covered coals, uncovered, until the vegetables are soft. (Approx. 12 to 13 minutes)
- Grill the beef kabobs, covered, until the meat it medium rare. (Approx. 8 minutes)
- Remove the vegetables and fruit from the skewers and chop until coarse.
- In a large bowl, mix the balance marinade, ½ tsp. of salt and lime peel.
- Use salt and pepper to season the beef.
- Serve the beef kebabs with the pineapple salsa.

Sweet Potato & Turkey Chowder
Ingredients:

- 1 large potato, peeled if desired and chopped (about 1-1/2 cups) 1 14-oz. can

- reduced-sodium chicken broth
- 2 small ears frozen corn-on-the-cob, thawed, or 1 cup loose-pack frozen
- whole kernel corn 12 oz. cooked low sodium turkey breast, cut into 1/2-inch
- cubes (about 2-1/4 cups) 1-1/2 cups fat-free milk
- 1 large sweet potato, peeled and cut into 3/4-inch cubes (about 1-1/2 cups)
- 1/8 to 1/4 tsp. ground black pepper
- 1/4 cup coarsely snipped fresh flat-leaf parsley

Instructions:

- Add the broth and potato to a saucepan and bring to a boil.
- Reduce heat to a lower setting and simmer, uncovered until the potato is tender. (Approx. 11 minutes)
- Remove the pan from the heat.
- Mash the potato until it is nearly smooth.
- If you wish to use corn-on-the-cob, cut the kernels; set aside.
- Add the turkey milk, kernels, sweet potato and pepper into the saucepan with
- the potato mixture; bring to a boil.
- Reduce to a lower heat setting, cover and cook until the sweet potato is soft. (Approx. 15 minutes)
- Serve into bowls and sprinkle with parsley if desired.

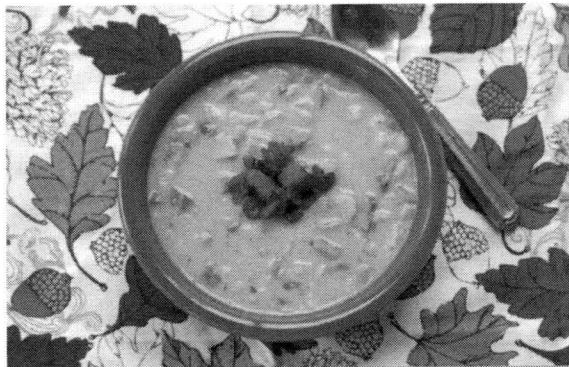

Brazilian Sausage & Black Beans
Ingredients:

173

- 2 tsps. vegetable oil
- 8 oz. low-fat polish kielbasa sausage, cut into small pieces
- 1 large onion, chopped
- 1 clove garlic, minced, or 1/8 tsp. garlic powder
- 1 red bell pepper, chopped
- 1 tsp. ground cumin
- 1 cup brown uncooked rice
- 1 can (15 oz.) black beans, drained and rinsed
- 2 cups water

Instructions:

- In a saucepan, heat the vegetable oil over a medium high heat.
- Sauté the onion and sausages in the pan until the onion is tender.
- Add the garlic, bell pepper, cumin, uncooked rice, black beans and water to the saucepan and bring to a boil over a high heat setting.
- Reduce heat and allow to simmer, covered, for 40 to 25 minutes.

Nectarine & Turkey Salad
Ingredients:

- 2/3 cup buttermilk
- 2 Tbsps. light mayonnaise dressing or salad dressing 2 to 3 tsps. snipped
- fresh dill or 1/4 to 1/2 tsp. dried dillweed 1/8 tsp. salt
- 1/8 tsp. onion powder
- 1/8 tsp. garlic powder
- 6 cups torn mixed greens
- 8 oz. boneless cooked low sodium turkey breast, thinly sliced 2 medium
- nectarines, pitted and sliced or 2 medium peaches, peeled, pitted, and sliced
- 1/4 cup chopped red sweet pepper Coarsely ground black pepper (optional)
- Snipped Fresh Dill (Optional)

Instructions:

- For the dressing; stir in the buttermilk slowly with the mayonnaise dressing or salad dressing, in a mixing bowl.
- Add the salt, dill, garlic powder and onion powder to the bowl and stir it in.
- On 4 serving dishes, arrange the greens and top with the turkey.
- Garnish with the nectarines, (or peaches) and sweet pepper.
- Pour the buttermilk dressing over the salad and sprinkle with additional chili and black pepper if desired.

Tangy Yogurt Sauce Over Broiled Halibut
Ingredients:

- Two 5 oz. halibut fillets
- 1 cup nonfat plain yogurt
- 1 large clove garlic, peeled and crushed
- ¼ tsp. ground black pepper
- ¼ cup freshly squeezed lemon juice
- ¼ tsp. salt

Instructions:

- Preheat the broiler.
- In a small bowl mix in the lemon juice, yogurt, salt and pepper.
- Use aluminum foil to line a broiler pan.
- Place the fish in the pan, skin side facing down.
- Pour the yogurt mix over the fish.
- Cook in broiler until the fish flakes easily and the top is golden in color. (Approx. 10 to 12 minutes)
- Serve warm on a dish with the yogurt sauce on the side.

Veggie Tortellini Salad
Ingredients:

- 1 9-oz. package refrigerated cheese tortellini
- 6 cups torn mixed greens
- 1-1/2 cups sliced fresh mushrooms 1 medium yellow or red sweet pepper, cut

- into bite-size strips (1 cup) 1/4 cup snipped fresh basil
- 1/4 cup white wine vinegar or white vinegar 2 Tbsps. water
- 2 Tbsps. olive oil
- 2 tsps. sugar
- 2 cloves garlic, minced
- 1/4 tsp. ground black pepper
- 1/2 cup fat-free toasted garlic-and-onion croutons

Instructions:

- Use the instructions on the package to cook the tortellini.
- Drain the tortellini, rinse, and drain again.
- Mix the mushrooms, sweet pepper, tortellini, basil and mixed greens in a large bowl.
- For the salad dressing, mix the water, white wine vinegar, sugar, oil, garlic and black pepper in a screw top jar, cover, and shake.
- Pour the dressing over the tortellini mixture.
- Toss well to coat.
- Take 4 dishes and divide the tortellini mix equally among them.
- Garnish with croutons.

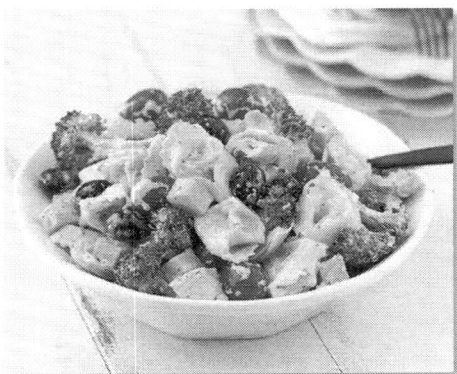

Rice Burgers
Ingredients:

- 2 cups cooked brown rice
- ½ cup parsley, chopped
- 1 cup carrot, finely grated

- ½ cup onion, finely chopped
- 1 clove garlic, minced
- 1 tsp salt
- ¼ tsp ground black pepper
- 2 eggs, beaten
- ½ cup whole wheat flour
- 2 tbsp vegetable oil for cooking

Instructions:

- In a medium bowl, mix the brown rice, parsley, carrot, onion, garlic, salt, black pepper, eggs and wheat flour.
- Form the rice mix into 12 patties; press down with hands, firmly.
- In a skillet, heat the vegetable oil over a medium heat.
- Add the patties to the oil and heat for 4 minutes on each side until it turns brown.

Chili Pan Fry & Butternut Squash
Ingredients:

- 1 medium butternut squash, about 1 1/2 to 2 lbs.
- 1 lb. fresh green Poblano chilies
- 1 1/2 Tbsps. olive or vegetable oil
- 1 medium onion, chopped
- 1 tsp. salt
- 1/2 tsp. chili powder
- 1 Cup Grated Cheese (Try Monterey Jack)

Instructions:

- Peel the butternut squash, cut it into half, and remove the seeds.
- Cut the butternut squash into small pieces.
- Roast the pepper (over a stovetop or an oven broiler) until all sides of the pepper are black and charred. (Approx. 8 minutes)
- Remove the peppers from heat and place in a small plastic bag; allow to cool for 15 to 20 minutes.
- Remove the stems and seeds of the peppers, and chop into small pieces.

- In a saucepan, heat the oil over a medium heat.
- Stir in the onions and cook until tender. (Approx. 3 to 4 minutes)
- Add the chili powder, salt and squash to the pan, cover, and cook; stir frequently. (Approx. 10 to 11 minutes)
- Add the chopped chilies to the pan and stir it in for 3 to 4 minutes.
- Sprinkle the pan with cheese, cover and cook until the cheese has melted. (Approx. 1 ½ to 2 minutes)
- Serve warm.
- If any leftovers, refrigerate within 2 hours.

Feta & Edamame with Tabbouleh
Ingredients:

- 2-1/2 cups water
- 1-1/4 cups bulgur
- 1/4 cup lemon juice
- 3 Tbsps. purchased basil pesto 2 cups fresh or thawed frozen shelled sweet
- soybeans (edamame)
- 2 cups cherry tomatoes, cut up
- 1/3 cup crumbled feta cheese
- 1/3 cup thinly sliced green onions 2 Tbsps. snipped fresh parsley 1/4 tsp.
- ground black pepper
- Fresh parsley sprigs (optional)

Instructions:

- Bring the water to a boil in a medium saucepan over a medium heat.
- Add the uncooked bulgur to the pan and return to a boil.
- Reduce the heat, cover, and let simmer until a majority of the liquid has been absorbed. (Approx. 15 to 16 minutes)
- Remove the pan from heat and pour into a large bowl.
- Whisk the pesto and lemon juice together in a small bowl.
- Add the lemon juice mix, soy beans, feta cheese, cherry tomatoes, parsley, green onions and pepper to the bowl containing the bulgur; toss gently.

- Garnish with parsley sprigs if desired.

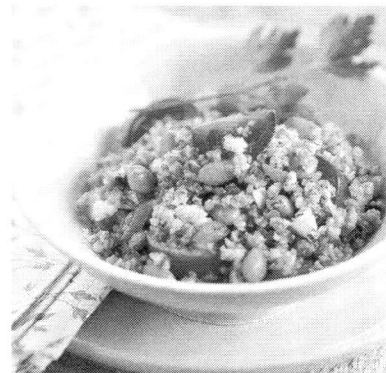

Tomatoes Stuffed with Wild Rice & Chicken
Ingredients:

- 1 cup uncooked wild rice (will yield 2-2 ½ cups cooked rice)
- 1 cup low sodium vegetable broth
- 1 cup water
- 1 chicken breast
- 4 large red tomatoes
- 2 Tbsps. fresh basil
- 2 cloves garlic, minced
- ½ cup shredded parmesan cheese
- 2 Tbsps. olive oil

Instructions:

- Use the Instructions on the package to cook the wild rice, adding the cup of low-sodium vegetable broth and cup of water to do so.
- Preheat the oven at 350°F.
- Grill the chicken until heated through.
- Slice the chicken into small pieces.
- Cut the top off each tomato.
- Scoop out the insides of the tomatoes, leaving a ½ to ¾ inch thick wall.
- Mix in the chicken, garlic, basil, and parmesan cheese (reserving a handful to garnish the tomatoes) once the rice is cooked.
- Use the rice filling to stuff the tomatoes.
- Sprinkle to tomatoes with the reserved parmesan cheese.

- Brush the tomatoes with olive oil and bake in oven for 22 to 25 minutes.

Cabbage & Chicken Stir Fry
Ingredients:

- 3 chicken breast halves
- 1 tsp. vegetable oil
- 3 cups green cabbage, shredded
- 1 Tbsp. cornstarch
- ½ tsp. ground ginger
- ¼ tsp. garlic powder
- ½ cup water
- 1 Tbsp. low-sodium soy sauce

Instructions:

- Heat the vegetable oil in a frying pan over a medium heat.
- Cut the chicken breast into strips, add to the pan, and stir fry until heated through.
- Add the cabbage to the pan and stir fry until the cabbage in tender-crisp. (Approx. 2 to 3 minutes)
- In a small bowl, mix the seasonings, cornstarch, water and soy sauce until smooth.
- Stir the mixture into the chicken mix.
- Cool well until the chicken is coated in the sauce. (Approx. 1 to 2 minutes)

Sweet Pepper Fish Salsa
Ingredients:

- 1 lb. fresh or frozen skinless fish fillets (3/4-inch-thick) 2 Tbsps. cooking oil
- 1-1/2 cups fresh mushrooms, quartered
- 1 cup coarsely chopped green and/or yellow sweet pepper 1 small onion,
- halved and sliced
- 1 cup salsa
- Fresh oregano (optional)

Instructions:

- If the fish is frozen, allow it to thaw.
- Cut and divide the fish fillets into 4 portions.

- Rinse the fish well with cold water and pat dry; set aside.
- Heat a Tbsp. of cooking oil in a large skillet.
- Add the green or yellow sweet pepper, onion and mushrooms to the skillet and cook until soft. (Approx. 5 to 6 minutes)
  • Remove the vegetables from the skillet and set aside.
- Add the balance cooking oil to the skillet, heat, and add the fish fillets.
- Cook the fish over a medium heat until it starts to flake. (Approx. 9 minutes)
- Place the cooked vegetables and salsa over the fish, cover, and cook on a low heat setting until heated through. (Approx. 2 to 3 minutes)
- Serve the fish fillets onto 4 serving plates and garnish each dish with oregano if desired.

Avocados, Oranges & Chicken
Ingredients:

- 1 cup Low-fat
- yogurt
- 1/4 cup Minced red onion
- 2 tbsp Chopped cilantro
- 1 tbsp Honey
- Salt
- Ground black pepper
- 4 Boneless, skinless chicken breasts - 4-6 oz each Garnish:
- 1 Avocado
- 1/4 cup Fresh lime juice
- 2 Oranges, peeled and sectioned
- 1 Small red onion, thinly sliced

Instructions:

- In a large bowl, mix the yogurt, red onion, cilantro, honey, salt and black pepper in a large bowl.
- Add the chicken to the yogurt mix, coat evenly, cover, and place in the refrigerator for at least 1 hour.
- Preheat the broiler or grill.
- Remove the chicken from the refrigerator and discard the marinade.

- Season the chicken with salt and pepper.
- Grill (or broil) the chicken until the juice runs clear.
- In the meantime, peel the avocado and chop it into small cubes.
- In a bowl, toss the avocado cubes with the lime juice (immediately after cutting so as to prevent the fruit from discoloring)
- Add the onion, cilantro and oranges to the bowl, and season with salt and pepper.
- Serve on the side, with the chicken.

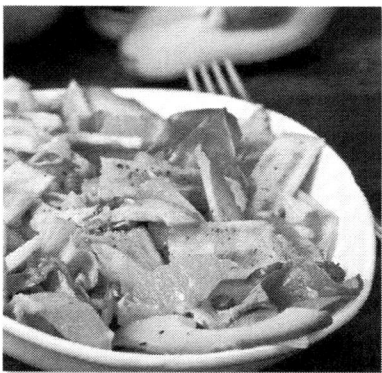

Revamped Chili Rellenos
Ingredients:

- 3 large bell peppers, any color, halved
- 2 eggs
- 4 Tbsps. mashed avocado
- 1 1/2 cups reduced fat Mexican style cheese, shredded
- 1/2 cup plain non-fat Greek yogurt
- 1-4oz can chopped green chilies, with juice

Instructions:

- Preheat the oven at 350°F.
- Wash the bell peppers, drain, and cut each into half.
- Remove the core and seeds from the bell peppers.
- Place the peppers snugly together in a 7.5 inch by 11-inch baking pan; set aside.

- Whisk the eggs, mashed avocado, cheese, yogurt and green chilies with juice together in a large bowl.
- Distribute the mixture equally over the bell peppers in the baking dish.
- Place the pan in the oven and cook until the cheese turns golden brown and the eggs are fully cooked. (Approx. 40 to 45 minutes)
- Once done, top the dish with salsa.

Buttermilk Dressing on Steak Salad
Ingredients:

- 1 recipe Buttermilk Dressing
- 8 cups torn, mixed salad greens
- 2 medium carrots, cut into thin bite-size strips 1 medium yellow sweet
- pepper, cut into thin bite-size strips 1 cup cherry or pear-shaped tomatoes,
- halved 8 oz. boneless beef top sirloin steak
- Nonstick cooking spray
- 1/4 cup finely shredded fresh basil

Instructions:

- Divide the salad greens, sweet pepper, carrots and tomatoes among 4 dinner plates; set aside.
- Use a knife to trim the fat off the meat.
- Cut the meat into small strips.
- Use cooking spray or oil to coat a large skillet, and heat over a medium high heat.
- Add the meat and cook until the meat is tender and slightly pink in the middle. (Approx. 3 minutes) • Remove the skillet from the heat and stir in the basil.
- Serve the meat mix over the green mix and drizzle with buttermilk dressing.
- Decorate the dishes with additional tomatoes if desired.
- Serve warm.

Bean & Spinach Salad
Ingredients:

- 1 15-oz. can black beans, rinsed and drained 1/2 cup snipped dried apricots
- 1/2 cup chopped red and/or yellow sweet pepper 1 green onion, thinly sliced
- 1 Tbsp. snipped fresh cilantro 1 clove garlic, minced
- 1/4 cup apricot nectar
- 2 Tbsps. salad oil
- 2 Tbsps. rice vinegar
- 1 tsp. soy sauce
- 1 tsp. grated fresh ginger
- 4 cups shredded fresh spinach

Instructions:

- Mix the apricots, black beans, sweet pepper, cilantro, green onion and garlic in a medium bowl.
- Mix the oil, vinegar, apricot nectar, soy sauce and ginger in a screw top jar, cover, and shake well.
- Pour the apricot nectar mix over the bean mixture and toss.
- Cover the bowl and refrigerate for at least 3 hours.
- Before serving, add spinach to the black bean mix and toss well to mix.
- Season with salt and pepper.

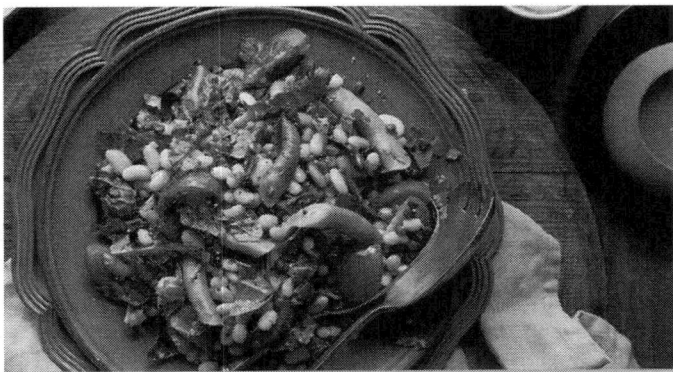

Black Eyed Pea Salad
Ingredients:

- 2 (15-oz.) cans black-eyed peas or black beans
- 1 (15-oz.) can corn
- 1 small bunch of cilantros, or to taste

- 1 bunch green onions (5 green onions)
- 3 medium tomatoes
- 1 avocado (optional)
- 1 Tbsp. canola or vegetable oil
- 2 Tbsps. vinegar or lime juice
- Salt and pepper to taste

Instructions:

- Rinse the corn and black-eyed peas or black beans well and drain. Chop the green onions and cilantro finely.
- Cut the tomatoes and avocados.
- In a large bowl mix the corn, black eyed peas (or black beans), cilantro, onions, tomatoes, and avocado.
- In a separate bowl, mix the vinegar or lime juice, oil, salt and pepper together.
- Pour the vinegar mix over the salad; toss gently.
- Serve as a snack or with a meal.

Easy Broccoli Pasta
Ingredients:

- 12 oz. uncooked pasta
- 6 ½ cups fresh broccoli florets, no stems
- 5 cloves garlic, smashed and chopped
- ¼ cup grated Parmesan or Romano cheese
- 2 Tbsps. olive oil, divided
- Salt and fresh cracked pepper, to taste

Instructions:

- Pour water into a pot, add a dash of salt and bring to the boil.
- Toss in the broccoli and the pasta and cook the pasta based on the instructions of the package.
- Once the pasta is cooked, remove 1 cup of the cooking water and set aside.
- Drain and remove the pasta and broccoli out of the pot.
- Return the empty pot onto the cooker and pour about 1 tbsp of the oil into the pot.

- Once the oil is hot, toss in the chopped garlic and sauté until golden in color.
- Lower the heat, place the pasta back in the pot and mix well.
- Mix in the balance olive oil and cheese and combine well.
- Smash the broccoli into tiny pieces using a back of a spoon if there are any large pieces left in the mixture.
- Pour the ½ cup of the left aside pasta water and combine well.
- Adjust seasonings and serve warm.

Honey Fried Chicken
Ingredients:

- 4 small red potatoes, quartered
- 2 tsps. olive oil
- 4 mugs (284 g) fresh broccoli florets
- One-Fourth mug (85 g) honey
- 1-pound boneless skinless chicken breast
- 2 tbsps. Spicy Brown Mustard
- 4 tbsps. dry bread crumbs
- 2 tbsps. low sodium chicken broth, or mineral water

Instructions:

- Switch on oven to 450°F (230°C, or gas mark 8). Cover a big baking sheet with nonstick vegetable oil Sprinkle. Butterfly chicken by cutting each piece in half horizontally, almost through to the other side, but not completely.
- Open chicken breast half to make one thin piece. Brush Spicy Brown Mustard over both sides. Put seasoned bread crumbs in a shallow dish; add chicken breasts and turn to Cover each side. Shift chicken to prepared baking sheet and Sprinkle the chicken breasts with nonstick vegetable oil Sprinkle.
- Bake 8 to 10 minutes until chicken is prepared through. Meanwhile, put red potatoes in a microwave-safe canister with a lid, add olive oil, and Roll to Cover potatoes. Cover and microwave

on high for 5 minutes until potatoes are ripe. Put broccoli in a microwave-safe canister with a lid, cover, and microwave on high for 3 minutes until broccoli is crisp-ripe. In a small dish, Whip together honey and chicken broth. Shift chicken to individual plates and Sprinkle honey mixture over Cover. Serve red potatoes and broccoli on the side.

Calories Free Macaroni with Chicken and Broccoli
Ingredients:

- 1 tsp. parched basil black pepper to taste
- One-Fourth mug white wine
- Third-Fourth mug low sodium chicken broth
- One-Fourth mug olive oil
- 2 garlic cloves, minced
- Half pound boneless skinless chicken breasts, cut in Half-inch shreds
- 1 Half mugs (107 g) broccoli florets
- Half pound whole warm up bow tie macaroni, prepared
- Parmesan cheese

Instructions:

- In a big frying pan, Warm up oil over medium-sized Warm up. Deep-fry garlic for about one minute, whisking constantly. Add the chicken and Prepare until well done. Add the broccoli and Prepare until crisp-ripe.
- Add basil, black pepper to taste; wine, and chicken broth. Prepare for about 5 minutes. Add the prepared and drained macaroni to the frying pan and Roll to Merge. Warm up for 1 to 2 minutes. Serve. Cover with grind Parmesan cheese if you want.

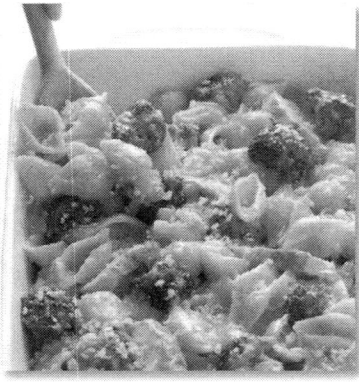

Chicken Shepherd's Pie
Ingredients:

- 1 mug Poblano pepper, Diced
- 1 mug red onion, Diced
- 20 ounces frozen combined veggies
- 20 ounces frozen broccoli
- 2 tbsps. cornstarch
- 1 mug low sodium chicken broth
- 3 mugs prepared chicken breast, chopped
- 3 mugs (610 g) mashed potatoes,
- Half mug (58 g) low fat cheddar cheese, cut into small pieces

Instructions:

- Combine cornstarch with broth. Warm up until thickened and bubbly. Whisk in chicken. Put in the base of a baking dish. Prepare veggies until almost ripe. Expand over chicken mixture. Cover with prepared mashed potatoes.
- Cover with cheddar cheese. Warm up under broiler until potatoes start to brown and cheese Defrosts.

Creamy Chicken and Stuffing Bake
Ingredients:

- Half tsp. black pepper
- Half tsp. garlic powder
- Half tsp. onion powder
- 4 Half mug broccoli florets, Brewed until crisp-ripe
- 6 ounces stuffing combine

- 1 Half pounds boneless skinless chicken breast, cut in bite-sized pieces
- 1 can low sodium cream of chicken soup
- One-Fourth mug fat-free sour cream

16 ounces frozen combined veggies, softened

Instructions:

- Switch on oven to 400°F. Prepare stuffing according to package directions. Combine chicken, soup, sour cream, and veggies. Put in a baking pan and sprinkle with black pepper, onion powder, and garlic powder.
- Cover the chicken mixture with the stuffing. Bake 30 to 40 minutes or until chicken is done. Serve with broccoli.

Delicious Chicken à la King
Ingredients:

- 1 mug onion, Diced
- 2 mugs (260 g) peas
- 1 mug Poblano pepper, Diced
- 8 ounces whole warm up macaroni
- 4 boneless skinless chicken breasts
- 2 mugs celery, Diced
- 2 mugs broccoli florets
- 1 can low sodium cream of mushroom soup

Instructions:

- Prepare macaroni according to package directions. Cut chicken breasts into small cubes and brown in a nonstick pan and set aside.
- Chop veggies and Deep-fry until they just start to turn soft. Add the mushroom soup and one can of mineral water to the veggies. Add the chicken and Prepare until chicken is done. Add the macaroni and Warm up through.

Really Low in Calories Roasted Veggie Pizza
Ingredients:

- One-Eighth tsp. salt
- One-Eighth tsp. cracked black pepper
- 1 (1-pound) whole warm up pizza dough
- 2 plum tomatoes, thinly diced
- 2 medium-sized portobello mushrooms about 4 inches in diameter
- 1 small yellow cucumber, cut in half longitudinally
- 1 small red onion, cut into rounds
- 4 tbsps. extra-virgin olive oil
- Half mug cut into small pieces skim mozzarella cheese
- One-Fourth mug fresh basil leaves, coarsely Diced

Instructions:

- Switch on the oven to 400°F. Warm up a Roast or Roast pan over medium-sized Warm up. Wipe the mushrooms with a damp towel, snap the stems off, scoop the gills out with a metal tbsp., and cut into Half-inch shreds. Brush the mushrooms, cucumber, and onion with 2 tbsps. of the oil, and sprinkle on salt and pepper. Put the herbs on the Roast, and Prepare covered for about 6 minutes, turning once, until ripe and browned. Take away from the Roast, and set apart the onion rings.
- Cover a Prepare sheet with olive oil Sprinkle. Stretch the pizza dough with your hands onto the Prepare sheet, or roll out the dough on a floured surface to prevent sticking. Pierce the dough with a fork in several spots so it does not fluff up when it bakes. Sprinkle the dough with the left-over 2 tbsps. olive oil, expanding with your fingers or a spatula, and bake 12 to 15 minutes, or until crispy.
- Take away the pizza crust from the oven, and quickly Cover with the herbs and cheese. Put back to the oven just until the cheese Defrosts, 5 to 6

minutes. Take away from the oven, cover with basil, and serve.

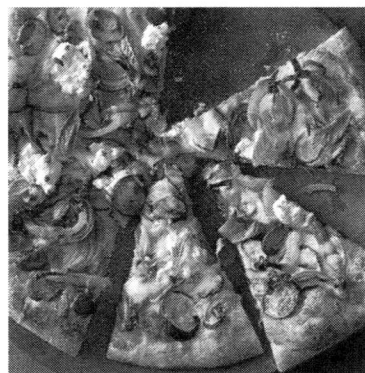

Amazing Barbecue Chicken
Ingredients:

- 20 ounces frozen combined veggies
- 2 mugs brown prepared rice, prepared
- 4 tbsps. diced almonds
- 4 boneless skinless chicken breasts
- One-Fourth mug barbecue dip sauce
- 1 tbsp. olive oil

Instructions:

- Roast chicken breast until chicken is done, about 8 minutes, brushing with barbecue dip sauce while Preparing.
- Deep-fry veggies in olive oil until ripe, about 8 minutes. Add brown rice and Warm up until warm through. Cover with almonds.

Stuffed Cucumber
Ingredients:

- 2 mugs no-salt-added tomatoes
- 1 Half mugs (293 g) brown mugs no rice, prepared or (236 g) small whole warm up macaroni
- 1 tsp. parched basil
- 3 big cucumbers
- 1 One-Fourth pounds ground turkey
- 1 mug onion, Diced
- 1 tsp. garlic, crushed

- 3 ounces (85 g) Cheddar Cheese, cut into small pieces

Instructions:

- Cut the cucumber is half longitudinally. Scrape out the center, leaving a thickness of about a half inch (1.3 cm). Discard the seeds and chop the remainder. Prepare the ground turkey, onion, and garlic in a big frying pan until meat is done.
- Whisk in tomatoes, brown rice or macaroni, and basil. Prepare the cucumber in boiling mineral water until it begins to soften. Drain and Put in baking pan. Cut up the filling between the cucumber. Put a Half ounce of cheese on Cover of each. Put under broiler until cheese is Defrosted and bubbly.

Tasty Chicken Stew
Ingredients:

- 10 ounces frozen corn
- 2 mugs no-salt-added tomatoes, chopped
- 1 tsp. ground cumin
- 5 boneless skinless chicken breasts
- 16 ounces warm sauce
- 4 mugs (688 g) black beans, prepared
- 3 ounces (85 g) fat-free cream cheese

Instructions:

- Put chicken breasts in base of slow Oven. Add left-over ingredients except cream cheese. Cover and Prepare on low for 8–10 hours. Add cream cheese, prepare on low setting for 30 minutes, and then whisk.

Really Low in Calories Chicken and Bean Frying pan
Ingredients:

- 1 mug onion, Diced
- One-Third mug Poblano pepper, Diced
- Third-Fourth tsp. garlic, crushed
- 10 ounces kidney beans, drained
- 2 mugs no-salt-added stewed tomatoes, undrained
- black pepper to taste
- Half mug (88 g) whole warm up couscous
- 2 tsps. olive oil
- Half-pound boneless chicken breast, cut in cubes
- Third-Fourth tsp. ground cumin
- Half tsp. cinnamon
- 10 ounces navy beans, drained

Instructions:

- Deep-fry onion, Poblano pepper, and garlic in oil in medium-sized dip saucepan 2 to 3 minutes. Add chicken, cumin, and cinnamon; Prepare over medium-sized-high Warm up until chicken is lightly browned, about 3 to 4 minutes.
- Add beans and tomatoes; Warm up to boiling. Decrease Warm up and simmer, Unwrapped, until slightly thickened, about 5 to 8 minutes. Season to taste with black pepper. Prepare couscous according to package directions. Serve chicken and bean mixture over couscous.

Delicious Chicken Cassoulet
Ingredients:

- 2 mugs navy beans, parched
- 4 mugs (950 ml) mineral water
- 1 tbsp. Worcestershire dip sauce
- Half tsp. parched basil
- Half tsp. parched oregano
- Half tsp. paprika
- 8 boneless skinless chicken breasts, cut up
- 2 tbsps. olive oil
- 1 mug (130 g) carrot, finely Diced
- 1 mug celery, Diced
- 1 mug onion, Diced

- 1 Half mugs (355 ml) low sodium tomato juice

Instructions:

- In big dip sauce pan, bring beans and 4 mugs (950 ml) mineral water to boiling. Decrease Warm up and simmer, covered, for 1 Half hours. Spill beans and liquid into dish. Brown chicken in the oil. In slow Oven, Put chicken, carrot, celery, and onion.
- Drain beans; combine with left-over ingredients. Spill over meat mixture. Cover; Prepare on low-Warm up setting for 8 hours. Mash bean mixture slightly, if you want.

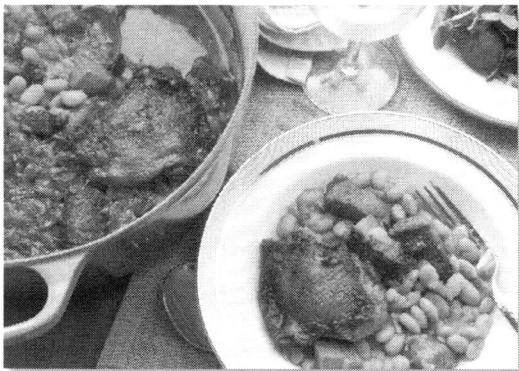

Healthy Chicken Noodles Stew

Ingredients:

- 1 mug (130 g) carrot, Peel offed and chopped
- One-Fourth mug shallot, diced
- 1 mug onion
- 4 boneless skinless chicken breasts, quartered
- 2 tbsps. Without salt butter
- 1 tbsp. olive oil
- 1 mug dry white wine
- 1-pound mushrooms, washed and minced
- 1 mug nonfat evaporated milk
- 1-ounce Calvados
- One-Fourth mug egg alternative
- 2 mugs egg noodles, prepared

- 1 mug mineral water
- 1 clove garlic, minced
- 1 tsp. parched thyme
- 2 bay leaves
- black pepper, to taste
- 1 Half mugs (188 g) apples (pippin), Peel offed and Diced

Instructions:

- In a cast iron meal or substantial Dutch broiler, softly earthy colored the chicken down the middle the margarine and a large portion of the oil. At the point when all the pieces are brilliant, add the carrot, shallots, and the diced onion and Prepare for a couple of moments. Spill the white wine and 1 cup of mineral water over the chicken and afterward add the garlic. Add some thyme leaves and inlet leaves and season with dark pepper.
- Cover and stew over low Warm awake for 40 minutes. Remove the chicken from the Warm up, Sort the bits of chicken in an ovenproof serving dish, and keep warm. Pass the Preparing fluid through a sifter.
- Put the veggies in a safe spot and keep warm. Then, Defrost the left-over spread in a griddle with the oil, add the apples, and Prepare until just softly earthy colored on all sides. Remove the apples from the skillet and Sort them around the chicken. Keep the dish warm in the broiler. Profound fry the mushrooms until they have lost every one of their juices. Put aside to add to the plunge sauce.
- To make the plunge sauce: Spill the stressed Preparing fluid into a plunge pot and set over medium-evaluated Warm. With a Whip, Stir in the dissipated milk, the Calvados, and the egg elective in a specific order. Stew until it has thickened to a light cream.

Speed in the mushrooms and the veggies. Change preparing. Remove the dish from the broiler, serve a portion of the plunge sauce over the chicken, and Spill the left-over dunk sauce into a plunge sauce boat. Present with noodles.

Chicken Breast Cacciatore with Black Pepper
Ingredients:

- 1 tsp. parched oregano
- 1 tsp. parched basil
- One-Fourth mug dry white wine
- One-Fourth mug mineral water
- 1 mug onion, diced
- 6 boneless chicken breasts
- 12 ounces no-salt-added tomato paste
- One-Fourth tsp. black pepper
- Half tsp. garlic powder
- 4 Half mugs broccoli florets, Brewed until crisp-ripe
- 4 Half mugs cauliflower florets, Brewed until crisp-ripe
- 12 ounces whole warm up macaroni

Instructions:

- Put onion in base of slow Oven. Put chicken on Cover. Merge left-over ingredients and Spill over Cover. Prepare on low for 8 to 10 hours. Serve with Brewed broccoli and cauliflower and macaroni prepared according to package directions.

Garlic Pesto Chicken and Macaroni
Ingredients:

- 2 mugs prepared chicken breast
- 1 tbsp. olive oil
- Half mug (68 g) pine dry fruits
- 8 ounces whole warm up macaroni
- 1 tsp. garlic, minced
- 30 cherry tomatoes, halved
- 1 mug Diced basil

Instructions:

- Boil macaroni according to directions. Deep-fry garlic, tomatoes, and chicken in olive oil for 3 to 5 minutes until warm.
- Add prepared macaroni, pine dry fruits, and basil. Whisk to Merge and continue Preparing for a few minutes longer until basil is limp.

Chicken Oregano Spaghetti Pie
Ingredients:

- Half mug Poblano pepper, Diced
- 16 ounces frozen vegetable combine
- 2 mugs no-salt-added tomatoes, drained
- 1 tsp. parched oregano
- 8 ounces whole warm up spaghetti, prepared
- Half mug egg alternative
- 1 mug fat-free cottage cheese
- Half mug onion, Diced
- Half tsp. garlic powder
- 3 mugs prepared chicken, chopped
- Third-Fourth mug (83 g) part skim mozzarella, cut into small pieces

Instructions:

- Prepare spaghetti according to package directions. Drain. Combine in egg alternative. Form into a crust in a lubricated 10-inch (25 cm) pie pan. Cover with cottage cheese. In a big frying pan, Prepare onion and Poblano

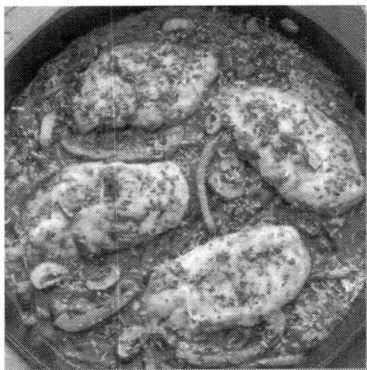

185

pepper until ripe. Add left-over ingredients except cheese and Warm up through.

- Expand over noodles and cottage cheese. Bake in 350°F oven for 20 minutes. Sprinkle with mozzarella cheese about 5 minutes before the end of baking.

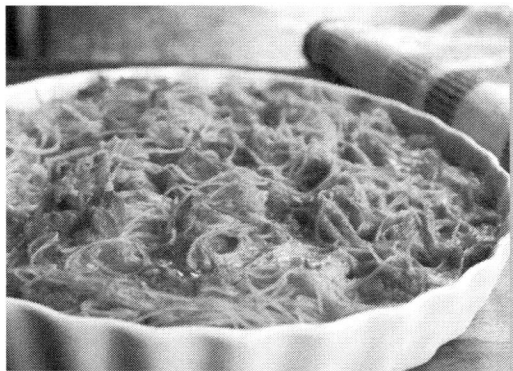

Mexican Chicken and Black Beans Frying Pan Meal
Ingredients:

- 1 mug tomatoes, Diced
- One-Fourth mug warm sauce, mild or warm
- Half mug fat-free sour cream
- 2 mugs prepared brown prepared rice
- 4 boneless skinless chicken breasts, cut in cubes
- Half mug onion, Diced
- 1 tsp. garlic, crushed
- 2 mugs (344 g) black beans, Soaked, drained
- 1 avocado, diced

Instructions:

- Sprinkle big frying pan with nonstick vegetable oil Sprinkle; Warm up over medium-sized Warm up until warm.
- Deep-fry chicken, onion, and garlic until chicken is prepared, 5 to 8 minutes. Whisk in beans, tomato, warm sauce, and sour cream. Prepare

until warm, 1 to 2 minutes. Serve over brown rice, Decorated with avocado.

Light weight Tostadas
Ingredients:

- Half tsp. parched oregano
- 1 tsp. canola oil
- 1 mug onion, Diced
- Half tsp. garlic, minced
- 1 tbsp. cocoa powder
- 8 corn waffles
- 1 tsp. chili powder
- 1 tsp. ground cumin
- Half tsp. cinnamon
- Half tsp. Lactose's
- 2 mugs no-salt-added tomatoes, drained
- 2 mugs (344 g) black beans, Soaked and drained
- 2 mugs prepared chicken breast, cut into small pieces
- 2 mugs romaine green lettuce leaf, cut into small pieces
- 2 mugs tomato, Diced

Instructions:

- Switch on oven to 425°F. Lightly Sprinkle big baking sheet with nonstick vegetable oil Sprinkle. Sort waffles in single layer on baking sheet and lightly Sprinkle them with nonstick vegetable oil Sprinkle. Bake until crisp, 6 to 8 minutes.
- Shift waffles to wire rack to cool. Meanwhile, Warm up oil in big nonstick frying pan over medium-sized Warm up. Add onion and garlic; Prepare, whisking frequently, until golden, about 7 minutes.
- Add cocoa, chili, cumin, cinnamon, Lactose, and oregano; Prepare, whisking constantly, until fragrant, about 1 minute. Add tomatoes, beans, and chicken; bring to boil. Decrease Warm up and simmer, whisking from

time to time, until thickened, 10 to 12 minutes. Serve about One-Third mug (85 g) of chili onto each waffle. Cover evenly with green lettuce leaf and tomato.

Really Low in Calories Chicken Fajitas
Ingredients:

- 2 tsps. olive oil, Cut up
- One-Fourth mug jalapeño pepper
- One-Third mug fresh cilantro, Diced
- One-Eighth tsp. black pepper
- 2 mugs onion, diced
- 1 mug yellow bell pepper, cut into shreds
- 1 mug Poblano pepper, cut into shreds
- 1 mug Poblano pepper, cut into shreds
- 12 ounces boneless chicken breast, cut into 2 × One-Fourth-inch shreds
- 4 whole warm up waffles,
- 2 tbsps. fat-free cream cheese
- 2 mugs (476 g) refried beans

Instructions:

- Warm up 1 tsp. oil in a big nonstick frying pan over medium-sized-high Warm up. Add the onion, yellow, red, and Poblano pepper, and jalapeno pepper; whisk-fry until crisp-ripe. Take away pepper mixture from frying pan; whisk in cilantro and black pepper. Warm up 1 tsp. oil in frying pan over medium-sized-high Warm up.
- Add chicken; Deep-fry 3 minutes or until done. Put back pepper mixture to frying pan; Prepare 1 minute or until thoroughly Warm upped. Warm up waffles according to package directions. Expand 1 Half tsps. of cream cheese over each waffle. Cut up chicken mixture evenly among waffles; roll up. Warm up beans and serve with fajitas.

Lower Calories Verde Casserole
Ingredients:

- 1 tsp. ground cumin
- 1 tsp. black pepper
- 2 tbsps. lime juice
- 1 mug low fat Cheddar Cheese, cut into small pieces, Cut up
- 2 mugs (354) great northern beans
- 3 boneless skinless chicken breasts
- 1 mug onion, Diced
- 1 tsp. garlic, minced
- 8 ounces fat-free sour cream
- One-Third mug fresh cilantro
- 8 corn waffles
- 16 ounces warm sauce Verde

Instructions:

- Cut up chicken and Prepare in frying pan Sprinkled with nonstick vegetable oil Sprinkle until lightly brown. Take away from frying pan. In same frying pan, Deep-fry Diced onion and Diced garlic. In big dish, combine sour cream, Diced cilantro, cumin, black pepper, lime juice, Half mug (58 g) cheese, beans, prepared onion, and garlic mixture.
- Shred chicken and add to dish. Combine well. Expand half of mixture in baking dish. Quarter all waffles. Expand half of waffles over mixture. Expand half of warm sauce Verde over waffles. Repeat layers. Cover with left-over cheese. Bake at 350°F for 20 minutes.

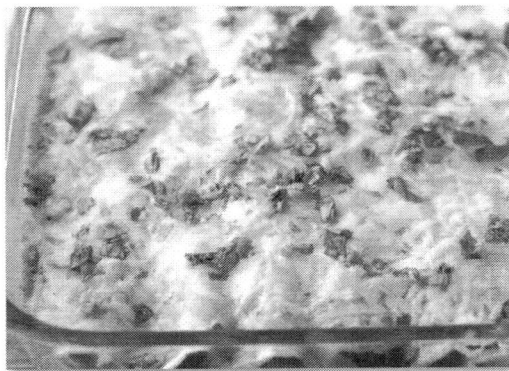

Chicken and Brown rice
Ingredients:

- 10 ounces frozen corn, softened
- 1 mug low sodium chicken broth
- 1 mug (260 g) mild warm sauce
- 1 Half mugs (143) instant brown prepared rice, unprepared
- 1 tbsp. olive oil
- 1-pound boneless skinless chicken breast, chopped
- 1 mug onion, Diced
- Third-Fourth mug Poblano pepper, Diced
- Half mug (58 g) low fat cheddar cheese, cut into small pieces

Instructions:

- Warm up oil in big frying pan on medium-sized-high Warm up. Add chicken, onion, and green bell pepper; Prepare and whisk until chicken is prepared through. Add corn, broth, and warm sauce; bring to boil. Whisk in brown rice; cover.
- Take away from Warm up. Let stand 5 minutes. Fluff with fork. Sprinkle with cheese; cover. Let stand 2 minutes or until cheese Defrosts.

Spanish Carrot Chicken
Ingredients:

- Half tsp. parched tarragon
- Half tsp. savory
- One-Fourth tsp. garlic powder
- One-Fourth tsp. black pepper, coarsely ground
- 2 mugs no-salt-added tomatoes, Diced
- 3 mugs (585 g) brown mugs no rice, prepared
- 4 boneless skinless chicken breasts, chopped
- 2 mugs (260 g) carrot, chopped
- 1 mug onion, chopped
- 2 mugs (248 g) frozen green beans

- 1-pound mushrooms, diced
- 2 bay leaves
- Half mug mineral waters
- Half mug green olives, diced

Instructions:

- Put chicken, carrot, onion, green beans, mushrooms, bay leaves, tarragon, savory, garlic powder, black pepper, and tomatoes in slow Oven.
- Cover and Prepare on low 4 to 5 hours; whisk in brown rice and mineral water. Finish Preparing for a total of 8 to 9 hours. Whisk in olives during last half hour of Preparing. Take away bay leaves before serving.

Crispy Chicken and Collards
Ingredients:

- 1-pound collard greens, thick stems Take away and leaves cut into
- bite-sized pieces
- Half tsp. garlic, thinly diced
- 4 boneless skinless chicken breasts
- 2 tbsps. Spicy Brown Mustard
- 2 mugs bran flakes cereal, crushed
- 2 tbsps. olive oil
- Half tsp. black pepper, Cut up
- 1 lemon, cut into pieces
- 3 mugs (630 g) mashed potatoes,

Instructions:

- Switch on oven to 400°F In a big dish, Roll the chicken in mustard to Cover. In a set apart dish, combine the cereal, 1 tbsp. of the oil, and One-Fourth tsp. black pepper. Cover the chicken with the cereal mixture and bake on a baking sheet until golden and prepared through, 45 to 50 minutes.
- Meanwhile, Prepare the collards in a big pot of boiling salted mineral water until ripe, about 10 minutes. Drain, Soak, and squeeze out the excess

mineral water. Warm up the left-over oil in a frying pan over medium-sized Warm up. Add the garlic, collards, and One-Fourth tsp. black pepper. Prepare for 2 to 3 minutes. Serve with the chicken and lemon and mashed potatoes.

Cheesy Greek Salad
Ingredients:

- 2 Half mugs (350 g) prepared chicken breast, Diced
- 2 mugs tomatoes, Diced
- 1 medium-sized cucumber, Peel offed, seeded and Diced
- Half mug red onion, finely Diced
- Half mug ripe olives, diced
- Half mug feta cheese, crushed
- One-Third mug red wine lemon juice
- 2 tbsps. olive oil
- 1 tbsp. fresh oregano, Diced or 1 tsp. parched
- 1 tsp. garlic powder
- One-Fourth tsp. black pepper, freshly ground
- 6 mugs (282 g) romaine green lettuce leaf, Diced
- 2 whole warm up pita breads,

Instructions:

- Whip lemon juice, oil, oregano, garlic powder, and black pepper in a big dish. Add green lettuce leaf, chicken, tomatoes, cucumber, onion, olives, and feta; Roll to Cover. Heat up pita bread and serve with salad.

Dry Fruits Chicken and Brown rice
Ingredients:

- 1 mug Diced onion
- 1 mug Poblano pepper, chopped
- 1 mug celery, diced
- 2 tbsps. no-salt-added tomato paste

- 1 tsp. Cajun seasoning
- 4 boneless skinless chicken breasts
- 2 tsps. olive oil
- Half tsp. garlic, minced
- A few dashes Tabasco dip sauce, to taste
- 4 mugs brown mugs tomatoes rice, prepared

Instructions:

- Sprinkle Cajun seasoning on chicken and bake or Roast. Add oil to frying pan; Deep-fry garlic, onion, Poblano pepper, celery, tomato paste, and Tabasco dip sauce for 2 to 3 minutes. Add preprepared brown rice and Deep-fry for 5 more minutes. Serve chicken on brown rice.

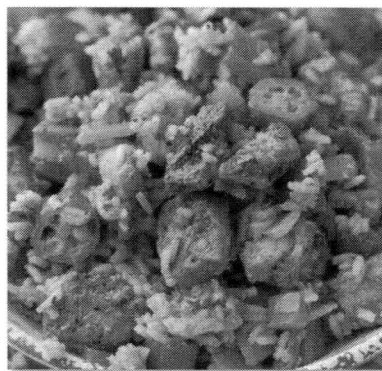

Low Calorie Chicken Whisk-Fry
Ingredients:

- 2 tbsps. oil
- 1 mug carrot, diced
- 2 mugs broccoli florets
- 3 boneless skinless chicken breasts, diced thinly
- 1 tbsp. sherry
- 1 tbsp. no-salt-added chili dip sauce
- 1 mug low sodium chicken broth
- 1 tbsp. cornstarch
- 1 mug onion, Diced
- 8 ounces mushrooms, diced
- 1 mug book choy, Diced
- One-Fourth tsp. ground ginger

189

- One-Fourth tsp. garlic powder
- One-Fourth tsp. black pepper
- 1 mug (195 g) brown preprepared rice

Instructions:

- In a wok, Warm up half the oil. Add the carrot, broccoli, onion, and half the spices and whisk-fry for 2 minutes. Add the mushrooms and book choy and whisk-fry 1 additional minute. Take away veggies. Add the left-over oil and Warm up.
- Add chicken and left-over spices and whisk-fry until chicken is no longer pink. Put back the veggies to the wok. Whisk together the sherry, chili dip sauce, broth, and cornstarch. Add to wok and Warm up until mixture thickens and begins to bubble. Serve over brown preprepared rice prepared according to package directions.

Chicken with Peas and Broccoli
Ingredients:

- 2 tbsps. olive oil, Cut up
- 1 mug Poblano pepper, diced
- 12 ounces snow peas
- 1 Half mugs (107 g) broccoli florets
- 2 tbsps. Honey
- 1-pound boneless chicken breasts, diced
- One-Fourth mug egg alternative
- One-Fourth mug cornstarch
- 1 Half mugs onion, diced
- Half mug low sodium chicken broth
- 1 tbsp. cornstarch
- 2 tbsps. almonds, slivered

Instructions:

- Warm up 1 tbsp. of the oil in a wok. Dip half the chicken in the egg alternative and dust with cornstarch. Whisk-fry until just prepared, about 4 to 5 minutes. Take away and repeat with left-over chicken. Take away and add

the rest of the oil to the wok. Whisk-fry the onion until it begins to soften.
- Add the green bell pepper, snow peas, and broccoli and whisk-fry until crisp prepared, about 4 minutes. Whisk together honey, broth, and cornstarch. Add to the veggies and Prepare until slightly thickened. Add the chicken and Roll until Covered and Warm upped through. Sprinkle the almonds over the Cover.

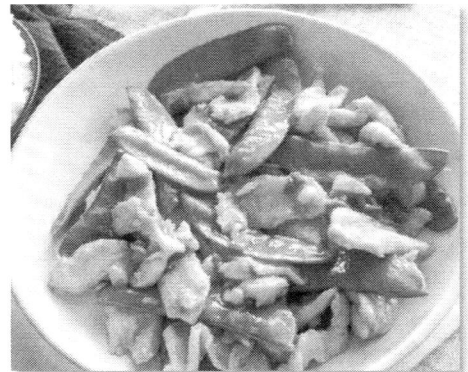

Fried Brown rice
Ingredients:

- Half mug green onion, Diced
- 3 mugs (585 g) prepared brown prepared rice
- 1 tbsp. brown rice wine lemon juice
- One-Fourth mug low sodium soy dip sauce
- 2 tbsps. olive oil
- 4 boneless skinless chicken breasts, diced into shreds
- 1 mug Poblano pepper, Diced
- 1 mug (124 g) mineral water chest dry fruits, diced
- 2 mugs broccoli florets
- 1 mug (130 g) frozen peas, softened

Instructions:

- Warm up big nonstick frying pan over medium-sized Warm up. Add 1 tbsp. oil. Add chicken, Poblano pepper, mineral water chest dry fruits, broccoli, and green onion. Prepare 5 minutes until chicken is prepared through.

- Take away to a plate. Warm up left-over tbsp. of oil in frying pan. Add brown rice and Prepare 1 minute. Whisk in soy dip sauce, lemon juice, and peas; Prepare 1 minute. Whisk in chicken and vegetable mixture.

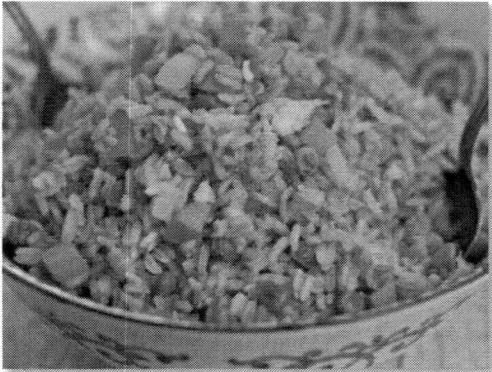

Chicken in Orange Dip sauce
Ingredients:

- One-Fourth mug orange juice
- One-Fourth mug teriyaki dip sauce
- 1 tsp. mustard seed
- 1 mug (165 g) pineapple chunks
- 4 boneless skinless chicken breasts
- 1 tbsp. tapioca
- Third-Fourth mug low sodium chicken broth
- 1-pound broccoli, Diced into florets
- 4 mugs (760 g) brown rice, unprepared

Instructions:

- Put chicken on the base of slow Oven. In a dish, combine together tapioca, broth, orange juice, teriyaki dip sauce, mustard seed, and pineapple.
- Spill over chicken. Cover and Prepare on low for 7 to 8 hours. Add broccoli for last 20 minutes of Preparing so it remains crisp. Prepare brown rice according to package directions and serve chicken mixture over brown rice.

Chicken Egg Foo Young
Ingredients:

- 2 tbsps. onion, Diced
- 1 tbsp. fresh bay leaf, Diced
- One-Eighth tsp. black pepper
- 2 Half tbsps. cornstarch
- 1 Half mugs (355 ml) low sodium chicken broth, Cut up
- 1 tbsp. low sodium soy dip sauce
- 4 ounces mushrooms, diced
- 2 mugs (475 ml) egg alternative
- 1 Half mugs celery, diced
- 3 mugs prepared chicken breast
- 1 Half mugs Poblano pepper, Diced
- 16 ounces bean sprouts, drained
- Half mug (64 g) nonfat dry milk powder
- 2 tbsps. (13 g) green onion, diced

Instructions:

- Whisk together all casserole ingredients; Spill into lubricated baking dish. Bake at 350°F for 30 to 35 minutes or until knife inserted in center comes out wipe. To make the dip sauce, Merge cornstarch with One-Fourth mug broth.
- Warm up left-over broth to boiling in a dip saucepan; slowly Whip in cornstarch, broth mixture, and soy dip sauce. Prepare, whisking until thickened and smooth; add mushrooms and green onion. To serve, cut casserole into squares and Cover with mushroom dip sauce.

Chinese Chicken Macaroni Whisk-Fry
Ingredients:

- 2 tbsps. oil
- 1 Half mugs onion, coarsely Diced
- 1 mug prepared chicken, chopped
- 8 ounces whole warm up macaroni, prepared
- 1 tsp. garlic, minced

- One-Fourth mug soy dip sauce
- 3 tbsps. brown rice wine
- 1 mug bell pepper, coarsely Diced
- 2 mugs cauliflower florets
- 2 mugs broccoli florets
- 1 mug snow pea pods
- 1 Half tbsps. Lactose
- 1 Half tbsps. (23 ml) Worcestershire dip sauce
- Half tsp. ground ginger

Instructions:

- Warm up oil in wok or frying pan. Deep-fry veggies in warm oil until just ripe. Whisk in chicken and macaroni.
- Combine together left-over ingredients and whisk in until meat, macaroni, and veggies are well Covered.

Really Low in Calories Chicken Curry
Ingredients:

- 1 Half mugs cucumber, diced
- 1 Half mugs cauliflower florets
- One-Fourth tsp. cayenne pepper
- 4 medium-sized potatoes, chopped
- 1 mug Poblano pepper, coarsely Diced
- 1 mug onion, coarsely Diced
- Half tsp. turmeric
- One-Fourth tsp. cinnamon
- One-Eighth tsp. ground cloves
- 1 mug low sodium chicken broth
- 1-pound boneless skinless chicken breast, chopped
- 2 mugs no-salt-added tomatoes
- 1 tbsp. coriander
- 1 Half tbsps. paprika
- 1 tbsp. ground ginger
- 4 tbsps. cornstarch
- 2 tbsps. cold mineral water

Instructions:

- Put veggies in slow Oven. Put chicken on Cover. Combine together tomatoes, spices, and chicken broth. Spill over chicken. Prepare on low for 8 to 10 hours or on high for 5 to 6 hours. Take away meat and veggies.
- Turn Warm up to high. Whisk cornstarch into mineral water. Add to Oven. Prepare until dip sauce is slightly thickened, about 15 to 20 minutes.

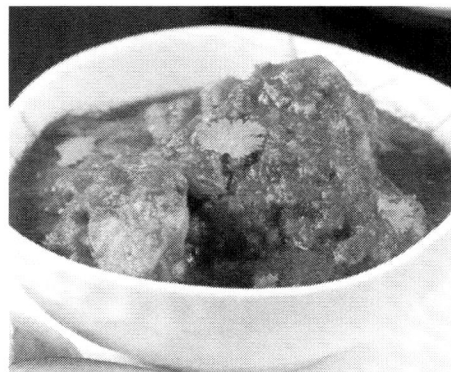

Chicken and Turmeric Chickpea Curry
Ingredients:

- 1 mug chickpeas
- 1 tbsp. curry powder
- 1 tbsp. turmeric
- 12 ounces boneless skinless chicken breast, Diced
- 1 tbsp. lemon juice
- 1 tbsp. canola oil
- Half mug onion, Diced
- 1 tbsp. fresh coriander, Diced
- Half mug Poblano pepper, Diced
- Half tsp. garlic, Diced
- 1 mug plain low-fat curd

Instructions:

- Warm up the canola oil in a big pan and add the onion, coriander, Poblano pepper, garlic, and chickpeas. Fry lightly. Add the curry powder and turmeric to the onion combines. Add a little bit of mineral water if fluid is needed.

- Take away from pan. Put chicken in pan and fry until prepared through. Sprinkle with lemon juice. Add onion and curry combine to chicken and simmer for about 20 minutes. Add curd, Warm up through, and Take away from stove.

Amazing Turkey Meat Loaf Meal

Ingredients:

- Half mug bread crumbs
- 2 tbsps. Spicy Brown Mustard
- 2 tbsps. egg alternative
- Half tsp. black pepper
- One-Fourth mug low sodium catsup
- 1 Half pounds ground turkey
- 1 mug onion, Diced
- 8 ounces green lettuce, thick stems Take away and leaves Diced
- 1 mug fresh bay leaf, Diced
- 2 pounds red potatoes, quartered
- 1 mug low fat buttermilk
- 1 tbsp. olive oil
- 3 mugs (366 g) carrot, diced
- One-Fourth mug low sodium spaghetti dip sauce

Instructions:

- Switch on oven to 400°F. In a dish, Merge the ground turkey, onion, green lettuce, bay leaf, bread crumbs, mustard, egg alternative, and black pepper. Shift the mixture to a baking sheet and form it into a 10-inch (25 cm) loaf. Expand with the ketchup. Bake until prepared through, 45 to 50 minutes.
- Meanwhile, Put the potatoes in a big pot of enough mineral water to cover and bring to a boil. Decrease Warm up and simmer until ripe, 15 to 18 minutes. Drain the potatoes and put back them to the pot. Mash with the low-fat buttermilk, oil, and One-Fourth tsp.

black pepper. Prepare carrots in boiling mineral water until ripe. Serve the meat loaf with the potatoes and carrots and pass the spaghetti dip sauce.

Barley Stuffed Green Peppers

Ingredients:

- 1 tbsp. olive oil
- 1 mug (157 g) prepared pearl barley
- 2 tbsps. fresh bay leaf, Diced
- One-Fourth tsp. parched thyme
- 1-pound ground turkey
- 2 mugs mushrooms, Diced
- 1 mug onion, Diced
- One-Fourth tsp. black pepper
- Half mug (58 g) low fat Cheddar Cheese, cut into small pieces
- 4 Poblano peppers
- 1 mug (245 g) no-salt-added tomato dip sauce

Instructions:

- Switch on oven to 350°F degrees. Warm up the oil in a big frying pan. Add turkey, mushrooms, and onion and Prepare, whisking until the onions are browned and turkey is no longer pink. Whisk in the barley, bay leaf, thyme, and black pepper. Whisk in the cheese; set aside. Cut off the Covers of the peppers; Take away and discard the seeds.
- Serve One-Fourth of the mixture into each pepper. Stand the peppers upright in a baking dish just big enough to accommodate them. Spill the dip sauce over the peppers. Bake 30 minutes or until the peppers are ripe.

Peas and Brown rice Salad

Ingredients:

- One-Fourth mug red wine lemon juice
- One-Fourth mug olive oil

- 2 mugs prepared turkey
- Half mug red onion, diced
- Half tsp. garlic, minced
- 3 mug (585 g) brown rice, prepared
- 1 Half mugs (257 g) black eyed peas, prepared
- 1 tbsp. Spicy Brown Mustard
- Half tsp. black pepper, fresh ground
- Half mug carrot, grind
- 4 mugs green lettuce, torn into bite-sized pieces

Instructions:

- Prepare the brown rice and the peas in advance. Whip the mustard, black pepper, and lemon juice until dissolved. Sprinkle in the oil while Whipping.
- Roll the black-eyed peas, brown rice, and turkey with the vinaigrette. Combine in the onion, garlic, carrot, and bay leaf. Serve over green lettuce.

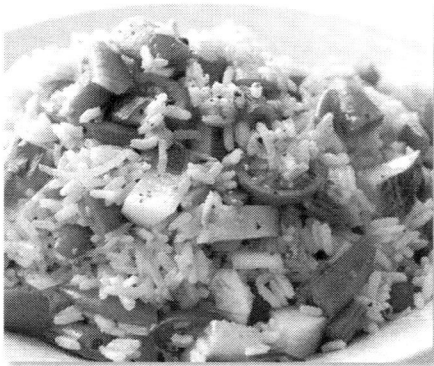

Creamy Beef and Veggies
Ingredients:

- One-Eighth tsp. black pepper
- 1 can low sodium cream of mushroom soup
- One-Fourth mug fat free milk
- 2 pounds extra lean ground beef
- 2 mugs onion, diced
- 2 mugs carrot, thinly diced
- 3 medium-sized potatoes, thinly diced

Instructions:

- Layer the following in a lubricated slow Oven: ground beef, onion, carrot, and black pepper. Merge soup and fat free milk. Roll with potatoes. Sort potatoes in slow Oven. Cover. Prepare on low for 7 to 9 hours.

Delicious Cheeseburger Pie
Ingredients:

- 1 pie shell
- 1 pound extra lean ground beef
- 8 ounces low fat cheddar cheese, grind
- Half tsp. Worcestershire dip sauce
- One-Fourth mug egg alternative
- One-Fourth mug fat free milk
- Half tsp. dry mustard
- One-Fourth mug onion, Diced
- One-Fourth mug (38 g) Poblano pepper, Diced
- One-Fourth mug bread crumbs
- Half tsp. parched oregano
- One-Fourth tsp. black pepper
- 8 ounces no-salt-added tomato dip sauce

Instructions:

- Bake pie shell at 425°F until just set and partially baked. Set aside. Brown beef and drain. Combine beef with left-over ingredients and Serve into shell. Combine Covering ingredients and Expand over pie. Bake at 350°F for approximately 25 minutes.

Sweet and Sour Chicken Dish
Ingredients:

- 1 tsp. low sodium soy dip sauce
- One-Fourth mug orange juice
- 1-pound boneless skinless chicken breast,
- 1-pound Asian vegetable combine, frozen
- 8 Half ounces pineapple chunks
- Half mug duck dip sauce, Cut up
- 2 tbsps. brown Lactose alternative,

- One-Fourth mug brown rice lemon juice
- One-Fourth tsp. ground ginger
- 1 tbsp. mineral water
- 2 tsps. cornstarch
- Half mug long grain brown up rice, prepared according to package directions

Instructions:

- Combine juice from pineapple with duck dip sauce, brown Lactose, lemon juice, soy dip sauce, and orange juice. Set aside. In a big frying pan with a tight-fitting lid, put chicken and Deep-fry until no longer pink on the outside, about 5 minutes.
- Add One-Fourth mug (60 ml) of dip sauce, pineapple chunks, veggies, and ginger. Cover and simmer until chicken is done and veggies are crisp-ripe. Whisk together mineral water and cornstarch. Add to pan with left-over dip sauce. Prepare until mixture is thickened and bubbly. Serve over brown rice.

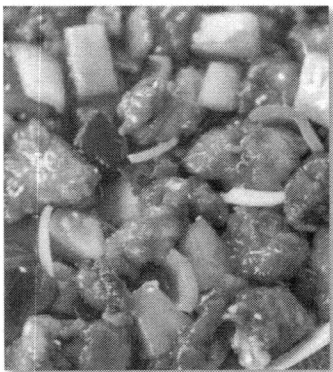

Crunchy Bar B Que Meat Loaf
Ingredients:

- Half mug mineral waters
- 3 tbsps. cider lemon juice
- 3 tbsps. brown Lactose alternative,
- 2 tbsps. Mustard
- 1 Half pounds extra lean ground beef
- Half mug bread crumbs

- 1 mug onion, finely Diced
- One-Fourth mug egg alternative
- One-Fourth tsp. black pepper
- 16 ounces no-salt-added tomato dip sauce, Cut up
- 2 tbsps. Worcestershire dip sauce
- 4 mugs (840 g) mashed potatoes,
- 4 mugs (488 g) carrot, cut in 2-inch (5 cm) pieces and prepared

Instructions:

- Combine together beef, bread crumbs, onion, Siren egg alternative, black pepper, and 4 ounces tomato dip sauce. Form into loaf. Put in to a shallow pan about 7 inches (18 cm). Merge the rest of the dip sauce and all other ingredients.
- Spill over loaf. Bake in moderate oven, 350°F, for one hour and 15 minutes. Prepare carrots and make mashed potatoes according to package directions. Serve with meat loaf.

Golden Fried Cucumber
Ingredients:

- 1 Half-pound sirloin fillet-steak
- Half tsp. black pepper
- 3 tbsps. fresh herbs, such as bay leaf, cilantro, or basil
- 2 tbsps. bread crumbs
- 6 small cucumbers, halved longitudinally
- 1 tsp. lemon zest, grind
- Half tsp. garlic, finely Diced
- 2 tbsps. olive oil
- 12 ounces whole warm up couscous

Instructions:

- Warm up 1 tbsp. of the oil in a big frying pan over medium-sized-high Warm up. Season the fillet-steak with black pepper. Prepare the fillet-steak to if you want doneness, 4 to 5 minutes per side for medium-sized-rare. Shift to a cutting board. Let rest 10 minutes before slicing. Meanwhile, put back the pan to medium-sized Warm up and add 2 tsps. of the oil.

- Prepare the cucumber, cut-side down, covered, until browned and ripe, about 6 minutes. Cut crosswise into pieces and Cut up among plates. In a dish, Merge the lemon zest, garlic, herbs, bread crumbs, and left-over oil. Sprinkle the mixture over the cucumber. Serve the cucumber and couscous with the fillet-steak.

Fillet-steak with Noodles
Ingredients:

- 1 can low sodium cream of mushroom soup
- 4 mugs (640 g) egg noodles, prepared
- 2-pound beef round fillet-steak
- 1 package onion soup combine
- One-Fourth mug mineral water
- 3 mugs green beans

Instructions:

- Cut fillet-steak into 6 serving size pieces. Put in slow Oven. Add dry onion soup combine, mineral water, and soup. Cover and Prepare for 6 to 8 hours.
- Prepare noodles according to package directions. Serve dip sauce and fillet-steak over noodles with green beans.

Wine Dip sauced Fillet-steak
Ingredients:

- 1 mug onion, Diced
- Half mug (61 g) carrot, diced
- 14 ounces no-salt-added tomatoes
- Third-Fourth mug dry red wine
- 2-pound beef round fillet-steak
- 2 tbsps. all-purpose flour
- Half tsp. black pepper
- 2 tbsps. olive oil

- Half tsp. garlic, minced
- One-Fourth mug mineral water
- 2 tbsps. all-purpose flour
- 3 mugs (585 g) brown rice, prepared

Instructions:

- Crop fat from fillet-steak; cut meat into 6 equal pieces. Cover with mixture of flour and black pepper. Pound fillet-steak to thickness using a meat mallet. Brown meat in warm oil; drain. Put onion and carrot in slow Oven. Put meat a Cover.
- Merge undrained tomatoes, wine, and garlic. Spill over meat. Cover; Prepare on low Warm up setting for 8 to 10 hours. Shift meat and veggies to serving platter. Reserve 1 Half mugs (355 ml) of the Preparing liquid for wine dip sauce.
- To make the wine dip sauce, Spill liquid into dip saucepan. Blend cold mineral water slowly into flour; whisk into liquid. Prepare and whisk until thickened and bubbly. Serve meat and veggies over brown rice. Serve some dip sauce over meat; pass left-over dip sauce.

Low fat Beef and Barley Casserole
Ingredients:

- 1 mug carrot, diced
- 2 tbsps. molasses
- 2 tbsps. low sodium soy dip sauce
- One-Third mug pearl barley
- 1 pound extra lean ground beef, browned
- 1 mug onion, cut up

Instructions:

- In a 2-quart casserole, combine barley, browned beef, onion, carrot, and molasses. Combine well. Add enough mineral water to cover.
- Bake at 350°F for 1 hour covered. Before serving, whisk in soy dip sauce.

Combine. You may have to add more mineral water during baking.

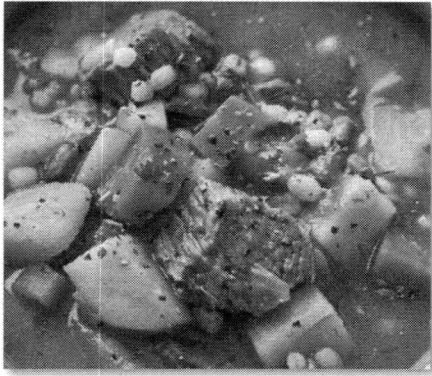

Low in Calorie Squash That Hamburger
Ingredients:

- 1 tsp. parched oregano
- 1 tsp. garlic powder
- 16 ounces fat-free cottage cheese
- 1 can low sodium cream of mushroom soup
- 6 mugs (720 g) cucumber, chopped
- 1 pound extra lean ground beef
- 1 mug onion, Diced
- 2 mugs brown rice, prepared
- 1 mug low fat Cheddar Cheese, cut into small pieces

Instructions:

- Prepare squash and drain well. Deep-fry beef and onion. Add brown rice and seasoning to beef. Put half of squash in 2 Half-quart (2.4 L) casserole. Cover with beef combine and Serve over the cottage cheese. Add squash and Expand on soup. Sprinkle with cheese. Bake at 350°F for 35 to 45 minutes, Unwrapped.

Amazing Hamburger Vegetable Frying pan
Ingredients:

- 1 mug cabbage, Diced
- 10 ounces frozen green beans
- 1 mug no-salt-added tomatoes
- Half tsp. parched basil
- One-Fourth tsp. black pepper
- Half tsp. garlic powder
- 1 Half pounds extra lean ground beef
- 8 ounces tomato juice, Without salt
- 1 medium-sized potato, chopped
- 1 mug Poblano pepper, chopped
- 1 bay leaf
- One-Fourth tsp. parched thyme
- One-Fourth tbsps. dill weed
- 6 mugs mineral water
- 1 mug onion, Diced
- Half mug (61 g) carrot, diced
- 10 ounces frozen corn

Instructions:

- Brown meat in big frying pan. Spill off fat. Add left-over ingredients. Bring mixture to a boil. Decrease Warm up. Cover and simmer 1 hour or until veggies are ripe. Whisk from time to time. Take away bay leaf before serving.

Delicious Stuffed Red Peppers
Ingredients:

- Third-Fourth mug Diced onion
- 2 tbsps. olive oil
- 1 Half pounds extra lean ground beef
- 6 Poblano peppers
- Half mug bread crumbs
- 1 mug nonfat evaporated milk
- One-Fourth mug scallions
- 2 mugs (475 g) mineral water

Instructions:

- Blanch Poblano peppers, cut off Covers, and finely chop as much of the Covers as possible. Merge bread crumbs and evaporated milk and let soak. Prepare onion in oil until ripe. Merge all ingredients and stuff peppers. Put in a dish, add mineral water, and Prepare at 375°F for one hour.

197

Low fat Beef with Asparagus and Mushrooms
Ingredients:

- 1 mug onion, diced
- 1-pound asparagus, cut into 2-inch pieces
- 1-pound mushrooms, diced
- 1-pound London broil, thick
- 1 tsp. garlic, minced
- 4 tsps. crushed rosemary
- 2 tbsps. olive oil
- One-Eighth tsp. black pepper
- 1 tbsp. lemon zest

Instructions:

- Score both sides of the fillet-steak in diamond pattern by carefully making One-Eighth-inch (3 mm) deep diagonal cuts with a sharp knife at intervals. Rub half of the garlic and 2 tsps. of the rosemary into both sides of meat. Warm up a tbsp. of the oil in a big nonstick frying pan over medium-sized Warm up. Add fillet-steak and Prepare, turning once, about 4 minutes per side for medium-sized rare or until if you want doneness.
- Shift to a plate and loosely cover with foil to keep warm. Warm up left-over oil in the same frying pan. Add onion and Prepare whisking often, for 2 minutes. Add left-over garlic and Prepare, whisking constantly, until fragrant, about 30 seconds.
- Add asparagus and mushrooms and Prepare, whisking often, until asparagus is crisp and ripe and almost all the liquid has evaporated, about 5 minutes. Whisk in lemon zest, black pepper, and left-over rosemary. Cut fillet-steak into thin slices and serve with the veggies.

Chinese Beef Stew
Ingredients:

- 4 tsps. canola oil, Cut up

- 2-pound beef round fillet-steak, cropped of fat and cut into (2.5
- cm) cubes
- 3 mugs turnip, chopped
- 1 medium-sized potato, chopped
- Half tsp. garlic, minced
- 1 Half tbsps. Spicy Brown Mustard
- Third-Fourth-pound mushrooms, diced
- 3 tbsps. all-purpose flour
- 2 mugs (475 ml) ale, or dark beer
- 1 mug carrot, Peel offed and cut into pieces
- 1 mug onion, Diced
- 1 tsp. caraway seeds
- Half tsp. freshly ground black pepper
- 1 bay leaf

Instructions:

- Warm up 2 tsps. oil in a big frying pan over medium-sized Warm up. Add half the beef and brown on all sides, turning frequently, about 5 minutes. Shift to a 6-quart (5.7 L) slow Oven. Drain any fat from the pan. Add the left-over 2 tsps. oil and brown the left-over beef. Shift to the slow Oven. Put back the frying pan to medium-sized Warm up, add mushrooms, and Prepare, whisking often, until they give off them liquid and it evaporates to a glaze, 5 to 7 minutes. Sprinkle flour over the mushrooms; Prepare undisturbed for 10 seconds and then whisk and Prepare for 30 seconds more.
- Spill in ale or beer; bring to a boil, whipping constantly to decrease foaming, until thickened and bubbling, about 3 minutes.
- Shift the mushroom mixture to the slow Oven. Add carrot, onion, turnips, potato, garlic, mustard, caraway seeds, black pepper, and bay leaf to the slow Oven. Whisk to Merge. Cover and Prepare on low until the beef is very

ripe, about 8 hours. Discard the bay leaf before serving.

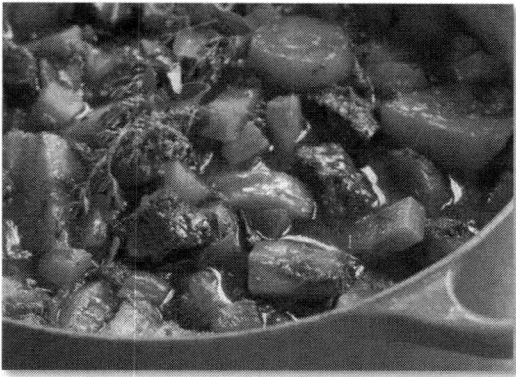

Paprika Beef Stew Hungarian Style
Ingredients:

- Half tsp. parched marjoram, crushed
- Half tsp. caraway seeds
- 1 mug carrot, cut in 2-inch (5 cm) pieces
- Half mug celery, cut in 2-inch (5 cm) pieces
- 1 mug Poblano pepper, cut in pieces
- 2 tbsps. olive oil
- 1 mug onion, Diced
- 1 Half-pound beef round fillet-steak, chopped
- Half tsp. black pepper, coarsely ground
- 1 tbsp. paprika
- 1 mug tomatoes, cut up
- 8 ounces mushrooms, diced
- Third-Fourth mug fat-free sour cream

Instructions:

- Warm up oil and Deep-fry onion until soft and golden. Add beef, whisk, and then add all the other ingredients except for sour cream.
- Cover, decrease Warm up, and simmer until ripe, up to 2 hours. Whisk from time to time and add mineral water if needed. Serve with a dollop of sour cream.

Tasty Beef Stew with Root Veggies
Ingredients:

- 1 tbsp. rosemary
- 2 tbsps. olive oil
- 12 ounces (355 ml) dark beer
- 1 quart (950 ml) low sodium beef broth
- Half mug crushed tomatoes
- 2 tbsps. Without salt butter
- 1 mug onions, Peel offed and chopped
- One-Fourth mug all-purpose flour
- 1 mug (130 g) carrots, Peel offed and chopped
- Half mug celery, chopped
- 2-pound beef round fillet-steak, cut into pieces
- 2 tsps. black pepper, freshly ground, Cut up
- 2 bay leaves
- 1 tbsp. thyme
- 1 mug rutabaga, Peel offed and chopped
- 1 mug (133 g) parsnips, Peel offed and chopped

Instructions:

- Season the beef with 1 tsp. black pepper. Tie the bay leaves, thyme, and rosemary into cheesecloth. In a big frying pan, Merge the oil and butter and Warm up until the butter bubbles. Add the beef in one flat and not-too-tightly-packed layer and brown the beef well on all sides. Take away the beef, set aside, and add the onions and Prepare to a golden-caramelized color.
- Sprinkle the onions with the flour and whisk to Merge well. Put back the beef to the pan, add the beer, broth, herbs, crushed tomatoes, and left-over 1 tsp. pepper. Bring to a boil and decrease the Warm up to a slow simmer. Cover and Prepare for Third-Fourth hour. Add the carrots, celery, rutabaga, and parsnips and continue to Prepare for 1 additional hour.

Brown Rice Pot Roast
Ingredients:

- 1 mug celery, Diced
- 1 mug Poblano pepper, Diced
- 2 tbsps. all-purpose flour
- 1 tsp. garlic, minced
- 28 ounces no-salt-added tomatoes
- 6 mugs brown rice, prepared
- 2 Half-pound (1.1 kg) beef round roast
- One-Fourth tsp. cayenne pepper
- Half tsp. black pepper
- 2 tsps. olive oil
- 1 mug onion, Diced
- 1 mug low sodium beef broth
- Half tsp. parched thyme
- Half tsp. basil 1 bay leaf

Instructions:

- Prepare brown rice according to package directions. Rub meat all over with cayenne pepper and black pepper. In Dutch oven, Warm up oil and brown meat. Take out meat and Deep-fry veggies. Add flour to veggies and Prepare 2 minutes, whisking constantly. Add garlic, tomatoes, broth, thyme, basil, and bay leaf.
- Whisk until well blended. Put meat back in Dutch oven. Bring liquid to boil on high Warm up. Decrease Warm up to simmer, cover, and Prepare 2 Half to 3 hours. Take away bay leaf. Slice meat and serve dip sauce and veggies over both meat and brown rice.

Low fat Beef and Cabbage Stew
Ingredients:

- 2 mugs onion, diced
- 2 Half mugs cabbage
- 2 mugs no-salt-added tomatoes
- 2 mugs turnips, Peel offed and chopped
- 2 mugs carrot, diced
- 2 tbsps. all-purpose flour

- One-Fourth tsp. black pepper
- 1 Half-pound beef round fillet-steak
- 2 tbsps. oil
- 1 medium-sized potato, Peel offed and chopped
- 1 mug low sodium beef broth
- 2 tbsps. lemon juice

Instructions:

- Merge flour and black pepper. Cover meat with mixture. Brown meat in oil on all sides. Put veggies in slow Oven and Cover with meat.
- Add broth and lemon juice to frying pan. Whisk, scraping up browned bits from base. Spill over beef and veggies in Oven. Cover and Prepare on low for 8 hours.

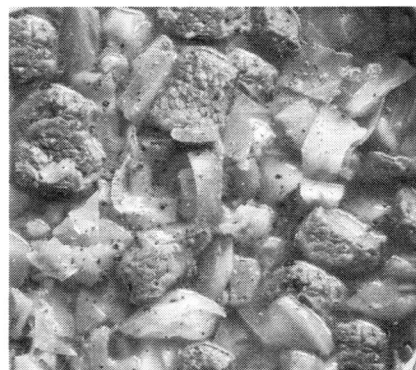

Mushrooms Eggplant Stew
Ingredients:

- 1 mug onion, Diced
- 2 tbsps. no-salt-added tomato paste
- One-Fourth tsp. red pepper
- 2-pound beef round fillet-steak, chopped
- 2 tbsps. olive oil
- 2 mugs no-salt-added tomatoes
- Half tsp. garlic powder
- 1 mug mineral water
- 1 medium-sized potato, Peel offed and chopped
- Half tsp. parched oregano
- Half tsp. parched basil

- Half tsp. ground cumin
- 1 mug white wine
- 2 eggplants, Peel offed and chopped
- 2 mugs cucumber, diced
- 8 ounces mushrooms, diced

Instructions:

- In a Dutch oven, brown half the beef at a time in the oil. Drain and put back all meat to the pan. Add tomatoes, onion, tomato paste, and spices. Whisk in mineral water. Bring to a boil. Decrease Warm up and simmer, covered, for 45 minutes.
- Add potato and wine. Cover and simmer 10 minutes more. Whisk in eggplant, cucumber, and mushrooms. Cover and simmer until meat and veggies are ripe, 15 to 20 minutes.

Garlic Smoked Roast
Ingredients:

- One-Fourth mug lemon juice
- 1 tbsp. garlic, minced
- 1 tbsp. Liquid Smoke
- 2 Half-pound (1.1 kg) beef round roast
- 2 mugs (475 ml) low sodium beef broth
- One-Fourth mug low sodium soy dip sauce
- 8 ounces egg noodles, prepared
- 6 mugs (600 g) green beans, prepared

Instructions:

- Put roast in roasting pan. Merge broth, soy dip sauce, lemon juice, garlic, and Liquid Smoke in dish. Combine well. Spill over roast.
- Marinate in fridge overnight. Bake covered at 300°F for 2 Half hours. Bake Unwrapped for 30 minutes longer. Serve with noodles and green beans.

Fillet-steak with Macaroni
Ingredients:

- 1 Half mugs onion, diced
- 1 mug Poblano pepper, cut in shreds
- 2-pound beef round fillet-steak
- One-Fourth tsp. black pepper
- 28 ounces low sodium spaghetti dip sauce
- 3 mugs cucumber, diced
- 12 ounces whole warm up macaroni, prepared

Instructions:

- Cut beef into serving sized pieces. Sprinkle with black pepper. Layer beef, onion, and Poblano pepper in slow Oven. Spill dip sauce over. Cover and Prepare on low for 8 to 10 hours. Whisk in cucumber, cover, turn Warm up to high, and Prepare for 15 to 20 minutes more until cucumber is ripe. While cucumber is Preparing, prepare macaroni according to package directions. Serve beef and vegetable mixture over macaroni.

Cheesy Spaghetti Bake
Ingredients:

- 16 ounces no-salt-added tomato dip sauce
- One-Fourth mug Parmesan cheese, grind
- 8 ounces mushrooms, Diced
- 1 tsp. parched oregano
- 1 pound extra lean ground beef
- Half mug Poblano pepper, Diced
- Half mug onion, Diced
- Half mug low fat mayonnaise
- Half tsp. black pepper
- Half tsp. garlic powder
- 7 ounces whole warm up spaghetti
- 1 mug low fat cheddar cheese, cut into small pieces,

Instructions:

- Switch on oven to 350°F. Brown meat with green bell pepper and onion; drain. Whisk in mayonnaise, tomato dip sauce, Parmesan cheese, mushrooms, oregano, black pepper, and garlic powder.

- Prepare 2 to 3 minutes over low Warm up or until thoroughly Warm upped. Put Half of the spaghetti in 2-quart casserole. Cover with Half of the meat mixture and Half mug (58 g) cheddar cheese. Repeat layers. Bake 30 minutes.

Low Sodium Poblano Macaroni
Ingredients:

- 2 mugs no-salt-added tomatoes, undrained
- 1 bay leaf
- 1 tsp. black pepper, or to taste dash cinnamon dash ground cloves
- Half tsp. parched basil
- Half tsp. parched oregano
- 2 slices bacon, low sodium
- Half pound extra lean ground beef, ground
- 1 mug Poblano pepper, Diced
- 8 ounces mushrooms, diced
- 1 mug onion, Diced
- 1 tsp. garlic, diced
- 6 ounces no-salt-added tomato paste
- One-Fourth mug red wine
- 6 ounces whole warm up spaghetti

Instructions:

- Deep-fry bacon in heavy frying pan. Crumble. Add beef, Poblano pepper, mushrooms, and onion. Prepare until meat is browned. Then add tomatoes (with juice), bay leaf, and seasonings. Simmer for 1 hour.
- Add tomato paste and wine and simmer for another 30 minutes. Take away bay leaf. Serve over macaroni.

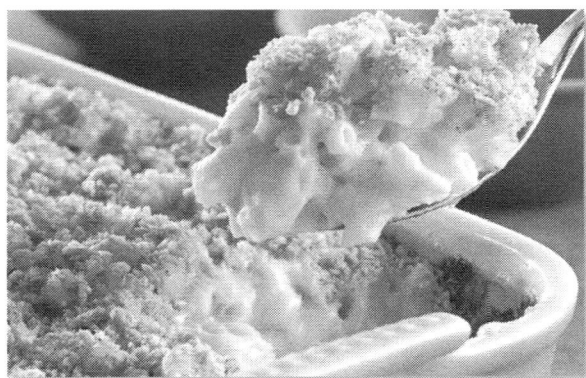

Cheddar Cheesy Lean Ground Beef Stacks
Ingredients:

- 5 ounces low fat cheddar cheese, grind
- 5 ounces low fat Cheddar Cheese, grind
- 4 ounces olives, diced
- 4 ounces green chilies, Diced
- 1 pound extra lean ground beef
- 1 package taco seasoning
- 5 whole warm up waffles,
- Half mug onion, Diced
- 1 tsp. olive oil

Instructions:

- Switch on oven to 350°F. Brown meat. Add taco seasoning according to directions on package. Layer waffles in pie pan Sprinkled with nonstick vegetable oil Sprinkle.
- Begin with waffles. Expand with One-Fourth of meat, cheeses, olives, chilies, and onion. Repeat 4 times. Brush Cover waffle with olive oil. Bake for 30 minutes or until Cover is golden brown.

Fajita Garlic Tacos
Ingredients:

- 1 Half mugs Poblano pepper
- 1 Half mugs Poblano pepper
- 1 mug onion, diced
- 8 corn waffles
- 2 tbsps. olive oil
- 2 tsps. ground cumin

- 1 tsp. garlic, minced
- 1-pound beef round fillet-steak, cut in shreds
- Half mug (130 g) warm sauce
- One-Fourth mug fat-free sour cream

Instructions:

- In a frying pan, Deep-fry olive oil, cumin, and garlic for 1 minute. Add fillet-steak shreds and Prepare about 5 minutes.
- Add green and Poblano pepper and onion slices and Prepare for another 8 minutes. Put mixture in waffles and fold. Cover with warm sauce and sour cream.

Kidney Beans Fillet-steak Salad
Ingredients:

- One-Fourth mug green onion, diced
- 8 ounces beef round fillet-steak, prepared and diced
- 1 small head iceberg green lettuce leaf, cut into small pieces
- 5 radishes, thinly diced
- Half mug sour cream
- Half mug (130 g) warm sauce
- 2 tbsps. cilantro, Cut up
- 1 mug (256 g) kidney beans, Soaked and drained
- Half mug (56 g) low fat Cheddar Cheese
- 1 avocado, Peel offed and diced
- 2 ounces waffle chips

Instructions:

- In a small dish, Merge sour cream, warm sauce, and 1 tbsp. cilantro; set aside. In a medium-sized dish, Merge beans, cheese, green onion, and left-over 1 tbsp. cilantro.
- To serve, Sort bean mixture, beef, green lettuce leaf, radishes, avocado, and waffle chips on four individual plates.

Serve Covered with the sour cream and warm sauce mixture.

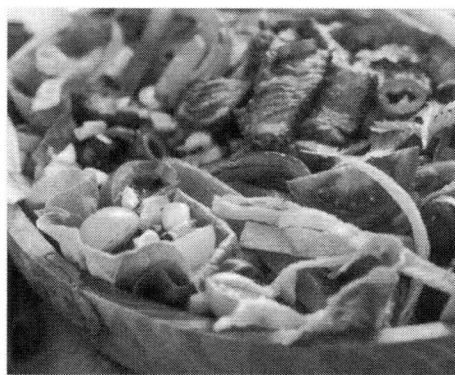

Asian Fillet-steak and Veggies
Ingredients:

- 2 tsps. parched bay leaf
- 1 tbsp. Worcestershire dip sauce
- 1 tbsp. dry mustard
- 1 tbsp. chili powder
- 4 mugs (720 g) no-salt-added tomatoes, Cut up
- 2 Half tsps. minced garlic, Cut up
- 1-pound beef round fillet-steak
- 1 mug onion, diced, Cut up
- Half mug celery, Diced, Cut up
- 1 mug Poblano pepper, diced in rings, Cut up
- 2 medium-sized baking potatoes
- 1-pound green beans, fresh

Instructions:

- Cut fillet-steak into serving-size pieces. Put fillet-steak pieces in ovenproof casserole. Cover with onion, celery, and Poblano pepper. Merge the bay leaf, Worcestershire dip sauce, dry mustard, chili powder, 2 mugs tomatoes, and 2 tsps. minced garlic. Spill over meat. Cover. Prepare at 350°F until fillet-steak is very ripe, about 1 Half hours.
- While fillet-steak is Preparing, bake or microwave the potatoes. Merge beans, 2 mugs tomatoes, and Half tsp. minced

garlic in a dip saucepan. Simmer until beans on done, about a half hour. Put One-Fourth of beans and fillet-steak and half of a potato on each plate. Serve dip sauce from fillet-steak over fillet-steak and potatoes.

Beef and Peppers Asian Style
Ingredients:

- 6 ounces no-salt-added tomato paste
- 6 mugs Poblano pepper, cut in cubes
- 2 mugs carrot, cut into 2-inch (5 cm) chunks
- 1 tbsp. caraway seed
- 1 Half mugs apple, Peel offed and chopped
- 2-pound beef round roast, cut to cubes
- 2 tbsps. all-purpose flour
- One-Fourth tsp. black pepper
- 2 tbsps. olive oil
- 3 mugs low sodium beef broth
- One-Third mug cider lemon juice
- One-Fourth mug fresh bay leaf, Diced
- 1 Half mugs gingersnaps, crushed
- 2 tbsps. brown Lactose alternative,

Instructions:

- Cover beef with flour combined with black pepper. In a big heavy dip sauce pot or Dutch oven, Warm up oil. Add beef; brown well on all sides, a few pieces at a time. Take away the browned beef and set aside. Whisk beef broth into the beef drippings in the dip sauce pots. Whisk in lemon juice and tomato paste.
- Prepare and whisk until mixture comes to a boil. Whisk well to get drippings off the base of the pot. Put back beef to pot. Bringing to a boil again. Decrease Warm up and simmer, covered, for 1 Half hours. Add Poblano pepper, carrot, and caraway seed. Bring mixture to a boiling point again.

- Decrease Warm up and simmer, covered, until meat and veggies are fork ripe, about 30 minutes. Whisk in apple, bay leaf, gingersnaps, and brown Lactose alternative. Cover and simmer for 5 minutes.

Pork Chops with Balsamic Glaze
Ingredients:

- Half tsp. kosher salt
- Half tsp. freshly ground black pepper
- Olive oil in a pump Sprinkler
- 4 (4-ounce) boneless pork loin chops, about Half inch thick
- 1 tbsp. finely Diced fresh rosemary
- One-Fourth mug balsamic lemon juice

Instructions:

- Sprinkle a big nonstick frying pan with oil and Warm up over medium-sized Warm up. Season the pork with the rosemary, salt, and pepper. Add to the frying pan and Prepare until the undersides are golden brown, about 3 minutes. Flip the pork and Prepare, adjusting the Warm up as needed so the pork Prepares steadily without burning, until the other sides are browned and the pork feels firm when pressed in the center with a fingertip, about 3 minutes more.
- Shift each chop to a dinner plate. Off Warm up, add the lemon juice to the frying pan. (Do not inhale the fumes, as they are strong.) Using a wooden Serve, scrape up the browned bits in the base of the frying pan. The residual Warm up of the frying pan should be enough to evaporate the lemon juice to about 2 tbsps. If mandatory, put back the frying pan to medium-sized Warm up to decrease the lemon juice slightly. Sprinkle the glaze over each chop and serve warm.

Sweet and Sour Beef Fillet
Ingredients:

- 2 tsp. Paprika
- One-Fourth mug Lactose alternative,
- Half mug cider lemon juice
- One-Fourth mug (85 g) molasses
- 2-pound beef round fillet-steak, cut into cubes
- 2 tbsps. olive oil
- 16 ounces no-salt-added tomato dip sauce
- 2 tsp. Chili Powder
- 2 mugs carrot, diced One-Fourth-inch (6 mm) thick
- 2 mugs onion, Diced
- 3 mugs Poblano pepper, cut into squares

Instructions:

- Brown meat in warm oil in frying pan; Shift to slow Oven. Add all left-over ingredients; combine well. Prepare for 6 to 7 hours on low setting. Serve immediately.

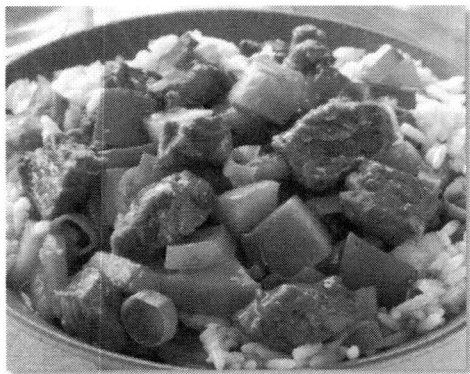

Steak Fillet and Vegetable Whisk-Fry
Ingredients:

- One-Fourth tsp. garlic, minced
- Half tsp. ground ginger
- Half mug low sodium beef broth
- 1 tbsp. cornstarch
- 1 Half-pound beef round fillet-steak
- 3 tbsps. low sodium soy dip sauce
- 2 tbsps. olive oil, Cut up

- One-Fourth tsp. black pepper
- 1 mug tomatoes, cut in pieces
- 1 mug Poblano pepper, cut in shreds
- 2 mugs mushrooms, diced
- 1 mug onion, diced
- 2 mugs brown rice, prepared

Instructions:

- Partially freeze beef. Slice diagonally into One-Fourth-inch (6 mm) thick slices. In a big dish, Merge soy dip sauce, 1 tbsp. oil (15 ml), and black pepper. Add beef. Roll to Cover well and marinate for several hours in the fridge. In a wok or big frying pan, whisk-fry the garlic and ginger in left-over oil for 1 minute.
- Add meat and whisk-fry until browned, about 4 minutes. Take away meat. Add all veggies except tomatoes and whisk-fry until crisp-ripe, about 2 minutes. Put back beef to wok. Merge left-over marinade, broth, and cornstarch. Spill over beef. Prepare and whisk until thickened. Add tomatoes and Warm up through. Serve over brown rice.

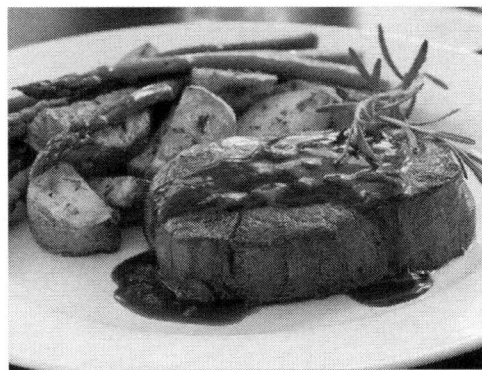

Roasted and Ginger Flank with Veggies
Ingredients:

- 3 tbsps. dry red wine
- 1 tbsp. honey
- 4 ears corn
- 4 Poblano peppers, halved

- 1-pound flank fillet-steak
- 1 tbsp. fresh ginger, minced
- 2 tsps. garlic, minced
- One-Fourth mug low sodium soy dip sauce
- 8 ounces mushrooms, whole

Instructions:

- Soak the meat and pat dry. Put fillet-steak in a 1-gallon (3.8 L) plastic freezer bag and add the left-over ingredients except the veggies. Seal bag and turn to Cover. Lightly oil a barbecue Roast and Switch on to very warm.
- Take away the fillet-steak from the bag, reserving marinade for veggies. Prepare fillet-steak, turning once, until done as you like it, about 15 minutes total for medium-sized-rare. To serve, slice diagonally across the grain into thin slices.
- Add husked corn, halved and seeded red bell peppers, and mushrooms to the marinade after removing the fillet-steak and then Prepare on the Roast, turning from time to time until slightly browned.

Chinese Pot Roast and Herbs
Ingredients:

- 2-pound beef chuck roast
- 1 tbsp. oil
- 2 tbsps. sherry
- Half tsp. garlic powder
- One-Fourth tsp. ground ginger
- 1 mug onion, diced into shreds
- 2 tsps. low sodium beef bouillon
- Half mug low sodium soy dip sauce
- 1 mug Poblano pepper, diced into shreds
- 1 mug carrot, diced
- Half pound green beans
- 3 tbsps. cornstarch
- 3 tbsps. cold mineral water

Instructions:

- Crop excess fat from roast. In a frying pan, brown beef on all sides in oil. Combine together broth, soy dip sauce, sherry, and spices.
- Put veggies in base of slow Oven. Put meat on Cover. Spill dip sauce over. Prepare on low for 8 to 10 hours or on high for 5 to 6 hours. Take away meat and veggies. Turn Warm up to high. Whisk cornstarch into mineral water.
- Add to slow Oven. Prepare until dip sauce is slightly thickened, about 15 to 20 minutes. Set apart meat into serving size pieces. Serve dip sauce over meat and veggies.

Low Calorie Beef and Tomato Curry
Ingredients:

- 1-pound beef round fillet-steak
- Half mug low sodium beef broth
- 1 Half mugs cucumber, diced
- 1 tsp. curry powder
- 1 tbsp. cornstarch
- 1 Half mugs tomatoes, coarsely Diced
- 1 mug Poblano pepper, cut in pieces
- 8 ounces mushrooms, diced
- 1 Half mugs onion, coarsely Diced
- 1 tbsp. mineral water
- 1 mug (195 g) brown rice, prepared according to package directions

Instructions:

- Cut meat into shreds. Sprinkle frying pan with nonstick vegetable oil Sprinkle. Prepare meat in broth until ripe. Add tomatoes, Peel offed and cut up, Poblano pepper, onion, mushrooms, cucumber, and curry powder and Warm up to boiling.
- Cover and Prepare on medium-sized for 3 to 5 minutes. Combine cornstarch and mineral water. Whisk into mixture and Prepare until thick and boiling. Serve over warm prepared brown rice.

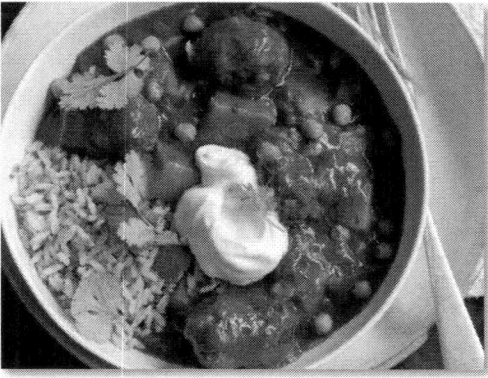

Corned Beef and Cabbage
Ingredients:

- 2 tbsps. olive oil
- 28 ounces no-salt-added stewed tomatoes
- One-Fourth tsp. cayenne pepper
- One-Fourth tsp. black pepper
- 1 big cabbage, diced in slices
- Half mug mineral waters
- 1 mug onion, cut in pieces
- 2 tbsps. Lactose alternative,
- 14 ounces corned beef

Instructions:

- In big pot, add diced cabbage and Half mug mineral water. Brew 10 minutes. In big frying pan, Deep-fry onion in oil until clear. Add stewed tomatoes.
- Add cayenne pepper, black pepper, and Lactose alternative. Prepare 20 minutes. Spill over cabbage. Prepare cabbage and tomato mixture 10 more minutes. Add corned beef and Prepare about 6 minutes longer or until cabbage is crisp-ripe.

Stuffed Pork Chops and Sweet Potatoes
Ingredients:

- 4 pork loin chops, thick
- 4 ounces corn bread stuffing combine
- 4 sweet potatoes
- 2 tbsps. (36 g) orange juice concentrate
- One-Fourth mug brown Lactose alternative,
- 2 tbsps. low sodium chicken broth
- One-Third mug orange juice
- 1 tbsp. pecans, finely Diced
- Half tsp. orange Peel off, grind

Instructions:

- With a sharp knife, cut a horizontal slit in side of each chop forming a pocket for stuffing. Merge stuffing with broth, orange juice, pecans and orange Peel off. Fill pockets with stuffing. Put in glass baking dish.
- Peel off sweet potatoes into cubes. Put in 8-inch (10 cm) square baking dish. Merge orange juice concentrate and brown Lactose alternative and Spill over sweet potatoes. Put both pans in a 350°F oven and bake until potatoes are ripe and pork chops are prepared through, about 45 to 60 minutes.

Dip Sauce Barbecued Chicken
Ingredients:

- 3 tbsps. Worcestershire dip sauce
- 1 tsp. dry mustard
- Half tsp. peppers
- 1 whole chicken, cut into pieces
- One-Fourth mug mineral water
- One-Fourth mug lemon juice
- 2 tbsps. onion, Diced

Instructions:

- Switch on oven to 350°F. Merge all ingredients except chicken in dip saucepan, Put over Warm up, and simmer for 5-10 minutes.
- Put chicken in a big baking pan. Spill half of the barbecue dip sauce over chicken and bake, Unwrapped, for about 45-60 minutes. Baste with left-over barbecue dip sauce every 15 minutes during Preparing.

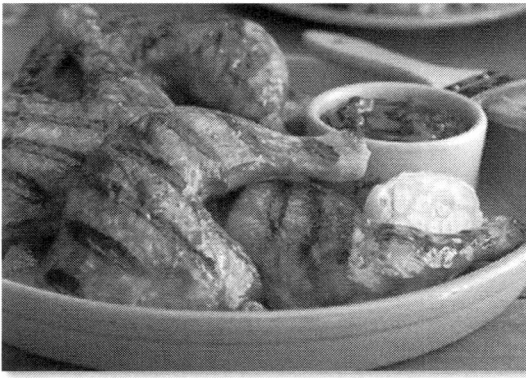

Chicken Crunchy Fingers

Ingredients:

- 1 tbsp. (1.3 g) bay leaf flakes
- One-Eighth tsp. garlic powder
- 12 ounces boneless skinless chicken breast halves, cut into 1 x 3-inch shreds
- One-Third mug cornflake crumbs
- Half mug pecans, finely Diced
- 2 tbsps. fat free milk

Instructions:

- In a shallow dish, Merge cornflake crumbs, pecans, bay leaf, and garlic powder. Dip chicken in milk and then roll in crumb mixture.
- Put in a baking pan. Bake in a 400°F oven for 7-9 minutes or until chicken is ripe and no longer pink.

Chicken Breasts Stuffed with Cheddar Cheese

Ingredients:

- One-Eighth tsp. black pepper, coarse ground
- 6 boneless skinless chicken breasts
- Third-Fourth mug (83 g) Cheddar Cheese, cut into small pieces
- Half mug ricotta cheese
- 1 tbsp. (4.3 g) thyme
- 2 tsps. Without salt butter

Instructions:

- In small dish, fold together Swiss and ricotta cheeses, thyme, and cracked black pepper. Put a chicken breast on flat surface. Cut a 21-inch (6 cm) horizontal slit into side of chicken breast to form a pocket.
- Repeat procedure with left-over breasts. Stuff each pocket with 2 tbsps. cheese mixture. Defrost butter in frying pan. Add chicken to frying pan and Prepare 6 minutes. Turn; decrease Warm up to medium-sized and Prepare 4-5 minutes until chicken is prepared through.

Curried Honey Chicken and Apples

Ingredients:

- 3 tbsps. oil
- Half mug celery, diced
- One-Fourth mug raisins
- 2 boneless skinless chicken breasts
- 2 tbsps. (42 g) honey
- 2 tsps. curry powder
- 2 apples, Peel offed and Diced
- 3 tbsps. fresh bay leaf

Instructions:

- Cut chicken into cubes and Put in dish. Merge honey and curry and combine with chicken. Whisk in apples.
- Warm up oil in heavy frying pan over high Warm up. Deep-fry celery for 1 minute. Add apple mixture and whisk-fry 3-4 minutes, just until chicken is no longer pink. Add raisins and bay leaf, whisk well, and serve over brown rice.

Chicken Breasts with Balsamic Dip sauce

Ingredients:

- 4 chicken breast halves
- 1 tbsp. shallots, finely Diced
- 3 tbsps. balsamic lemon juice
- Half tsp. salts

- One-Fourth tsp. black pepper
- 2 tbsps. butter, Cut up
- 1 tbsp. vegetable oil
- 1 Half mugs (355 ml) chicken broth
- 2 tsps. finely Diced fresh marjoram

Instructions:

- Sprinkle chicken with pepper. Warm up 1 tbsp. butter and the oil in big, heavy frying pan over high Warm up. Add chicken, skin side down, and Prepare until skin is crisp.
- Decrease Warm up to medium-sized-low; turn chicken breasts over and Prepare until chicken is no longer pink inside, about 12 minutes. Shift chicken to Warm upped platter and keep warm in oven. Spill off all but 1 tbsp. fat from frying pan.
- Add shallots and Prepare over medium-sized-low Warm up for 3 minutes or until translucent, scraping up any browned bits. Add lemon juice and bring to a boil. Boil for 3 minutes or until decreased to a glaze, whisking constantly. Add broth and boil until decreased to 2 mugs (120 ml), whisking from time to time. Season to taste with salt and pepper.
- Take away dip sauce from Warm up and Whip in left-over butter and marjoram. Whip in any juices from chicken. Serve dip sauce over chicken and serve instantly.

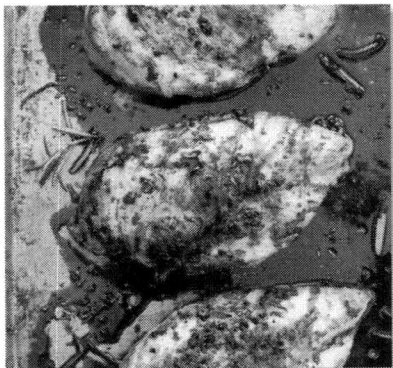

Mozzarella Lasagna Pie
Ingredients:

- 1 tbsp. fat free milk
- 1 mug cucumber, diced
- 1 mug Poblano pepper, diced
- 1 mug onion, diced
- 1 mug fresh mozzarella, grind
- 1 pound extra lean ground beef
- 1 mug (245 g) low sodium spaghetti dip sauce
- One-Third mug (85 g) ricotta cheese
- 3 tbsps. Parmesan cheese, grind
- Half mug all-purpose flour
- Third-Fourth tsp. baking powder
- 2 tbsps. Without salt butter
- 1 mug fat free milk
- Half mug egg alternative

Instructions:

- Switch on oven to 400°F. Grease a pie plate. Prepare beef in a 10-inch (25 cm) frying pan over medium-sized Warm up, whisking from time to time, until brown; drain. Whisk in Half mug (123 g) spaghetti dip sauce; Warm up until bubbly. Whisk together ricotta cheese, Parmesan cheese, and 1 tbsp. fat free milk.
- Expand half of the beef mixture in pie plate. Drop cheese mixture by Servetus's onto the beef mixture. Cover with veggies. Sprinkle with Half mug of the mozzarella cheese.
- Cover with left-over beef mixture. Whisk together flour and baking powder. Cut in butter. Whisk in fat free milk and egg alternative until blended. Spill into pie plate. Bake 30 to 35 minutes or until knife inserted in center comes out wipe. Sprinkle with left-over Half mug mozzarella cheese. Bake 2 to 3 minutes longer or until cheese is Defrosted.

Veggie Oregano Fajitas
Ingredients:

- 2 big portobello mushrooms about 6 inches in diameter
- 2 big white onions, diced
- 3 tbsps. Extra virgin olive oil
- 3 cloves garlic, minced
- 3 big Poblano peppers, cut into shreds
- 3 big Poblano peppers, cut into shreds
- 3 big yellow bell peppers, cut into shreds
- 2 big green cucumbers, cut into shreds
- 1 Half 210spas. Parched oregano
- One-Fourth tsp. ground cumin
- One-Eighth tsp. cracked black pepper
- One-Eighth tsp. sea salt
- 8 corn waffles

Instructions:

- Cut the bell peppers into Half-inch shreds. Cut the cucumber longitudinally into thin shreds, and then cut each shred in half. Wipe the mushrooms with a damp towel, snap the stems off, scoop the gills out with a metal tbsp., and cut into Half-inch shreds. Cut the onions into Half-inch slices. Warm up the oil in a big pot over medium-sized-high Warm up.
- Once the oil is warm, add the bell peppers, cucumber, mushrooms, onions, garlic, oregano, cumin, pepper, and salt. Prepare until the herbs are soft and the onions translucent, about 5 to 6 minutes. Warm the waffles in a flat pan over medium-sized Warm up, Serve in the herbs. Fold the waffle over and serve. Serving Suggestion: Serve with black beans and be creative with Coverings, such as plain Greek curd (in Put of sour cream), warm sauce, cut into small pieces green lettuce leaf, guacamole, or low-fat cut into small pieces cheese.

Spicy Chicken with Green Onions
Ingredients:

- 2 tbsps. vegetable oil
- 1 tbsp. Tabasco dip sauce
- 2 tsps. honey
- 1 tsp. paprika
- 7 green onions
- 2 chicken breasts, boned and skinned

Instructions:

- Prepare the Roast (medium-sized-high Warm up). Whip oil, Tabasco, honey, and paprika in a 9-inch (23 cm) glass pie dish to blend. Mince 1 green onion and combine into marinade. Shift 2 tbsps. (30 ml) of the marinade to a small dish and reserve.
- Add chicken to the pie dish marinade and turn to Cover. Let stand 10 minutes, turning from time to time. Roast chicken and whole onions until chicken is prepared through and onions soften, turning from time to time, about 10 minutes. Shift chicken and Roasted onions to plates and Sprinkle with 1 tbsp. each of the marinade.

Low Calories Chicken with Avocado and Tomato
Ingredients:

- 2 avocados
- 1 mug tomatoes, Diced
- 2 tbsps. (42 g) Without salt butter, Defrosted
- 4 boneless skinless chicken breasts
- Half mug sour cream
- Half mug (58 g) Cheddar Cheese cut into small pieces

Instructions:

- Slice chicken l/2-inch (1 cm) thick. In big frying pan, Warm up butter on medium-sized-high. Add chicken slices and Deep-fry 3-5 minutes, until they start to turn brown. Switch on oven to 350°F. Peel off, pit, and thinly slice avocado.

- In medium-sized casserole, layer chicken, avocado, and tomato. Cover with sour cream. Sprinkle with cheese. Bake 30 minutes.

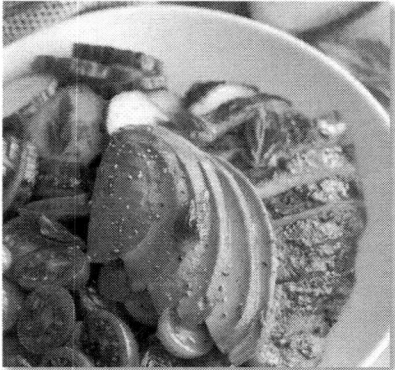

Delicious Roasted Roasting Chicken
Ingredients:

- 1 big roasting chicken, 5 to 6 pounds (2 to 2Third-Fourth kg)
- 2 tbsps. olive oil
- 1 tsp. paprika
- 1 tsp. onion powder
- Half tsp. black pepper
- Half tsp. thyme
- One-Fourth tsp. garlic powder
- 1 tsp. liquid smoke

Instructions:

- Split chicken in half along the backbone and breastbone. Combine together left-over ingredients and rub into both sides of chicken halves.
- Roast over indirect Warm up, turning from time to time, until done, 1 to 2 hours. Put over low Warm up for the last 15 minutes to brown skin.

Amazing Chicken in Sour Cream Dip sauce
Ingredients:

- 2 pounds boneless skinless chicken breast
- Half mug (2 g) Without salt butter
- 2 tbsps. fresh bay leaf
- Half tsp. thyme
- 1 tbsp. green pepper, finely Diced
- Half-pint fat-free sour cream
- Half mug sherry
- Half tsp. rosemary
- Pepper to taste
- Half mug slivered almonds

Instructions:

- Brown chicken in butter in frying pan. Put in casserole. Add sour cream and sherry to chicken drippings. Add left-over ingredients and simmer 10 minutes.
- Spill mixture over chicken pieces. Bake 350°F for 1 hour.

Tasty Chicken Breasts Baked in Creamy Herb Dip sauce
Ingredients:

- Half tsp. oregano
- One-Fourth tsp. celery seed
- One-Fourth tsp. garlic powder
- One-Fourth tsp. coriander
- 4 boneless skinless chicken breasts
- 1 mug plain curd
- One-Fourth mug sour cream
- Half tsp. lime Peel off, grind
- One-Fourth tsp. bay leaf
- One-Fourth tsp. thyme
- 3 tbsps. lime juice

Instructions:

- Switch on oven to 375°F Sprinkle roasting pan with nonstick vegetable oil Sprinkle, put chicken breasts in it, and set aside. Merge all other ingredients. Baste chicken breasts with mixture and bake for 20 minutes.

- Take away from oven. Turn chicken breasts, baste with dip sauce, and bake 15 minutes longer until meat is ripe. Turn off oven. Cover chicken with foil and let stand in oven 10 minutes. Take away aluminum foil, Sort chicken breasts on serving dish, and serve warm with any left-over dip sauce.

Chicken and Mushroom Risotto
Ingredients:

- Half mug carrot, diced
- 1 mug (185 g) long grain brown rice, unprepared
- 14Half ounces (410 g) low-sodium chicken broth
- 2 tbsps. Without salt butter, Cut up
- Third-Fourth pound boneless skinless chicken breasts, cut in cubes
- Half mug onion, finely Diced
- Half mug frozen peas

Instructions:

- In 3-quart dip saucepan over medium-sized-high Warm up, in 1 tbsp. Defrosted butter, prepare chicken until browned, whisking often. Take away; set aside. In same dip saucepan, add left-over butter.
- Decrease Warm up to medium-sized; Prepare onion, carrot, and brown rice until brown rice is browned, whisking constantly. Whisk in broth, soup, and pepper. Warm up to boiling. Decrease Warm up to low. Cover; Prepare 15 minutes, whisking from time to time. Add peas and chicken. Cover; Prepare 5 minutes or until chicken is no longer pink, brown rice is ripe, and liquid is absorbed, whisking from time to time.

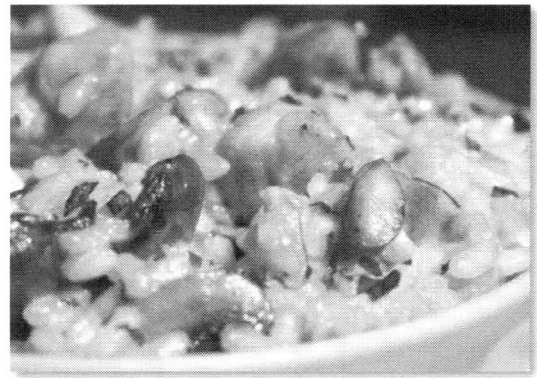

Basil Chicken Alfredo
Ingredients:

- 2 tbsps. Parched basil
- 1 slice low-sodium bacon, prepared and crushed
- 8 ounces no-salt-added tomato dip sauce
- 2 boneless chicken breasts, cut in chunks
- Half mug Diced tomato
- 1 mug diced mushrooms
- 2 cloves garlic, minced
- 2 tbsps. Grind Parmesan cheese
- 4 ounces half-and-half

Instructions:

- Deep-fry the chicken in olive oil until browned. Turn chicken and add tomato, mushrooms, and garlic and Prepare on medium-sized Warm up until the mushrooms start to darken. Add basil, bacon, tomato dip sauce, and Parmesan.
- Warm up on low for 15 minutes. Take away from Warm up. Add half-and-half to mixture. Combine well. Serve over macaroni.

White Wine Macaroni with Chicken and Broccoli
Ingredients:

- 2 garlic cloves, minced
- 1 Half mugs (107 g) broccoli florets
- 1 tsp. parched basil

- One-Fourth mug olive oil
- Half-pound boneless skinless chicken breasts, cut in l/2-inch (1 cm) shreds
- Half-pound (227 g) bow tie macaroni, prepared
- One-Fourth mug white wine
- Third-Fourth mug low-sodium chicken broth

Instructions:

- In a big frying pan, Warm up oil over medium-sized Warm up. Deep-fry garlic for about one minute, whisking constantly. Add the chicken and Prepare until well done. Add the broccoli and Prepare until crisp but ripe.
- Add basil. Add pepper to taste, wine, and chicken broth. Prepare for about 5 minutes. Add the prepared and drained macaroni to the frying pan and Roll to Merge. Warm up for 1 to 2 minutes. Serve. Cover with grind Parmesan cheese if prepare you want.

Asian Chicken Thighs
Ingredients:

- 1 tsp. garlic powder
- 1 tsp. paprika
- 1 tsp. bay leaf
- 4 chicken thighs
- 1 mug Diced onion
- 1 can (8 ounces or 225 g) no-salt-added tomato dip sauce
- One-Fourth mug mineral water
- 1 tsp. basil
- 1 tsp. black pepper

Instructions:

- Merge spices in a plastic bag. Add chicken pieces and shake to Cover evenly. Put chicken and onion in frying pan with a lid. Add mineral water.

- Cover and Prepare for 10 minutes. Turn and Prepare 10 minutes more. Spill tomato dip sauce over and continue Preparing until done through, about 10 more minutes. Serve with macaroni or brown rice. Serve dip sauce and onion mixture over Cover.

Thai Curried Veggies
Ingredients:

- 2 tbsps. coconut oil
- 1 tsp. curry powder
- Half tsp. ground cinnamon
- Half tsp. ground turmeric
- Half tsp. cracked black pepper
- 2 mugs unsweetened light coconut milk
- Half mug low-sodium vegetable broth
- 1 medium-sized onion, cut into One-Fourth-inch pieces
- 1 medium-sized Poblano pepper, coarsely Diced
- 1 medium-sized Poblano pepper, coarsely Diced
- 1 mug coarsely Diced broccoli
- 3–4 mugs chopped eggplant, Half-inch pieces
- 1 small jalapeño chile pepper, thinly diced (seeded for less Warm up)
- 1 tbsp. Diced fresh ginger
- 2 big cloves garlic, coarsely Diced
- 1 heaping tbsp. Without salt peanut butter
- 4 tbsps. coarsely Diced Thai basil

Instructions:

- Warm up a big pot over medium-sized Warm up, and add the coconut oil. Once it has Defrosted, add the onion, bell peppers, and broccoli, whisking constantly. Add the eggplant, chile pepper, ginger, garlic, curry powder, cinnamon, turmeric, and pepper. Whisk to incorporate the ingredients and spices and Prepare until the eggplant browns and the veggies soften a bit, about 4 to 5 minutes.

- Add the coconut milk, broth, and peanut butter. Whisk well to incorporate the peanut butter, and then cover the pot. Simmer on low for about 10 minutes. Then Take away the lid, and simmer Unwrapped for an additional 5 minutes, or until the dip sauce thickens to the if you want consistency. Whisk in the basil right before serving. Serving Suggestion: Scoop Half mug of prepared brown rice into individual dishes, and Cover each with a big ladleful of herbs and dip sauce.

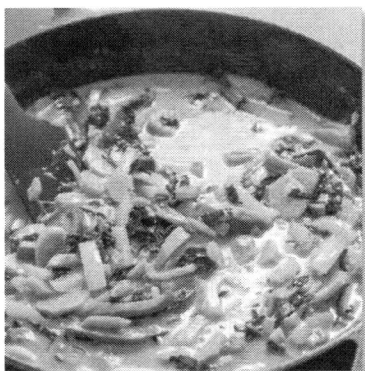

Mexican Crave Special Pizza
Ingredients:

- 1 (12-inch) prebaked 100% whole warm up thin-crust pizza
- 1 small cucumber, thinly diced in rounds
- Half mug thinly diced red onion
- Half mug diced Poblano pepper
- Half mug Soaked and drained canned black beans
- 1 tbsp. canned chipotle pepper dip sauce
- 3 tbsps. mineral water
- Half mug cut into small pieces skim mozzarella cheese
- Half tsp. parched oregano

Instructions:

- Switch on the oven to 400°F. In a blender or food processor, Merge the black beans, chipotle dip sauce, and mineral water. Puree until smooth.
- Evenly Expand the mixture on the pizza crust. Cover with cucumber rounds, then bell peppers and onions, and finally cheese. Sprinkle oregano on Cover, and bake for about 15 minutes, or until the cheese is bubbling and browning.

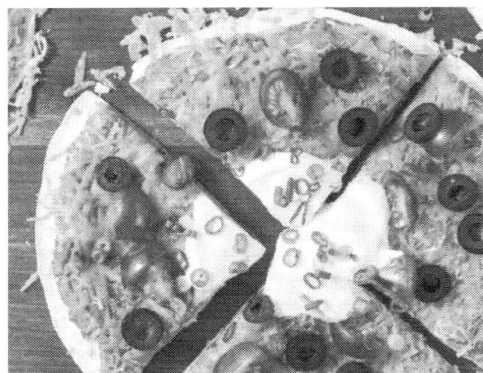

Cauliflower, Garlic and Carrot Soup
Ingredients:

- 1 mug Diced carrot
- 1 quart low-sodium vegetable broth
- Half tsp. sea salt
- 1 big head cauliflower, coarsely Diced (about 8 mugs)
- 2 tbsps. Extra virgin olive oil
- Half small white onion, Diced
- 2 big cloves garlic, Diced
- Half tsp. cracked black pepper
- One-Eighth tsp. chile pepper flakes
- One-Eighth tsp. parched basil

Instructions:

- Fill a big pot with mineral water, and bring it to a boil. Take away the outer leaves of the cauliflower head, and then cut out the core. Coarsely chop the cauliflower, and add it to the boiling mineral water. Cover the pot, and boil

214

for 6 or 8 minutes, or until a fork easily pierces the cauliflower pieces.

- Strain the cauliflower, and discard the mineral water. Warm up the oil in the same pot over medium-sized Warm up. Add the onion, garlic, and carrot, and Deep-fry until the onion is translucent. Add the cauliflower. Shift a ladleful of herbs to a blender.
- Add 1 mug of broth, and blend on low to Merge, then on high until smooth. Shift the blended herbs to another big pot, and repeat the process until all the herbs are blended. Warm up the blended herbs over medium-sized-high Warm up, and season with salt, pepper, chile pepper flakes, and basil. Bring to a boil, and serve warm.

Roasted Butternut Squash Soup
Ingredients:

- 2 Half liters low-sodium vegetable or chicken broth, Cut up
- One-Eighth tsp. cracked black pepper
- One-Fourth tsp. white pepper
- 1 big butternut squash or 2 (16-ounce) bags precut butternut
- squash (to skip the roasting)
- 2 tbsps. extra virgin olive oil
- 1 big clove garlic
- Half white onion, Diced
- 1 tbsp. Diced fresh bay leaf
- One-Fourth tsp. chile pepper flakes
- 1 tsp. finely Diced fresh rosemary
- 3–4 finely minced fresh sage leaves

Instructions:

- The squash can be roasted a day or two ahead. Just store the roasted squash in an airtight canister in the fridge. Switch on the oven to 400°F. Cut off the Cover of the squash, and then cut the squash in half longitudinally, and scoop out the seeds from the center with a metal

Serve until there are no strings or seeds left.

- Cover a Prepare sheet with olive oil Sprinkle, and Put the squash on it, cut sides down.
- Roast in the oven for about 30 minutes, or until the squash is soft to the touch. Take away from the oven, and let cool completely. In a big pot over medium-sized Warm up, add the oil, garlic, and onion. Deep-fry a few minutes, until the onion turns light brown. While the onion and garlic are Preparing, scoop out the roasted squash from its skin with a Serve, and add to the pot. Combine together, using a spatula to Split up big chunks of squash. Add 1 liter of broth, and bring to a boil.
- Decrease the Warm up to low, and Shift the herbs in batches to a blender, leaving most of the liquid in the pot.
- Blend the squash on low to combine, and then on high until smooth. If the squash won't blend easily, add a bit of the broth.
- Once all the squash has been blended, put back it to the pot, add the rest of the broth as well as the black pepper, white pepper, bay leaf, chili pepper flakes, rosemary and sage. Bring the soup to a boil and serve warm. Serving Suggestion: Swirl a tsp. of low-fat sour cream or curd into each dish of soup, and then sprinkle fresh bay leaf on Cover before serving.

Beef Salad with Beets and Horseradish
Ingredients:

- 1 big Rome apple, cored and cut into Pieces
- 1 scallion, white and green parts, finely Diced
- 4 medium-sized beets (1 pound),
- 2 tbsps. cider lemon juice

- 1 Half tbsps. pared and freshly grind horseradish
- 12 ounces thinly diced Spiced Roast Eye of Round

Instructions:

- Switch on the oven to 400°F. Wrap each beet in aluminum foil and Put-on a rimmed baking sheet. Bake until the beets are ripe when pierced with the tip of a small, sharp knife, about 1 One-Fourth hours.
- Unwrap and let cool. Peel off the beets and cut into Pieces. In a medium-sized dish, Whip together the lemon juice and horseradish, then Whip in the oil. Add the beets, apple, and scallion and combine well.
- Cover and freeze until cool downed, at least 1 hour or up to 1 day. Cut up the beet salad among four dinner plates and Cover with equal amounts of the diced roast beefs. Serve cool downed.

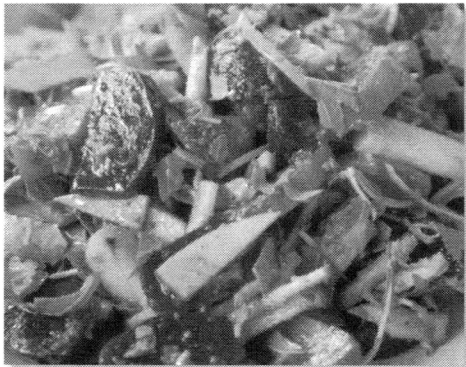

Low Fat Chicken Salad with Romaine
Ingredients:

- One-Eighth tsp. freshly ground black pepper
- 8 ounces Basic Roast Chicken Breast 101 or Classic Poached Chicken
- 1 scallion, white and green parts, finely Diced
- 2 tbsps. light mayonnaise
- 2 tbsps. plain low-fat curd
- One-Fourth tsp. kosher salt
- 4 romaine green lettuce leaf leaves, for serving

Instructions:

- In a medium-sized dish, Merge the mayonnaise, curd, salt (if using), and pepper. Add the chicken, celery, and scallion and combine well. (The salad can be freeze in a covered canister for up to 2 days.) Serve equal portions of the chicken salad onto two plates, add the green lettuce leaf, and serve.

Light Calories Chicken Salad with Grapes
Ingredients:

- 3 tbsps. plain low-fat curd
- One-Fourth tsp. freshly ground black pepper
- 8 ounces Basic Roast Chicken Breast
- 2 medium-sized celery ribs, thinly diced
- 2 tbsps. light mayonnaise
- 2 tsps. finely Diced fresh tarragon
- Pinch of kosher salt
- One-Fourth mug diced almonds; Heat upped 2 mugs (2 ounces) combined
- salad greens
- Lemon pieces, for serving

Instructions:

- In a medium-sized dish, Whip the curd, mayonnaise, tarragon, salt, and pepper. Add the chicken, grapes, celery, and almonds and combine well.
- Cut up the salad greens between two salad dishes. Cover each with half of the chicken mixture. Serve instantly with the lemon pieces for squeezing the juice over the salad.

Autumn Salad with Apples and Cranberries
Ingredients:

- 10 ounces prepared turkey breast
- Lemon, and Garlic Cloves, cut into Pieces (2 mugs) 2 sweet apples
- One-Fourth mug buttermilk
- 2 tbsps. light mayonnaise
- One-Fourth tsp. kosher salt
- One-Fourth tsp. freshly ground black pepper
- One-Fourth mug parched cranberries
- One-Fourth mug Without salt raw sunflower seeds
- 5 mugs (4 ounces) combined salad greens

Instructions:

- In a medium-sized dish, Whip together the buttermilk, mayonnaise, salt, and pepper. Add the turkey, apples, parched cranberries, and sunflower seeds and combine well. (The salad may be stored freeze in a covered canister for up to 1 day.) Cut up the greens among four salad dishes. Cover each with equal amounts of the salad and serve instantly.

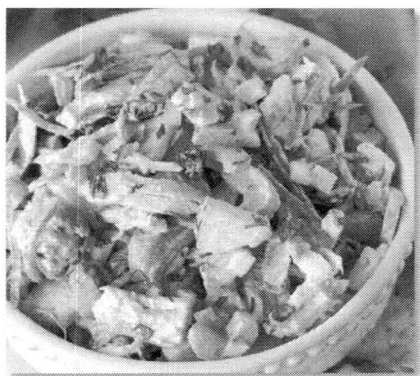

Old-style Sweet and Sour Chicken
Ingredients:

- One-Fourth mug brown rice lemon juice
- 4 tsps. cornstarch
- 1 tbsp. low sodium soy dip sauce
- 1-pound boneless skinless chicken breasts, cut in shreds
- 16 ounces frozen Asian vegetable combine

- two-thirds mug pineapple juice
- 2 mugs (330 g) pineapple chunks, in juice
- 2 mugs brown rice, prepared

Instructions:

- Sprinkle 10-inch (25 cm) frying pan with nonstick vegetable oil Sprinkle and whisk-fry chicken until done. Meanwhile, prepare veggies according to package directions. In small dish, Merge pineapple juice, brown rice lemon juice, cornstarch, and soy dip sauce.
- Add pineapple chunks to prepared chicken and then add prepared veggies. Spill in dip sauce mixture. Prepare over medium-sized Warm up until thick and bubbly. Serve over brown rice.

Smooth Macaroni with Chicken and Veggies
Ingredients:

- 10 ounces whole warm up linguine, or spaghetti
- 2 tbsps. olive oil
- 2 mugs cucumber, cut in shreds
- Half tsp. parched basil
- 1 mug fat free milk
- 2 mugs chicken breast, prepared and chopped
- One-Eighth tsp. black pepper
- 1 mug roam tomatoes, diced
- 12 ounces mushrooms, diced
- 2 mugs broccoli florets
- 1 mug onion, Diced
- Half tsp. garlic, minced
- One-Fourth mug Parmesan cheese

Instructions:

- Prepare linguini or spaghetti in step with package directions. In a frying pan, Warm up oil. Add cucumber, mushrooms, broccoli, onion, garlic, and basil. Prepare and whisk until cucumber is crisp-ripe, about two to 3 minutes.

- Drain macaroni and put back to dip saucepan. Whisk in fat free milk, chicken, cucumber mixture, and black pepper and Warm up through. Add tomatoes and cheese. Roll and serve.

Shrimp, Olive and Black Bean Salad
Ingredients:

- 2 ripe mangoes, pitted, Peel offed, and cut into Pieces 1 (15-ounce) can
- decreased-sodium black beans,
- 2 tbsps. olive oil, plus more in a pump Sprinkler
- ¾ pound big shrimp (16 to 20), Peel offed and deveined
- 2 tbsps. fresh lime juice
- Half jalapeño, seeded and minced
- 2 tbsps. finely Diced fresh cilantro or mint
- 2 tbsps. minced red onion

Instructions:

- Sprinkle a big ridged Roast pan with oil and Warm up over medium-sized Warm up. Add the shrimp to the pan. (Or position a broiler rack about 4 inches from the source of Warm up and Switch on the broiler.)
- Sprinkle the broiler rack with oil and Expand the shrimp on the rack.) Prepare, turning from time to time, until the shrimp are opaque throughout, 3 to 5 minutes. Freeze to cool completely, about 20 minutes. In a big serving dish, Whip together the lime juice and the 2 tbsps. oil. Add the shrimp, mango, beans, jalapeño, cilantro, and onion and Roll gently. Serve instantly.

Chicken with Avocado, Tomato and cauliflower florets
Ingredients:

- 4 boneless skinless chicken breasts
- 2 tbsps. olive oil, Defrosted
- 2 avocados
- 1 mug cauliflower florets, Brewed until crisp-ripe
- Half mug (61 g) carrot, diced and Brewed
- 1 mug tomatoes, Diced
- Half mug fat-free sour cream
- Half mug (58 g) low fat Cheddar Cheese, cut into small pieces
- 1 mug broccoli florets, Brewed until crisp-ripe

Instructions:

- Slice chicken thick. In big frying pan, Warm up oil on medium-sized-high. Add chicken slices and Deep-fry 3 to 5 minutes until they start to turn brown. Switch on oven to 350°F. Peel off, pit, and thinly slice avocado.
- Cut tomatoes into thin pieces. In medium-sized casserole, layer chicken, avocado, and tomato. Cover with sour cream. Sprinkle with cheese. Bake 30 minutes. Serve with Brewed veggies.

Healthy Watermelon, Basil, and Shrimp Salad
Ingredients:

- 6 mugs seedless mineral watermelon cubes, cut into squares, cool downed
- Half medium-sized red onion, cut into thin half-moons
- Olive oil in a pump Sprinkler
- 1-pound big shrimp (21 to 25), Peel offed and deveined
- 24 big basil leaves, cut into thin shreds (One-Fourth mug packed)

Instructions:

- Sprinkle a big nonstick frying pan with oil and Warm up over medium-sized-high Warm up. Add the shrimp and Prepare, whisking from time to time, until opaque throughout, about 3 minutes. Shift to a plate and let cool.

- Cover and freeze until cool downed, at least 1 hour. In a big serving dish, combine the mineral watermelon, onion, and basil. Add the shrimp and vinaigrette and Roll gently. Serve cool downed.

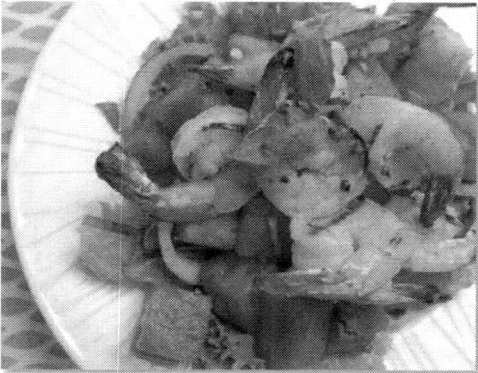

Delicious Tuna and Vegetable Salad
Ingredients:

- 1 small scallion, white part only, finely Diced
- 2 tbsps. light mayonnaise
- 1 (5-ounce) can low-sodium tuna in mineral water, drained
- 2 small celery ribs, finely chopped
- 1 small carrot, cut into small pieces
- 2 tsps. Diced fresh bay leaf or dill

Instructions:

- In a small dish, combine all of the ingredients, including the bay leaf, if using. (The salad can be freeze in a covered canister for up to 2 days.). Garnish with green chili and mint. Serve immediately.

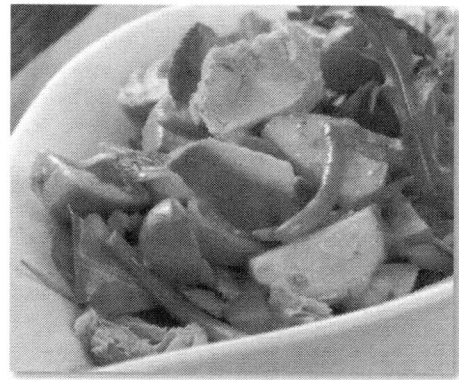

Pork Chops in Mustard Dip sauce
Ingredients:

- 2 tsps. cornstarch
- Half mug Homemade Chicken Broth or canned low-sodium chicken broth Half mug
- low-fat (1%) milk
- 1 tbsp. Spicy Brown Mustard
- Canola oil in a pump Sprinkler
- 6 (4-ounce) boneless pork loin chops, about Half inch thick
- Half tsp. kosher salt
- Half tsp. freshly ground black pepper
- 1 tbsp. Without salt butter
- 2 tbsps. minced shallots
- 2 tsps. Diced fresh tarragon, rosemary, or chives

Instructions:

- Sprinkle a big nonstick frying pan with oil and Warm up over medium-sized Warm up. Season the pork with the salt and pepper and add to the frying pan. Prepare until the undersides are golden brown, about 3 minutes. Flip the pork and Prepare until the other sides are golden brown and the meat feels firm when pressed in the thickest part with a fingertip, about 3 minutes more. Shift to a plate.
- Meanwhile, in a small dish Whip the cornstarch into the broth. Add the milk and mustard and Whip again; set aside.

- Defrost the butter in the frying pan over medium-sized Warm up. Add the shallots and Prepare, whisking often, until ripe, about 2 minutes. Whip the broth mixture again, Spill into the frying pan, and bring to a boil.
- Put back the pork and any juices on the plate to the frying pan and Prepare, turning from time to time, until the dip sauce thickens, about 1 minute. Shift the pork to a deep platter and cut each chop in half. Spill the dip sauce over the pork chops and sprinkle with the tarragon. Serve warm.

Pork with Sweet-and-Sour Cabbage
Ingredients:

- Red Cabbage
- 1 slice decreased-sodium bacon, coarsely Diced
- One-Fourth mug mineral water
- 3 tbsps. grade B maple syrup One-Fourth tsp. kosher salt
- One-Fourth tsp. freshly ground black pepper
- Pork Chops
- Canola oil in a pump Sprinkler
- 1 tsp. canola oil
- 1 medium-sized yellow onion, Diced
- 1 small red cabbage (1 One-Fourth pounds), cored and thinly diced
- One-Fourth mug cider lemon juice
- 2 Granny Smith apples, cored and cut into Pieces
- 4 (4-ounce) boneless center-cut pork chops, excess fat Cropped
- One-Fourth tsp. kosher salt
- One-Fourth tsp. freshly ground black pepper

Instructions:

- To prepare the red cabbage: In a medium-sized dip saucepan over medium-sized Warm up, Prepare the

bacon in the oil, whisking from time to time, until the bacon is crisp and brown, about 5 minutes. Add the onion and Prepare, whisking from time to time, until golden, about 5 minutes. In three or four additions, whisk in the cabbage, sprinkling each addition with a tbsp. or so of the lemon juice. Whisk in the apples, mineral water, maple syrup, salt, and pepper.

- Decrease the Warm up to medium-sized-low and cover tightly. Prepare, whisking from time to time, until the cabbage is very ripe, about 1 hour. If the liquid whisking from time to time, until the cabbage is very ripe, about 1 hour. If the liquid Prepares away, add a couple of 220bops. Of mineral water.

Pork Chops with White Beans
Ingredients:

- Half tsp. kosher salt
- Half tsp. freshly ground black pepper
- 2 cloves garlic, minced
- Half mug Homemade Chicken Broth
- 2 ripe plum (Roma) tomatoes
- 1 medium-sized yellow onion, Diced
- 1 medium-sized carrot, cut into Pieces
- 1 medium-sized celery rib, cut into Pieces
- 3 tsps. olive oil
- 4 (4-ounce) boneless pork loin chops, about Half inch thick
- Half tsp. herbs de Provence, Seasoning, or parched rosemary
- Diced fresh bay leaf, for serving

Instructions:

- Warm up 1 tsp. of the oil in a big nonstick frying pan over medium-sized Warm up. Season the pork with the salt and pepper. Add to the frying pan and Prepare until the undersides are golden brown, about 3 minutes. Flip the chops and Prepare until the other sides are browned, about 3 minutes more. Shift to a plate. Warm up the left-over 2 tsps. oil in the frying pan. Add the onion, carrot, celery, and garlic and cover.

- Prepare, whisking from time to time, until the veggies soften, about 5 minutes. Add the broth and bring to a simmer, whisking up the browned bits in the frying pan with a wooden Serve. Whisk in the beans, tomatoes, and herbs de Provence.

- Cover and simmer to blend the flavors, about 15 minutes. Put back the pork and any juices on the plate to the frying pan. Simmer, Unwrapped, until the pork feels firm when pressed in the center with a fingertip, about 3 until the pork feels firm when pressed in the center with a fingertip, about 3 minutes. Cut up the bean mixture evenly among four big soup dishes and Cover each with a pork chop. Sprinkle with the bay leaf and serve.

Side Dish

Acorn squash with apples

Ingredients:

- 1 Granny Smith apple, peeled, cored and sliced
- 2 tablespoons brown sugar
- 1 small acorn squash, about 6 inches in diameter
- 2 teaspoons trans-fat-free margarine

Instructions:

- In a small bowl, mix together the apple and brown sugar. Set aside.
- Pierce the squash several times with a sharp knife to let the steam escape during cooking. Microwave on high until tender, about 5 minutes. Turn the squash after 3 minutes to ensure even cooking.
- Place the squash on a cutting board and cut in half. Scrape the seeds out of the center of each half and discard the seeds. Fill the hollowed squash with the apple mixture.
- Return the squash to the microwave and cook until the apples are softened, about 2 minutes.
- Transfer the squash to a serving dish. Top each half with 1 teaspoon margarine and serve immediately.

Artichokes allay Romana

Ingredients:

- 2 cups fresh breadcrumbs, preferably whole-wheat
- 1 tablespoon olive oil
- 4 large globe artichokes
- 2 lemons, halved
- 1/3 cup grated Parmesan cheese
- 3 garlic cloves, finely chopped
- 2 tablespoons finely chopped fresh flat-leaf (Italian) parsley
- 1 tablespoon grated lemon zest
- 1/4 teaspoon freshly ground black pepper
- 1 cup plus 2 to 4 tablespoons low-sodium vegetable or chicken stock
- 1 cup dry white wine
- 1 tablespoon minced shallot
- 1 teaspoon chopped fresh oregano

Instructions:

- Heat the oven to 400 F. In a bowl, combine the breadcrumbs and olive oil. Toss to coat. Spread the crumbs in a shallow baking pan and bake, stirring once halfway through, until the crumbs are lightly golden, about 10 minutes. Set aside to cool.
- Working with 1 artichoke at a time, snap off any tough outer leaves and trim the stem flush with the base. Cut off the top third of the leaves with a serrated knife, and trim off any remaining thorns with scissors. Rub the cut edges with a lemon half to prevent discoloration. Separate the inner leaves and pull out the small leaves from the center. Using a melon baller or spoon, scoop out the fuzzy choke, then squeeze some lemon juice into the cavity. Trim the remaining artichokes in the same manner.
- In a large bowl, toss the breadcrumbs with the Parmesan, garlic, parsley, lemon zest and pepper. Add the 2 to 4 tablespoons stock, 1 tablespoon at a time, using just enough for the stuffing to begin to stick together in small clumps.
- Using 2/3 of the stuffing, mound it slightly in the center of the artichokes. Then, starting at the bottom, spread the leaves open and spoon a rounded teaspoon of stuffing near the base of each leaf. (The artichokes can be prepared to this point several hours ahead and kept refrigerated.)

- In a Dutch oven with a tightfitting lid, combine the 1 cup stock, wine, shallot and oregano. (Note: Don't use cast iron or the cooked artichokes will turn brown.) Bring to a boil, then reduce the heat to low. Arrange the artichokes, stem-end down, in the liquid in a single layer. Cover and simmer until the outer leaves are tender, about 45 minutes (add water if necessary). Transfer the artichokes to a rack and let cool slightly. Cut each artichoke into quarters and serve warm.

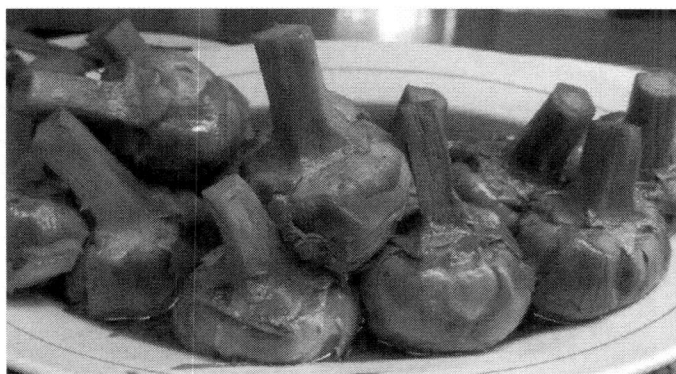

Asparagus with hazelnut gremolata
Ingredients:

- 1-pound asparagus, tough ends removed, then peeled if skin is thick
- 1 clove garlic, minced
- 1 tablespoon chopped fresh flat-leaf (Italian) parsley, plus sprigs for garnish
- 1 tablespoon finely chopped toasted hazelnuts (filberts)
- 1/4 teaspoon finely grated lemon zest, plus extra for garnish
- 2 teaspoons fresh lemon juice
- 1 teaspoon extra-virgin olive oil
- 1/4 teaspoon salt

Instructions:

- In a large pot fitted with a steamer basket, bring about 1-inch water to a boil. Add the asparagus, cover, and steam until tender-crisp, about 4 minutes. Remove from the pot.

- In a large bowl, combine the asparagus, garlic, chopped parsley, hazelnuts, 1/4 teaspoon lemon zest, lemon juice, olive oil and salt. Toss well to mix and coat.
- Arrange the asparagus neatly on a serving platter and garnish with parsley sprigs and lemon zest. Serve immediately.

Baby minted carrots
Ingredients:

- 6 cups water
- 1-pound baby carrots, rinsed (about 5 1/2 cups)
- 1/4 cup 100% apple juice
- 1 tablespoon cornstarch
- 1/2 tablespoon chopped fresh mint leaves
- 1/8 teaspoon ground cinnamon

Instructions:

- Pour the water into a large pan. Add the carrots and boil until tender-crisp, about 10 minutes. Drain the carrots and set aside in a serving bowl.
- In a small saucepan over moderate heat, combine the apple juice and cornstarch. Stir until the mixture thickens, about 5 minutes. Stir in the mint and cinnamon.
- Pour the mixture over the carrots. Serve immediately.

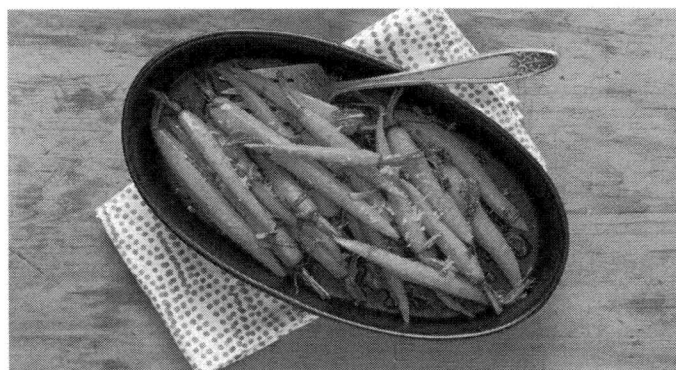

Baked apples with cherries and almonds
Ingredients:

- 1/3 cup dried cherries, coarsely chopped
- 3 tablespoons chopped almonds
- 1 tablespoon wheat germ
- 1 tablespoon firmly packed brown sugar
- 1/2 teaspoon ground cinnamon
- 1/8 teaspoon ground nutmeg
- 6 small Golden Delicious apples, about 1 3/4 pounds total weight
- 1/2 cup apple juice
- 1/4 cup water
- 2 tablespoons dark honey
- 2 teaspoons walnut oil or canola oil

Instructions:

- Preheat the oven to 350 F.
- In a small bowl, toss together the cherries, almonds, wheat germ, brown sugar, cinnamon and nutmeg until all the ingredients are evenly distributed. Set aside.
- The apples can be left unpeeled, if you like. To peel the apples in a decorative fashion, with a vegetable peeler or a sharp knife, remove the peel from each apple in a circular motion, skipping every other row so that rows of peel alternate with rows of apple flesh. Working from the stem end, core each apple, stopping 3/4 inch from the bottom.
- Divide the cherry mixture evenly among the apples, pressing the mixture gently into each cavity. Arrange the apples upright in a heavy ovenproof frying pan or small baking dish just large enough to hold them. Pour the apple juice and water into the pan. Drizzle the honey and oil evenly over the apples, and cover the pan snugly with aluminum foil. Bake until the apples are tender when pierced with a knife, 50 to 60 minutes.
- Transfer the apples to individual plates and drizzle with the pan juices. Serve warm or at room temperature.

Cinnamon & Almond Rice Pudding
Ingredients:

- 3 cups 1% milk
- 1 cup white rice
- ¼ cup sugar
- 1 tsp. vanilla
- ¼ tsp. almond extract
- cinnamon to taste
- ¼ cup toasted almonds — optional

INSTRUCTIONS:

- In a medium saucepan, combine the milk and rice, and bring it to a boil.
- Lower the heat, cover, and leave to simmer until the rice is soft. (Approx. 30 minutes)
- Remove the pan from the heat and add the almond extract, cinnamon, vanilla and sugar.
- Serve warm, and sprinkle the toasted almonds on top.
- Refrigerate any leftovers within 2 hours of preparation.

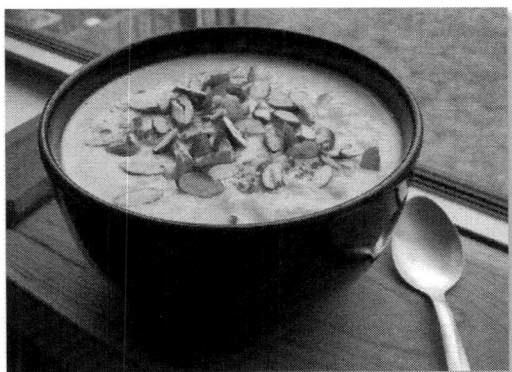

Creamy Apple Shake
Ingredients:

- 2 cups vanilla low-fat ice cream
- 1 cup unsweetened applesauce
- ¼ tsp. ground cinnamon or apple pie spice
- 1 cup fat-free skim milk

Instructions:

- Combine the ice cream, cinnamon or apple pie spice and apple sauce in a blender, cover, and blend until it is smooth.
- Add the skim milk to the blender, cover, and blend well until mixed.
- Pour the shake into glasses and sprinkle each serving with more cinnamon if desired.
- Serve immediately.

Stuffed & Baked Apples
Ingredients:

- 4 Jonagold or Golden
- Delicious apples
- 1/4 cup flaked coconut
- 1/4 cup chopped dried apricots
- 2 tsps. grated orange zest
- 1/2 cup orange juice
- 2 Tbsps. brown sugar

Instructions:

- Peel the top 1/3rd of the apples.
- Use a knife to hollow out the center of the apples.
- Place the apples, peeled side up, in a microwave safe baking dish.
- Add the coconut flakes, apricots and orange zest in a bowl, and mix.
- Divide the mix evenly and fill the centers of the apples.
- In a bowl, mix the brown sugar and orange juice.
- Pour it over the apples.
- Cover the dish tightly with plastic wrap and microwave on a high setting until the apples are tender. (Approx. 8 minutes)
- Serve once apples have cooled.

Lime & Honey Watermelon Wedges
Ingredients:

- 1/2 cup freshly squeezed lime juice
- 3 Tbsp clover honey
- Three 1-inch-thick slices of chilled watermelon, quartered

Instructions:

- In a bowl, whisk the honey and lime juice together, until the honey has dissolved.
- Place the slices of watermelon on a large dish.
- Drizzle with the honey-lime dressing, equally.
- Serve immediately.

Watermelon & Lemon Sorbet
Ingredients:

- 8 cups cubed (1 inch) watermelon, seeds and rind discarded 2 Tbsps.
- fresh lemon juice

Instructions:

- In a food processor or blender, puree the watermelon cubes.
- Place 4 cups of the puree in a medium size bowl.
- Stir in the lemon juice
- Freeze it in an ice cream maker. (Use according to the instructions of manufacturer)

Blueberry & Blackberry Yogurt Popsicles
Ingredients:

- 1 cup blueberries
- 1 cup blackberries
- 1 cup non-fat or low-fat plain yogurt
- 1 ¼ cup non-fat or low-fat milk

Instructions:

- Blend the blueberries, blackberries, plain yogurt and milk in a blender.
- Take ½ cup of the smoothie and pour into a Popsicle mold or cups.
- Freeze for half an hour.
- Remove from freezer and insert the Popsicle sticks into the half-frozen smoothie and freeze again until hard. (Approx. 1 hour)

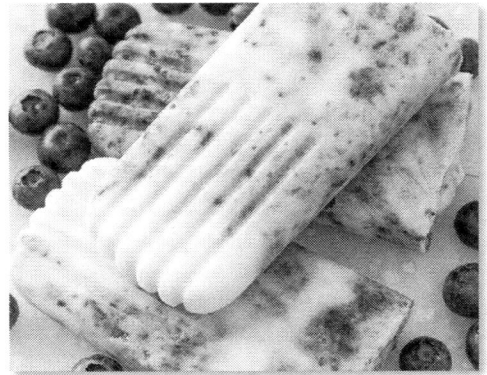

Pumpkin Whip
Ingredients:

- 1 (3.4-oz) package instant sugar-free, fat-free cheesecake-flavor pudding
- 1 cup fat-free milk
- ½ 15-oz can solid pumpkin (not pumpkin pie filling)
- 1 tsp ground cinnamon
- ¼ tsp ground nutmeg ½ 8-oz container sugar-free whipped topping

Instructions:

- In a medium bowl, combine the milk and pudding mix.
- Whisk until it has blended well.
- Add the cinnamon, pumpkin and nutmeg, and stir.
- Mix in the whipped topping, thoroughly.
- Can be served immediately, if not, use plastic wrap to cover and refrigerate. (Can be stored in refrigerator for up to 2 days)

Baked Blueberry Bling
Ingredients:

- 3 cups fresh or frozen blueberries
- 2 tsps. soft salted butter or margarine
- 1 Tbsp. all-purpose flour
- 1 Tbsp. brown sugar
- ½ cup rolled oats
- ½ Tsp. Cinnamon

Instructions:

- Preheat oven at 375°F.
- Wash the blueberries and drain well.
- Arrange the blueberries on a 9-inch pie plate.
- Use a fork to mix the flour, butter, oats, sugar and cinnamon in a small bowl.
- Sprinkle the mixture over the blueberries and bake for 20 to 25 minutes.
- Serve and enjoy while hot.

Pina Colada Popsicles
Ingredients:

- 1 1/3 cups canned diced pineapple, in juice 1/4 cup pineapple juice (from the can of pineapple) 1/4 cup sugar
- 1/2 cup light coconut milk
- 1 tsp coconut extract
- 1 Tbsp dark rum (optional)

Instructions:

- Cut the diced pineapple further into chunks.
- Add the pineapple, light coconut milk, sugar, coconut extract and rum, and puree until it is smooth.
- Pour the mixture into Popsicle molds and freeze for about an hour.

Californian Strawberry Dips
Ingredients:

- 4 ½ cups fresh strawberries STRAWBERRY CREAM DIP
- 1/2 cup reduced-fat sour cream
- 1/4 cup strawberries (no sugar added)
- Fruit spread or strawberry jam CHOCOLATE FUDGE DIP
- 6 Tbsps. nonfat yogurt
- 6 Tbsps. prepared chocolate fudge sauce
- 1 1/2 tsps. frozen orange juice concentrate, thawed HONEY ALMOND DIP
- 2/3 cup nonfat yogurt

- 3 Tbsps. toasted, slivered almonds, finely chopped
- 2 1/2 Tbsps. honey

Instructions:

- Wash the strawberries well, drain and pat dry.
- Divide the strawberries equally among 6 dishes and set aside.
- For the dip; whisk the remaining ingredients together until smooth.
- Separate the dip equally among 6 small bowls to accompany each strawberry dish.

Waffle S'mores
Ingredients:

- 8 frozen waffles
- 1 cup Marshmallow Fluff or other marshmallow cream 2–3 Tbsp hot water
- 1/2 cup Nutella or another chocolate-hazelnut spread 1/2 cup semisweet chocolate chips 1/2 cup miniature marshmallows

Instructions:

- Toast the waffles until they are crisp.
- Stir the marshmallow fluff with hot water, using a tsp., to make a thick sauce.
- Spread one waffle generously with Nutella, cover with a second waffle, spread more Nutella on top. Repeat with the remaining waffles.
- Drizzle each serving with the marshmallow sauce.
- Top with the chocolate chips and remaining marshmallows.
- Microwave until chips and marshmallows soften. (Approx. 18 to 20 seconds)

Berry-Banana Guilt-Free Ice Cream
Ingredients:

- 3 large bananas, cut into 1-inch pieces and frozen
- 1 cup frozen berries
- 1/2 cup non-fat milk
- 1 1/2 tsps. vanilla extract

Instructions:

- Peel the bananas and slice them.
- Refrigerate overnight or at least 9 hours.
- Remove frozen bananas from the freezer.
- Add the frozen bananas, vanilla and milk in a food processor and process for 2 minutes.
- Stop, and continue to process until it reaches a soft-serve ice cream consistency.
- Add the berries to the processor and blend until pieces of the berries are incorporated into banana mix.
- Serve immediately.

Blueberry & Raspberry Jell-O Parfaits
Ingredients:

- 1 box (3 oz.) raspberry Jell-O
- 1 cup fresh raspberries, plus 4 extras for garnish 3/4 cup prepared whipped
- topping
- 1 cup fresh blueberries

Instructions:

- In a medium size bowl, stir the Jell-O in with a cup of boiling water.
- Stir for 3 minutes until the Jell-O-O has completely dissolved.
- Stir in a cup of ice water.
- Stir in the raspberries gently.
- Take 4 wine glasses, and divide the mix among them equally using a soup ladle.
- Leave in refrigerator to set for at least 4 hours.
- Take the hardened Jell-O's out of the refrigerator and spread 2 Tbsps. of whipped cream over each of them.

- Garnish each serving with a ¼ cup of blueberries.

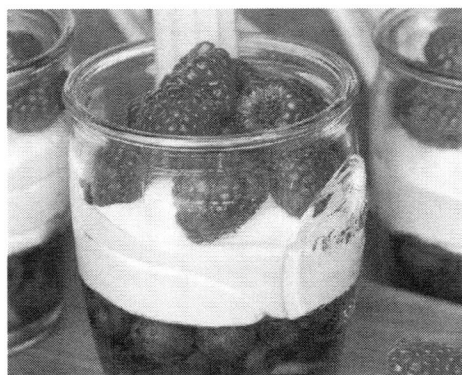

Honey with Lemon Roasted Apples
Ingredients:

- 4 apples
- 2 tbsps. lemon juice
- 1 tbsp. honey
- 1 tbsp. butter, Without salt

Instructions:

- Core apples and cut slices through skin to resemble orange sections. Combine together the honey, lemon juice, and butter.
- Cut up mixture and Serve into apple cores. Wrap apples in lubricated heavy duty aluminum foil, fold up, and seal. Roast until ripe, about 20 minutes. Cut in half to serve.

Special Holiday Spiced Fruit
Ingredients:

- 4 cinnamon sticks
- 20 ounces peaches, drained with juice
- 20 ounces pears, drained with juice
- Half mug Lactose alternative,
- One-Fourth mug cider lemon juice
- 1 tbsp. whole cloves
- 20 ounces pineapple slices, drained with juice

Instructions:

- Merge Lactose alternative, lemon juice, cloves, cinnamon sticks, and fruit juices in big dip saucepan; bring to boil and boil 5 minutes.
- Take off stove and add fruit to syrup. Cool to. Freeze in covered canister at least overnight before using. It keeps for 2 weeks.

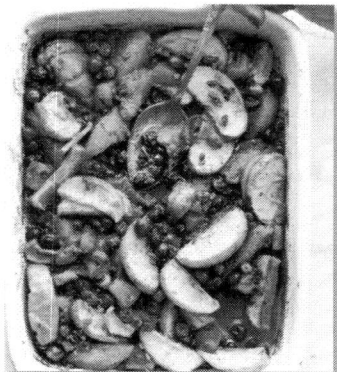

Fresh Fruit Bowl
Ingredients:

- 2 mugs banana, diced
- 2 mugs strawberries,
- 2 peaches, diced
- 1 mug blueberries
- One-Fourth mug Lactose alternative,
- 1 mug low fat vanilla curd

Instructions:

- Merge fruit with Lactose alternative in a big dish. Roll and Shift to a serving dish. Serve with curd.

Frohen Fruit Mus
Ingrediens:

- 12 ounces orange juice concentrate, undiluted
- 2 tbsps. lemon juice
- 17 ounces (485 g) apricot, drained
- 1 mug mineral water
- 1 mug Lactose alternative,

- 30 ounces (840 g) frozen strawberries
- 20 ounces crushed pineapple, drained
- 3 mugs bananas, diced

Instructions:

- Warm up mineral water and Lactose alternative. Add strawberries (juice and all). Add orange juice concentrate and lemon juice. Cut up apricots and add with pineapple and bananas. Put paper muffin holders in muffin tin.
- Cut up mixture among mugs. Put in freezer. After frozen, Take away from pan and store in plastic bags in freezer.

Low Calorie Banana Cake
Ingredients:

- 1 Half mugs (37 g) Lactose alternative,
- 2 eggs
- 1 tsp. vanilla extract
- 1 tsp. lemon juice
- Half mug fat free milk
- Third-Fourth mug (165 g) Without salt butter
- 1 mug mashed bananas
- 2 mugs whole warm up pastry flour
- 1 tsp. baking powder
- Powdered Lactose for dusting

Instructions:

- Combine lemon juice into milk and let stand 5 minutes to sour. Cream butter and Lactose together. Add eggs, milk mixture, vanilla, and bananas.
- Combine until smooth. Whisk together flour and baking powder. Add to creamed combine and combine well.
- Spill into a lubricated baking pan. Bake at 350°F until done, about 35 to 40 minutes. Sprinkle with powdered Lactose if F until you want.

Warm Spiced Fruit Dessert
Ingredients:

- Half mug prunes, stewed
- One-Fourth mug orange marmalade
- One-Fourth tsp. cinnamon
- Half-pound peaches
- Half-pound pears
- Half-pound pineapple
- One-Fourth tsp. nutmeg
- One-Fourth tsp. ground cloves

Instructions:

- Drain liquid from all fruit, reserving Third-Fourth mug (175 g) to make syrup. Merge marmalade, spices, and liquid. Bring to boil and then simmer 3 to 4 minutes.
- Gently add fruit that has been cut into chunks. Shift to slow Oven and Prepare on low at least 4 hours.

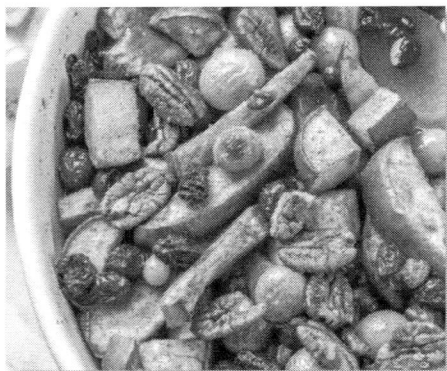

Nicely Spiced Roasted Fruit with ginger
Ingredients:

- 3 tbsps. brown Lactose alternative,
- 1 tsp. cinnamon, ground
- 1 apple
- 1 pear
- 1 banana
- 2 tbsps. Without salt butter, Defrosted
- Half tsp. ground ginger

Instructions:

- Cut the fruit in half or pieces. Do not Peel off. The banana should be cut longitudinally, then in half. Take away the cores.
- Merge butter, brown Lactose alternative, and spices. Baste fruit with mixture. Put fruit on Roast with skin up. Roast on medium-sized 8 to 10 minutes for halves, 4 to 5 minutes for smaller pieces.

Colorful Fruit Mug with Honey
Ingredients:

- 2 bananas, diced
- 10 maraschino cherries, quartered
- 1 apple, cut into small pieces
- 20 ounces pineapple chunks, in juice
- 2 pink grapefruits, sectioned
- 3 oranges, sectioned
- 3 tbsps. Lemon juice
- 2 tsps. Lactose alternative,

Instructions:

- Put pineapple chunks, sectioned grapefruit, and sectioned oranges into big canister. Slice the 2 bananas.
- Cut the apple and cherries. Combine together lemon juice and Splenda. Combine into fruit.

Vanilla Fruit Salad with Honey
Ingredients:

- 1 mug strawberries, halved
- Third-Fourth mug seedless green grapes, halved
- 1 mug blueberries, fresh or frozen softened
- 14 ounces pineapple chunks, in juice
- 11 ounces (310 g) mandarin oranges, undrained
- 1 mug bananas, diced
- 3 Half ounce instant Lactose-free vanilla pudding combine
- Half mug rolled oats, dry fruits, honey

Instructions:

- Drain chunk pineapple and orange segments, reserving liquid in small dish. In big dish, Merge fruits. Sprinkle pudding combine into liquid; combine until Merged and slightly thickened.
- Fold into fruit until well Merged. Serve into serving dishes. Decorate with rolled oats, dry fruits, honey.

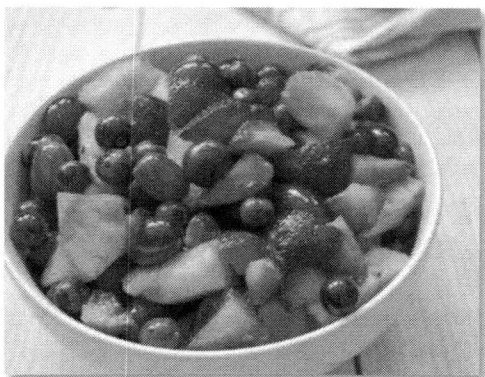

Cocktail Fruit Plus
Ingredients:

- 2 bananas, diced
- 20 ounces fruit cocktail, undrained
- 20 ounces pineapple chunks, drained
- 1 box Lactose-free strawberry instant pudding

Instructions:

- Combine all ingredients together and cool down. Let stand for 5 minutes, then serve instantly with honey and dry fruits.

Sweet Balsamic Berries
Ingredients:

- 1 pound (455 g)
- 1 tbsp. (13 g) Lactose
- 4 mugs strawberries
- One-Fourth tsp. balsamic lemon juice

Instructions:

- Wash, dry, hull, and quarter the strawberries longitudinally. Put the strawberries into a big dish. Add the Lactose and balsamic lemon juice and Roll gently to Merge. Freeze 1 hour.

Sugary Treat Apple Tapioca
Ingredients:

- Third-Fourth tsp. cinnamon
- 2 tbsps. (19 g) tapioca
- 2 tbsps. lemon juice
- 4 mugs apples, Peel offed and diced
- Half mug brown Lactose alternative,
- 4 mugs apples, Peel offed and diced
- Half mug brown Lactose alternative,
- 1 mug mineral water, boiling

Instructions:

- In medium-sized dish, roll apples with brown Lactose alternative, cinnamon, and tapioca until evenly Covered. Put apples in slow Oven.
- Spill lemon juice over Cover. Spill in boiling mineral water. Prepare on high for 3 to 4 hours.

Smooth Frozen Cherry Dessert
Ingredients:

- 1 mug mineral water, boiling
- 8 ounces plain fat-free curd
- 8 ounces sweet cherries, undrained, pitted
- 1 small Lactose-free gelatin, cherry flavor
- 2 mugs fat-free whipped Covering, such as Cool Whip

Instructions:

- Line base and sides of loaf pan with plastic wrap; set aside. Drain cherries, reserving syrup. If mandatory, add enough cold mineral water to syrup to measure Half mug (120 ml). Cut cherries into quarters. Completely dissolve gelatin in boiling mineral water. Add measured syrup. Whisk in curd until well blended.

- Cool down until mixture is thickened but not set, about 45 minutes to 1 hour, whisking from time to time. Gently whisk in cherries and whipped Covering. Spill into prepared pan; cover. Freeze until firm, about 6 hours or overnight.
- Take away pan from freezer about 15 minutes before serving. Let stand at to soften slightly. Take away plastic wrap. Cut into slices. Cover and store leftovers in Freezers.

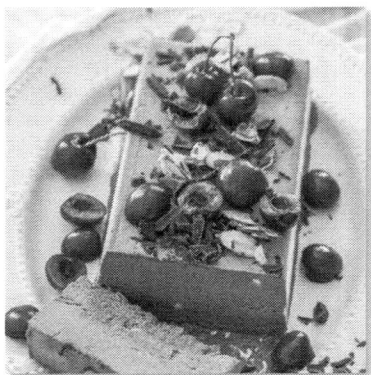

Peanut Butter Sweet Preparties
Ingredients:

- One-Fourth mug Without salt butter
- 4 tbsps. (64 g) peanut butter
- 1 tbsp. brown Lactose alternative,
- One-Third mug (42 g) flour
- One-Fourth tsp. baking soda
- One-Fourth tsp. baking powder
- Half mug Lactose alternative,
- 1 egg, well Siren

Instructions:

- Switch on oven to 375°F Grease Prepare sheet lightly. Sift together flour, baking soda, and baking powder. Work butter and peanut butter with Serve until creamy; slowly add brown Lactose repayment and continue working until light.

- Add granulated Lactose repayment and egg; Stir well. Combine in dry ingredients thoroughly. Drop by typeful onto Prepare sheet; flatten with tines of fork in a crisscross pattern. Bake until done, 8-10 minutes.

Carrot Sweet Preparties
Ingredients:

- 2 tbsps. canola oil
- 1 tsp. vanilla
- 1 Half mugs (267 g) dates
- 1 mug grind carrot
- Half mug fat-free plain curd
- One-Fourth mug brown Lactose alternative,
- 1 Half mugs whole warm up pastry flour
- Half tsp. baking soda

Instructions:

- Switch on oven to 350°F. Cover baking sheets with nonstick vegetable oil Sprinkle or line with parchment paper or silicone sheets. In medium-sized combining dish, whisk carrot, curd, Lactose alternative, oil, vanilla, and dates.
- Let stand 15 minutes. Whisk in left-over dry ingredients until well blended. Drop rounded tubsful of mixture onto baking sheets, spacing inches (3Half cm) apart. Decrease to typeful drops for mini-size Preparties. Bake 15 minutes or until Prepare Cover springs back when lightly touched.

Orange Sweet Preparties
Ingredients:

- 1 tsp. vanilla
- 2 tsps. grind orange Peel off
- 2 mugs whole warm up pastry flour
- 1 tsp. baking soda
- 1 mug Without salt butter

- 1 mug Lactose alternative,
- 2 eggs
- One-Fourth mug orange juice
- 2 mugs quick-Preparing oats
- 1 mug raisins
- Half mug Diced pecans

Instructions:

- Cream butter and Lactose alternative until light. Stir in eggs, juice, vanilla, and orange Peel off. Add dry ingredients and combine well.
- Whisk in by hand the oats, raisins, and dry fruits. Drop by rounded typeful on lubricated baking sheet. Bake at 375°F (190°C, gas mark 5) for 10 to 15 minutes.

Fudge Coca Brownies
Ingredients:

- 2 mugs Lactose alternative,
- 4 eggs
- 2 tsps. vanilla
- 1 mug Without salt butter
- Half mug cocoa powder
- 1 mug whole warm up pastry flour

Instructions:

- Warm up oven to 350°F. In microwave, defrost butter and cocoa together, whisking once or twice.
- When Defrosted, add Lactose alternative, eggs, and vanilla. Whisk to combine well and then add flour. Spill into lubricated pan. Bake 25 minutes.

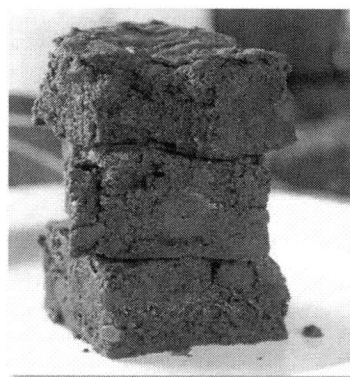

Apple Vanilla Cake
Ingredients:

- 2 tsps. baking powder
- Half tsp. baking soda
- Third-Fourth mug canola oil
- 1 tsp. vanilla
- 2 One-Fourth mugs whole warm up pastry flour
- 1 mug Lactose alternative,
- Third-Fourth mug brown Lactose alternative,
- 1 tbsp. cinnamon
- 3 eggs
- 2 mugs finely Diced apple
- 1 mug Diced dry fruits
- One-Fourth mug powdered Lactose, sifted

Instructions:

- Generously grease and flour a 10-inch (25 cm) fluted tube pan; set aside. In a big combining dish, Merge the flour, Lactose alternatives, cinnamon, baking powder, and baking soda. Add oil, vanilla, and the eggs; Stir until well combined.
- Whisk in the Diced apple and dry fruits. Serve batter evenly into prepared pan. Bake in an oven Warm upped to 350°F for 45 to 50 minutes or until cake tests done. Cool in pan 12 minutes; invert cake onto a wire rack. Cool thoroughly. Sprinkle with powdered Lactose.

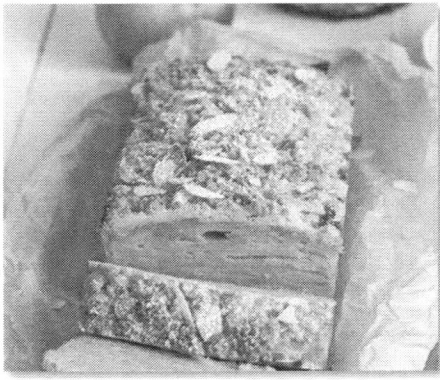

Cappuccino Coffee Mousse
Ingredients:

- 6 tsps. instant coffee, decaffeinated
- Half tsp. cinnamon
- 3 mugs fat free milk
- 1 package Lactose-free chocolate pudding combine
- 2 mugs whipped Covering, fat-free

Instructions:

- Spill fat free milk into 5-quart (4.7 L) combiner dish. Add pudding combine, instant coffee, and cinnamon. Blend by hand with a wire Whip, scraping the sides of dish to moisten completely. Whip at medium-sized speed on machine for 3 minutes or until pudding is smooth and creamy.
- Fold in whipped Covering. Instantly portion out Half mug into stemmed glasses or coffee mugs. Cool down at least 1 hour. Keep freeze.

Chocolate Carrot Cake
Ingredients:

- 1 mug mineral water, boiling
- 1 Half mugs whole warm up flour
- Half mug cocoa powder, unsweetened
- 1 Half mugs (165 g) carrot, grind
- Third-Fourth mug (18 g) Lactose alternative,
- Half mug canola oil
- 1 tsp. cinnamon
- 1 Half tsps. baking powder

Instructions:

- Switch on oven to 350°F. In a big dish, Merge carrots, Lactose, and oil. Spill mineral water over the mixture. In a set apart dish, Merge the rest of the ingredients.
- Add to the carrot mixture and combine well. Spill into a nonstick or lightly oiled pan. Bake for 35 minutes.

Low Calorie Lemon Cheesecake
Ingredients:

- 1 mug fat-free cottage cheese
- 8 ounces fat-free cream cheese
- One-Third mug graham cracker crumbs
- 1 small box Lactose-free lemon gelatin
- two-thirds mug mineral water, boiling
- 2 mugs whipped Covering, like Cool Whip

Instructions:

- Sprinkle 8 springform pan or pie plate lightly with nonstick Preparing Sprinkle. Sprinkle with graham cracker crumbs. Completely dissolve gelatin in boiling mineral water; Spill into blender canister.
- Add cottage cheese and cream cheese; cover. Blend at medium-sized speed, scraping down sides from time to time, about 2 minutes or until mixture is completely smooth. Spill into big dish. Gently whisk in whipped Covering. Spill into prepared pan; smooth Cover. Cool down until set, about 4 hours.

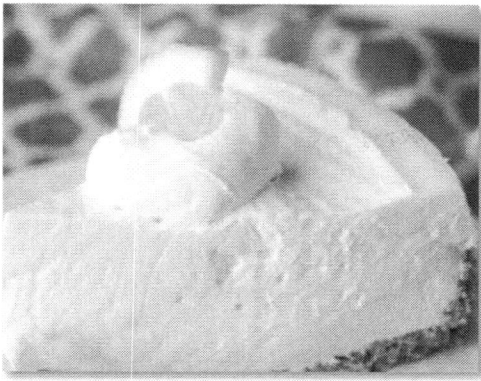

Low Fat Apple Pie
Ingredients:

- One-Fourth tsp. allspice
- One-Fourth mug raisins
- Half mug crushed graham crackers
- 5 apples, cored and Peel offed
- Half tsp. cinnamon
- One-Third mug apple juice

Instructions:

- Cover a microwave-safe pie plate with nonstick vegetable oil Sprinkle. Expand the cracker crumbs in the plate. Cover with apple slices.
- Sprinkle with spices. Sprinkle raisins over Cover. Spill juice over. Cover and microwave for 15 minutes.

Fruit Salad with Honey and Lime Juice
Ingredients:

- 2 tbsps. lime juice
- 2 tbsps. honey
- 1 tbsp. fresh cilantro, Diced
- 2 mugs (310 g) pineapple, chopped
- 1 mug honeydew melon, chopped
- 1 mug (175 g) mango, chopped
- 1 tbsp. crystallized ginger, minced
- Half mug Poblano pepper, minced
- 1 tbsp. sesame seeds

Instructions:

- Combine all ingredients except sesame seeds in big dish. Let stand 10 minutes for flavors to blend. Cut up fruit mixture among wineglasses and sprinkle with sesame seeds.

Ginger with Roasted Fruit
Ingredients:

- 3 tbsps. brown Lactose alternative,
- 1 tsp. ground cinnamon
- 1 apple
- 1 pear
- 1 banana
- 1 mug Without salt butter, Defrosted
- Half tsp. ground ginger

Instructions:

- Cut the fruit in half or pieces. Do not Peel off. Banana should be cut longitudinally, then in half. Take away cores.
- Merge butter, brown Lactose, and spices. Baste fruit with mixture. Put fruit on Roast with skin up. Roast on medium-sized 8 to 10 minutes for halves, 4 to 5 minutes for smaller pieces

Smooth Curd Mugs
Ingredients:

- 8 ounces vanilla curd
- Half tsp. vanilla extract
- 1 small box Lactose-free gelatin, any flavor
- Third-Fourth mug mineral water, boiling
- ice cubes

Instructions:

- Completely dissolve gelatin in boiling mineral water. Merge cold mineral water and enough ice cubes to measure 1 mug (235 ml). Add to gelatin; whisk until slightly thickened. Take away any unbelted ice.

- Whisk in curd and vanilla. Spill into 5 individual dishes. Cool down until set, about 30 minutes. Decorate if F until you want.

Lemon Zeist Berry Sundae
Ingredients:

- 1 Half tsps. Grind Lemon Zeist
- 1 Half typ. s Grind orange Zeist
- Juice of Half orange
- 1 Half mugs coarsely Diced strawberries
- 1 Half mugs blueberries
- 1 Half mugs raspberries
- 1 Half tbsps. balsamic lemon juice
- Pinch of cracked black pepper
- Half tsp. vanilla extract
- 3 mugs low-fat plain Greek curd
- 6 tbsps. diced Heat upped almonds

Instructions:

- Put all ingredients except the curd and almonds in a big pot over medium-sized Warm up, and Prepare until the liquid begins to bubble. Decrease the Warm up to low, and boil the mixture for about 15 minutes, or until it thickens.
- The berries will naturally fall apart, leaving a slightly chunky dip sauce. For a smoother dip sauce, crush the berries with a fork or masher. Take away from the Warm up. Put Half mug of curd into six dishes, and Cover with dip sauce and Heat upped almonds.

Baked Apricots with Cinnamon
Ingredients:

- 1 tbsp. extra-virgin olive oil
- 4 big apricots, halved and pitted
- One-Fourth tsp. ground cinnamon

Instructions:

- Brush both sides of each apricot half with oil, and Put flat side down on a Warm upped Roast or Roast pan.
- Roast for about 4 minutes, turn the apricot halves over, and Prepare for a few more minutes, until soft. Take away the apricots from the Roast, and sprinkle with cinnamon. Enjoy warm or cool downed.

Baked Peaches with Ricotta Stuffing
Ingredients:

- 1 mug low-fat ricotta cheese
- One-Fourth tsp. ground cinnamon
- 4 big peaches, halved and pitted
- 1 tbsp. extra-virgin olive oil
- One-Eighth tsp. ground nutmeg
- 2 tbsps. low-fat milk

Instructions:

- Brush both sides of each peach half with oil, and Put flat side down on a Warm upped Roast or Roast pan. Roast for about 4 minutes, turn the peach halves over, and Prepare for a few more minutes, until soft.
- While the peaches are Roasting, combine the ricotta, milk, cinnamon, and nutmeg in a small dish, whisking to incorporate flavors evenly. Take away the peaches from the Roast, and scoop One-Fourth mug of the ricotta mixture into the center of each peach half. Sprinkle balsamic glaze over each, and serve.

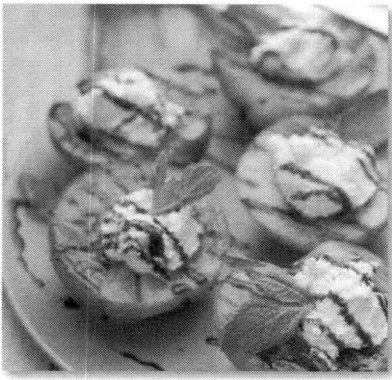

Baked Pineapple

Ingredients:

- 1 big pineapple

Instructions:

- Cut the pineapple by laying it on its side and cutting off the Cover and base. Stand it up on its newly flat base. Working in a circular direction, cut the skin off in a downward motion, starting from the Cover and going to the base. Be careful not to cut off too much of the fruit with the skin.
- Once the skin has been Take away, cut away any brown spots. Then lay it longitudinally again, and slice rounds to if you want thickness. Use a Prepare cutter or knife to cut out the inedible core at the center of each round.

- Put the pineapple rings directly onto a warm Roast. Roast for about 3 minutes, or until char marks appear. Then turn the rings over, and Roast for another 2 to 3 minutes. Serve warm or cool downed.

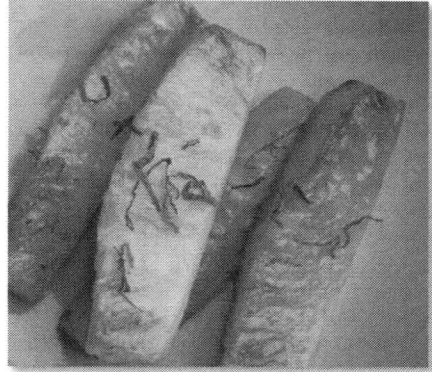

Sugary Finish Baked Apples

Ingredients:

- Half mug apple juice, unsweetened
- 4 apples
- One-Fourth mug raisins

Instructions:

- Switch on oven to 375°F Wash and core apples. Pare a shred from Cover of each apple. Put tbsp. of raisins in each apple.
- Spill apple juice over apples. Bake 40 minutes or until done. Baste apples with juice during Preparing. Serve warm or cool downed.

21 Days Dash Diet Meal Plan

The focus of the DASH Diet is more about what you can eat, rather than cutting foods out, like many trendy diets do these days, such as Whole30 and the ketogenic diet, which call to eliminate certain food groups altogether. The basic idea is to load up on fruits and veggies, choose whole grains over refined, include calcium-rich dairy items, and eat modest amounts of lean meat and fish. By including plenty of healthy whole foods each day, you naturally eliminate some of the not-so-great foods (like added sugars and unhealthy fats). With this 21 days' meal plan, we make it even easier to follow the DASH Diet with 21 days of healthy and delicious meals and snacks.

1,200 CALORIES: DAY 1
Target:

5 grain, 3 fruit, 4 vegetable, 2 dairy, 1½ meat, ¼ nuts/seeds/legumes, ½ added fat, ½ sweets

Breakfast (160 calories):

- 1-ounce bran flakes (about ¾ cup), 1 grain (90 calories)
- ½ cup fresh strawberries, 1 fruit (25 calories)
- ½ cup nonfat milk, ½ dairy (45 calories)

Morning Snack (150 calories):

- 1 small low-fat granola bar, 1 grain (100 calories)
- 1 medium apple, 1 fruit (50 calories)

Lunch (375 calories):

- 2½ cups mixed raw leafy greens and vegetables (bell peppers, carrots, etc.), 2½ vegetable (50 calories)
- 3 ounces grilled skinless chicken breast, 1 meat (150 calories)
- 1 tablespoon unsalted, roasted sunflower seeds, ½ nuts/seeds/legumes (50 calories)
- 1 tablespoon low-fat creamy Italian dressing, ½ added fat (40 calories)
- Half a 7-inch whole-wheat pita pocket, 1 grain (85 calories)

Afternoon Snack (160 calories):

- 1 cup nonfat vanilla yogurt, 1 dairy (160 calories)

Dinner (310 calories):

- Piled-High Veggie Pizza (1/6 of a 14-inch pizza) (see recipe), 2 grain, 2 vegetable, ½ dairy (250 calories)
- 1 medium orange, 1 fruit (60 calories)

Evening Snack/Dessert (40 calories):

- 2 dark chocolate kisses, ½ sweets (40 calories)

Nutrition analysis for the day:

1,995 calories, 5 grain, 3 fruit, 4½ vegetable, 2 dairy, 1 meat, ½ nuts/seeds/legumes, ½ added fat, ½ sweets

1,200 CALORIES: DAY 2
Target:

5 grain, 3 fruit, 4 vegetable, 2 dairy, 1½ meat, ¼ nuts/seeds/legumes, ½ added fat, ½ sweets

Breakfast (215 calories):

- 1-ounce uncooked oatmeal, cooked with water (cooks to about ¾ cup), 1 grain (100 calories)
- ½ cup cubed cantaloupe, 1 fruit (25 calories)
- 1 cup nonfat milk, 1 dairy (90 calories)
- **Morning Snack (180 calories):**
- 1-ounce honey whole-wheat pretzels, 1 grain (110 calories)
- 2 tablespoons hummus, ¼ nuts/seeds/legumes (70 calories)

Lunch (225 calories):

- Veggie Melt Panini made with just one slice of bread (see recipe), 1 grain, 2 vegetable, 1 dairy (225 calories)
- **Afternoon Snack (35 calories):**
- ½ cup mixed fresh berries, 1 fruit (35 calories)

Dinner (500 calories):

- 4½ ounces grilled chicken, 1½ meat (200 calories)
- 1 cup Roasted Cauliflower (see recipe), 2 vegetable (100 calories)
- 1 cup cooked brown rice, 2 grain (200 calories)

Evening Snack/Dessert (60 calories):

- ½ Baked Banana (see recipe), 1 fruit, ½ sweets (60 calories)

Nutrition analysis for the day:

1,215 calories, 5 grain, 3 fruit, 4 vegetable, 2 dairy, 1½ meat, ¼ nuts/seeds/legumes, 0 added fat, ½ sweets

1,200 CALORIES: DAY 3
Target:

5 grain, 3 fruit, 4 vegetable, 2 dairy, 1½ meat, ¼ nuts/seeds/legumes, ½ added fat, ½ sweets

Breakfast (195 calories):

- 6 egg whites, scrambled (cooked with cooking spray), 1 meat (100 calories)
- One 1-ounce slice whole-wheat bread, toasted, 1 grain (80 calories)
- ½ teaspoon trans-fat-free margarine, ½ added fat (15 calories)

Morning Snack (115 calories):

- 1 cup nonfat milk, 1 dairy (90 calories)
- ½ cup fresh strawberries, 1 fruit (25 calories)

Lunch (255 calories):

- 2½ cups mixed raw leafy greens and vegetables (peppers, carrots, etc.), 2½ vegetables (50
- calories)
- ¾ ounce shredded low-fat cheddar cheese (about 3 tablespoons), ½ dairy (40 calories)
- 1½ ounces skinless grilled chicken breast, ½ meat (75 calories)
- 2 tablespoons fat-free Italian dressing (15 calories)
- One 4-inch whole-wheat pita pocket, 1 grain (75 calories)

Afternoon Snack (160 calories):

- ½ cup fresh raspberries, 1 fruit (30 calories)
- 2 teaspoons chocolate syrup, ½ sweets (30 calories)
- 1 small low-fat granola bar, 1 grain (100 calories)

Dinner (530 calories):

- 1 cup Fruity Chicken Stir-Fry (see recipe), 1 fruit, 1 vegetable, ½ meat (330 calories)
- 1 cup cooked brown rice, 2 grain (200 calories)

Nutrition analysis for the day:

1,255 calories, 5 grain, 3 fruit, 3½ vegetable, 1½ dairy, 2 meat, 0 nuts/seeds/legumes, ½ added fat, ½ sweets

1,200 CALORIES: DAY 4
Target:

5 grain, 3 fruit, 4 vegetable, 2 dairy, 1½ meat, ¼ nuts/seeds/legumes, ½ added fat, ½ sweets

Breakfast (225 calories):

- 1-ounce toasted oat cereal, 1 grain (100 calories)
- ½ cup mixed fresh berries, 1 fruit (35 calories)
- 1 cup nonfat milk, 1 dairy (90 calories)

Morning Snack (25 calories):

- ½ cup sliced melon, 1 fruit (25 calories)

Lunch (345 calories):

- 3 ounces sliced roasted turkey breast, 1 meat (115 calories)
- One 4-inch whole-wheat pita pocket, 1 grain (75 calories)
- 4 slices tomato, 1 vegetable (20 calories)
- 4 leaves romaine lettuce, 1 vegetable (20 calories)
- 1 teaspoon deli mustard (5 calories)
- One 1-ounce snack bag pretzels, 1 grain (110 calories)

Afternoon Snack (110 calories):

- 1 medium apple, 1 fruit (60 calories)

- 1½ teaspoons peanut butter, ¼ nuts/seeds/legumes (50 calories)

Dinner (395 calories):

- 1 Chicken Caesar Wrap (see recipe), 2 vegetable, ½ meat, 2 grain, ½ dairy, 1 added fat (395 calories)

Evening Snack/Dessert (60 calories):

- 1 snack-size peppermint patty, ½ sweets (60 calories)

Nutrition analysis for the day:

1,160 calories, 5 grain, 3 fruit, 4 vegetable, 1½ dairy, 1½ meat, ¼ nuts/seeds/legumes, 1 added fat, ½ sweets

1,200 CALORIES: DAY 5
Target:

5 grain, 3 fruit, 4 vegetable, 2 dairy, 1½ meat, ¼ nuts/seeds/legumes, ½ added fat, ½ sweets

Breakfast (250 calories):

- 1 Low-Fat Blueberry Muffin (see recipe), 2 grain (200 calories)
- 1 medium apple, 1 fruit (50 calories)

Morning Snack (75 calories):

- ½ cup sliced nectarine, 1 fruit (35 calories)
- ¾ ounce (1 small slice) low-fat cheddar cheese, ½ dairy (40 calories)

Lunch (310 calories):

- 1 Cobb Salad (see recipe), 4 vegetable, ½ dairy, ½ meat, 1 added fat (225 calories) Half a 7-inch whole-wheat pita pocket, 1 grain (85 calories)

Afternoon Snack (105 calories):

- 4 celery sticks (5 inches each), 1 vegetable (5 calories) 1 tablespoon peanut butter, ½ nuts/seeds/legumes (100 calories)

Dinner (345 calories):

- Shrimp Scampi, 3 ounces shrimp with sauce (see recipe), 1 meat (145 calories)
- 1 cup cooked whole-wheat linguine, 2 grain (200 calories)

Evening Snack/Dessert (165 calories):

- ½ cup low-fat frozen yogurt, 1 dairy (140 calories)
- ½ cup fresh strawberries, 1 fruit (25 calories)

Nutrition analysis for the day:

1,250 calories, 5 grain, 3 fruit, 5 vegetable, 2 dairy, 1½ meat, ½ nuts/seeds/legumes, 1 added fat, 0 sweets

1,200 CALORIES: DAY 6
Target:

5 grain, 3 fruit, 4 vegetable, 2 dairy, 1½ meat, ¼ nuts/seeds/legumes, ½ added fat, ½ sweets

Breakfast (170 calories):

- 1 medium low-fat granola bar, 2 grain (140 calories)
- 1 medium peach, 1 fruit (30 calories)

Morning Snack (130 calories):

- 1 cup nonfat plain Greek-style yogurt, 1 dairy (130 calories)

Lunch (340 calories):

- Hummus sandwich with fresh tomatoes
- Half a 7-inch whole-wheat pita pocket, 1 grain (85 calories)
- ¾ ounce (1 thin slice) low-fat swiss cheese, ½ dairy (40 calories)
- 2 tablespoons hummus, ¼ nuts/seeds/legumes (70 calories)
- 3 thick slices tomato, 1 vegetable (15 calories)
- ½ cup bean sprouts, ½ vegetable (15 calories)
- 2 cups Simple Spinach Salad (see recipe), 2 vegetable, ¼ dairy, 1 added fat (115 calories)

Afternoon Snack (110 calories):

- 1-ounce unsalted mini pretzels (about ½ cup), 1 grain (110 calories)

Dinner (370 calories):

- 4 ounces Poached Salmon (see recipe), 11/3 meat (195 calories)
- ½ cup Roasted Brussels Sprouts (see recipe), 1 vegetable (50 calories)
- 2/3 cup Quinoa, Corn, and Black Bean Salad (see recipe), 1 grain, ¼ vegetable, ¼ nuts/seeds/legumes (125 calories)

Evening Snack/Dessert (75 calories):

- 1 cup fresh strawberries, 2 fruit (50 calories)
- 1½ teaspoons sugar, ½ sweets (25 calories)

Nutrition analysis for the day:

1,195 calories, 5 grain, 3 fruit, 4¾ vegetable, 1¾ dairy, 11/3 meat, ½ nuts/seeds/legumes, 1 added fat, ½ sweets

1,200 CALORIES: DAY 7
Target:

5 grain, 3 fruit, 4 vegetable, 2 dairy, 1½ meat, ¼ nuts/seeds/legumes, ½ added fat, ½ sweets

Breakfast (280 calories):

- 1½ ounces shredded wheat squares, 1½ grain (150 calories)
- 1 cup nonfat milk, 1 dairy (90 calories)
- ½ cup blueberries, 1 fruit (40 calories)

Morning Snack (160 calories):

- 1-ounce unsalted pretzels, 1 grain (110 calories)

- ½ cup grapes, 1 fruit (50 calories)

Lunch (240 calories):

- Toasted cheese sandwich:
- Half a 7-inch whole-wheat pita pocket, 1 grain (85 calories)
- 1½ ounces low-fat cheddar cheese (2 slices), 1 dairy (75 calories)
- 1 cup baby carrots, 2 vegetable (50 calories)
- 2 tablespoons fat-free ranch dressing (30 calories)

Afternoon Snack (80 calories):

- 2 dark-chocolate-covered strawberries, 1 fruit, ½ sweets (80 calories)

Dinner (310 calories):

- 4 ounces baked cod, * 11/3 meat (120 calories)
- Place fish on a baking sheet sprayed with cooking spray. Bake at 425°F for 15 minutes or until fish flakes with a fork.
- ½ cup (5–6 small spears) Roasted Asparagus (see recipe), 1 vegetable (40 calories)
- ½ small (2-ounce) whole-wheat dinner roll, 1 grain (75 calories)
- 1 cup mixed raw leafy greens, 1 vegetable (15 calories)
- 1 tablespoon Lemon Caper Vinaigrette (see recipe), 1 added fat (60 calories)

Evening Snack/Dessert (100 calories):

- 1 small low-fat granola bar, 1 grain (100 calories)

Nutrition analysis for the day:

1,170 calories, 5½ grain, 3 fruit, 4 vegetable, 2 dairy, 11/3 meat, 0 nuts/seeds/legumes, 1 added fat, ½ sweets

1,400 CALORIES: DAY 8
Target:

5 grain, 4 fruit, 4 vegetable, 2 dairy, 1½ meat, ¼ nuts/seeds/legumes, ½ added fat, ½ sweets

Breakfast (205 calories):

- 1-ounce bran flakes (about ¾ cup), 1 grain (90 calories)
- ½ cup sliced banana, 1 fruit (70 calories)
- ½ cup nonfat milk, ½ dairy (45 calories)

Morning Snack (150 calories):

- 1 small low-fat granola bar, 1 grain (100 calories)
- 1 medium apple, 1 fruit (50 calories)

Lunch (465 calories):

- 2½ cups mixed raw leafy greens and vegetables (bell peppers, carrots, etc.), 2½ vegetable (50 calories)
- 4 ounces grilled skinless chicken breast, 11/3 meat (160 calories)
- 1 hard-boiled egg, 1/3 meat (80 calories)

- 1 tablespoon unsalted roasted sunflower seeds, ½ nuts/seeds/legumes (50 calories)
- 1 tablespoon low-fat creamy Italian dressing, ½ added fat (40 calories)
- Half a 7-inch whole-wheat pita pocket, 1 grain (85 calories)

Afternoon Snack (220 calories):

- 1 cup nonfat vanilla yogurt, 1 dairy (160 calories)
- 1 medium orange, 1 fruit (60 calories)

Dinner (305 calories):

- Piled-High Veggie Pizza (1/6 of a 14-inch pizza) (see recipe), 2 grain, 2 vegetable, ½ dairy (250
- calories)
- ½ cup sliced mango, 1 fruit (55 calories)

Evening Snack/Dessert (40 calories):

- 2 dark chocolate kisses, ½ sweets (40 calories)

Nutrition analysis for the day:

1,385 calories, 5 grain, 4 fruit, 4½ vegetable, 2 dairy, 12/3 meat, ½ nuts/seeds/legumes, ½ added fat, ½ sweets

1,400 CALORIES: DAY 9
Target:

5 grain, 4 fruit, 4 vegetable, 2 dairy, 1½ meat, ¼ nuts/seeds/legumes, ½ added fat, ½ sweets

Breakfast (250 calories):

- 1-ounce uncooked oatmeal cooked with water (cooks to about ¾ cup), 1 grain (100 calories)
- 1 medium orange, 1 fruit (60 calories)
- 1 cup nonfat milk, 1 dairy (90 calories)

Morning Snack (230 calories):

- 1-ounce whole-wheat snack crackers, 1 grain (130 calories)
- 1 tablespoon peanut butter, ½ nuts/seeds/legumes (100 calories)

Lunch (335 calories):

1 Veggie Melt Panini (see recipe), 2 grain, 2 vegetable, 1 dairy (335 calories)

Afternoon Snack (115 calories):

- ½ cup nonfat vanilla yogurt, ½ dairy (80 calories)
- ½ cup fresh berries, 1 fruit (35 calories)

Dinner (365 calories):

- 4½ ounces grilled skinless chicken breast, 1½ meat (165 calories)
- 1 cup Roasted Cauliflower (see recipe), 2 vegetable (100 calories)
- ½ cup cooked brown rice, 1 grain (100 calories)

Evening Snack/Dessert (120 calories):

- 1 Baked Banana (see recipe), 2 fruit, 1 sweet (120 calories)

Nutrition analysis for the day:

1,415 calories, 5 grain, 4 fruit, 4 vegetable, 2½ dairy, 1½ meat, ½ nuts/seeds/legumes, 0 added fat, 1 sweet

1,400 CALORIES: DAY 10
Target:

5 grain, 4 fruit, 4 vegetable, 2 dairy, 1½ meat, ¼ nuts/seeds/legumes, ½ added fat, ½ sweets

Breakfast (180 calories):

- 6 egg whites or ¾ cup egg substitute, scrambled (cooked with cooking spray), 1 meat (100 calories)
- One 1-ounce slice whole-wheat bread, toasted, 1 grain (80 calories)

Morning Snack (130 calories):

- 1 medium peach, 1 fruit (30 calories)
- 1 small low-fat granola bar, 1 grain (100 calories)

Lunch (350 calories):

- 3 cups mixed raw leafy greens and vegetables, 3 vegetables (60 calories)
- 1½ ounces reduced-fat cheddar cheese (about 1/3 cup shredded), 1 dairy (120 calories)
- 1½ ounces skinless grilled chicken breast, ½ meat (55 calories)
- 1 tablespoon reduced-fat ranch dressing, ½ added fat (40 calories)
- One 4-inch pita pocket, 1 grain (75 calories)

Afternoon Snack (270 calories):

- 1-ounce unsalted mini pretzels (about ½ cup), 1 grain (110 calories)
- ½ cup low-fat cottage cheese, 1 dairy (80 calories)
- 1 cup pineapple chunks, 2 fruit (80 calories)
- **Dinner (430 calories):**
- 1 cup Fruity Chicken Stir-Fry (see recipe), 1 fruit, 1 vegetable, ½ meat (330 calories)
- ½ cup cooked brown rice, 1 grain (100 calories)

Evening Snack/Dessert (60 calories):

- 5 Tootsie Rolls, ½ sweets (60 calories)

Nutrition analysis for the day:

1,420 calories, 5 grain, 4 fruit, 4 vegetable, 2 dairy, 2 meat, 0 nuts/seeds/legumes, ½ added fat, ½ sweets

1,400 CALORIES: DAY 11
Target:

5 grain, 4 fruit, 4 vegetable, 2 dairy, 1½ meat, ¼ nuts/seeds/legumes, ½ added fat, ½ sweets

Breakfast (260 calories):

- 1-ounce toasted oat cereal, 1 grain (100 calories)
- ½ cup sliced banana, 1 fruit (70 calories)
- 1 cup nonfat milk, 1 dairy (90 calories)

Morning Snack (105 calories):

- 1 cup unsweetened applesauce, 2 fruit (105 calories)

Lunch (345 calories):

- 3 ounces sliced roasted turkey breast, 1 meat (115 calories)
- One 4-inch whole-wheat pita pocket, 1 grain (75 calories)
- 4 slices tomato, 1 vegetable (20 calories)
- 4 leaves romaine lettuce, 1 vegetable (20 calories)
- 1 teaspoon deli mustard (5 calories)
- One 1-ounce snack bag unsalted pretzels, 1 grain (110 calories)

Afternoon Snack (110 calories):

- 1 medium apple, 1 fruit (60 calories)
- 1½ teaspoons peanut butter, ¼ nuts/seeds/legumes (50 calories)

Dinner (395 calories):

- 1 Chicken Caesar Wrap (see recipe), 2 vegetable, ½ meat, 2 grain, ½ dairy, 1 added fat (395 calories)

Evening Snack/Dessert (130 calories):

- ¼ cup low-fat frozen yogurt, ½ dairy (70 calories)
- 1 snack-size peppermint patty, ½ sweets (60 calories)

Nutrition analysis for the day:

1,345 calories, 5 grain, 4 fruit, 4 vegetable, 2 dairy, 1½ meat, ¼ nuts/seeds/legumes, 1 added fat, ½ sweets

1400 CALORIES: DAY 12
Target:

5 grain, 4 fruit, 4 vegetable, 2 dairy, 1½ meat, ¼ nuts/seeds/legumes, ½ added fat, ½ sweets

Breakfast (290 calories):

- 1 Low-Fat Blueberry Muffins (see recipe), 2 grain (200 calories)
- 1 cup nonfat milk, 1 dairy (90 calories)

Morning Snack (110 calories):

- 1 cup sliced mango, 2 fruit (110 calories)

Lunch (365 calories):

- 1 Cobb Salad (see recipe), 4 vegetable, ½ dairy, ½ meat, 1 added fat (225 calories)

- ½ cup low-fat vanilla yogurt, ½ dairy (80 calories)
- 1 medium orange, 1 fruit (60 calories)

Afternoon Snack (180 calories):

- One 1-ounce slice whole-wheat bread, toasted, 1 grain (80 calories)
- 1 tablespoon peanut butter, ½ nuts/seeds/legumes (100 calories)

Dinner (345 calories):

- Shrimp Scampi (see recipe), 3 ounces shrimp with sauce (see recipe), 1 meat (145 calories)
- 1 cup whole-wheat linguine, 2 grain (200 calories)

Evening Snack/Dessert (105 calories):

- 1 medium apple, 1 fruit (50 calories)
- 2 tablespoons low-fat caramel sauce, ½ sweets (55 calories)

Nutrition analysis for the day:

1,395 calories, 5 grain, 4 fruit, 4 vegetable, 2 dairy, 1½ meat, ½ nuts/seeds/legumes, 1 added fat, ½ sweets

1,400 CALORIES: DAY 13
Target:

5 grain, 4 fruit, 4 vegetable, 2 dairy, 1½ meat, ¼ nuts/seeds/legumes, ½ added fat, ½ sweets

Breakfast (255 calories):

- 1 small low-fat granola bar, 1 grain (100 calories)
- 1 cup sliced peaches, 2 fruit (65 calories)
- 1 cup nonfat milk, 1 dairy (90 calories)

Morning Snack (110 calories):

- 3 cups air-popped popcorn, 1 grain (110 calories)
- Sparkling water with a squeeze of orange (0 calories)

Lunch (290 calories):

- Hummus sandwich with fresh tomatoes:
- Half a 7-inch whole-wheat pita pocket, 1 grain (85 calories)
- 2 tablespoons hummus, ¼ nuts/seeds/legumes (50 calories)
- 3 thick slices tomato, 1 vegetable (15 calories)
- ½ cup bean sprouts, ½ vegetable (15 calories)
- ½ cup mixed raw leafy greens, ½ vegetable (10 calories)
- 2 cups Simple Spinach Salad (see recipe), 2 vegetable, ¼ dairy, 1 added fat (115 calories)

Afternoon Snack (270 calories):

- 1-ounce unsalted mini pretzels (about ½ cup), 1 grain (110 calories)
- 1 cup nonfat vanilla yogurt, 1 dairy (160 calories)

Dinner (340 calories):

- 4½ ounces Poached Salmon (see recipe), 1½ meat (215 calories)
- 2/3 cup Quinoa, Corn, and Black Bean Salad (see recipe), 1 grain, ¼ vegetable, ¼ nuts/seeds/legumes (125 calories)

Evening Snack/Dessert (75 calories):

- 1 cup fresh strawberries, 2 fruit (50 calories)
- 1½ teaspoon sugar, ½ sweets (25 calories)

Nutrition analysis for the day:

1,340 calories, 5 grain, 4 fruit, 4¼ vegetable, 2¼ dairy, 1½ meat, ½ nuts/seeds, 1 added fat, ½ sweets

1,400 CALORIES: DAY 14
Target:

5 grain, 4 fruit, 4 vegetable, 2 dairy, 1½ meat, ¼ nuts/seeds/legumes, ½ added fat, ½ sweets

Breakfast (320 calories):

- 1½ ounces shredded wheat squares, 1½ grain (150 calories)
- 1 tablespoon flaxseeds, ½ nuts/seeds/legumes (40 calories)
- 1 cup nonfat milk, 1 dairy (90 calories)
- ½ cup blueberries, 1 fruit (40 calories)

Morning Snack (210 calories):

- 1-ounce unsalted pretzels, 1 grain (110 calories)
- ¼ cup dried cherries, 1 fruit (100 calories)

Lunch (240 calories):

- Toasted cheese sandwich:
- Half a 7-inch whole-wheat pita pocket, 1 grain (85 calories)
- 1½ ounces low-fat cheddar cheese (about 2 slices), 1 dairy (75 calories)
- 1 cup sliced carrots, 2 vegetable (50 calories)
- 2 tablespoons fat-free ranch dressing (30 calories)

Afternoon Snack (50 calories):

- ½ cup grapes, 1 fruit (50 calories)

Dinner (455 calories):

- 5 ounces baked cod, * 12/3 meat (150 calories)
- 1 cup (10–12 small spears) Roasted Asparagus (see recipe), 2 vegetable (80 calories)
- 1 small (2-ounce) whole-wheat dinner roll, 2 grain (150 calories)
- 1 cup mixed raw leafy greens, 1 vegetable (15 calories)
- 1 tablespoon Lemon Caper Vinaigrette (see recipe), 1 added fat (60 calories)
- Place fish on a baking sheet sprayed with cooking spray. Bake at 425°F for 15 minutes or until fish flakes with a fork.

Evening Snack/Dessert (80 calories):

- 2 dark-chocolate-covered strawberries, 1 fruit, ½ sweets (80 calories)

Nutrition analysis for the day:

1,355 calories, 5½ grain, 4 fruit, 5 vegetable, 2 dairy, 12/3 meat, ½ nuts/seeds, 1 added fat, ½ sweets

1600 CALORIES: DAY 15
Target:

6 grain, 4 fruit, 4 vegetable, 2 dairy, 1½ meat, ¼ nuts/seeds/legumes, 1 added fat, ½ sweets

Breakfast (350 calories):

- 1 cup low-fat fruited yogurt, 1 dairy (200 calories)
- 1-ounce low-fat granola (about ¼ cup), 1 grain (110 calories)
- ½ cup blueberries, 1 fruit (40 calories)

Morning Snack (150 calories):

- 1 small low-fat granola bar, 1 grain (100 calories)
- 1 medium apple, 1 fruit (50 calories)

Lunch (525 calories):

- 2½ cups mixed raw leafy greens and vegetables (bell peppers, carrots, etc.), 2½ vegetable
- (50 calories)
- 4 ounces grilled skinless chicken breast, 11/3 meat (200 calories)
- 1 hard-boiled egg, 1/3 meat (80 calories)
- 1 tablespoon unsalted, roasted sunflower seeds, ½ nuts/seeds/legumes (50 calories)
- 2 tablespoons low-fat balsamic vinaigrette, 1 added fat (60 calories)
- Half a 7-inch whole-wheat pita pocket, 1 grain (85 calories)

Afternoon Snack (185 calories):

- ½ cup low-fat cottage cheese, 1 dairy (80 calories)
- 1 medium (7-inch) banana, 2 fruit (105 calories)

Dinner (250 calories):

- Piled-High Veggie Pizza (1/6 of a 14-inch pizza) (see recipe), 2 grain, 2 vegetable, ½ dairy (250 calories)

Evening Snack/Dessert (170 calories):

- 2 dark chocolate kisses, ½ sweets (50 calories)
- 2 graham cracker rectangles, 1 grain (120 calories)
- Nutrition analysis for the day: 1,630 calories, 6 grain, 4 fruit, 4½ vegetable, 2½ dairy, 12/3
- meat, ½ nuts/seeds/legumes, 1 added fat, ½ sweets

1,600 CALORIES: DAY 16
Target:

6 grain, 4 fruit, 4 vegetable, 2 dairy, 1½ meat, ¼ nuts/seeds/legumes, 1 added fat, ½ sweets

Breakfast (315 calories):

- 1-ounce uncooked oatmeal cooked with water (cooks to about ¾ cup), 1 grain (100 calories)
- ¼ cup raisins, 1 fruit (110 calories)
- 1 cup low-fat milk, 1 dairy (110 calories)

Morning Snack (200 calories):

- 1-ounce unsalted whole-wheat mini pretzels (about ½ cup), 1 grain (100 calories)
- 1 tablespoon peanut butter, ½ nuts/seeds/legumes (100 calories)

Lunch (335 calories):

- 1 Veggie Melt Panini (see recipe), 2 grain, 2 vegetable, 1 dairy (335 calories)
- Afternoon Snack (25 calories)
- ½ cup cubed melon, 1 fruit (25 calories)

Dinner (555 calories):

- 4½ ounces grilled chicken, 1½ meat (165 calories)
- 1 small (3-inch) baked potato, 1 vegetable (150 calories)
- ½ cup grilled zucchini, 1 vegetable (15 calories)
- 1 teaspoon trans-fat-free margarine, 1 added fat (25 calories)
- 1 cup cooked brown rice, 2 grain (200 calories)

Evening Snack/Dessert (120 calories):

- 1 Baked Banana (see recipe), 2 fruit, 1 sweet (120 calories)

Nutrition analysis for the day:

1,550 calories, 6 grain, 4 fruit, 4 vegetable, 2 dairy, 1½ meat, ½ nuts/seeds/legumes, 1 added fat, 1 sweet

1,600 CALORIES: DAY 17
Target:

6 grain, 4 fruit, 4 vegetable, 2 dairy, 1½ meat, ¼ nuts/seeds/legumes, 1 added fat, ½ sweets

Breakfast (280 calories):

- 6 egg whites or ¾ cup egg substitute, scrambled (cooked with cooking spray), 1 meat (100 calories)
- 1½ ounces shredded low-fat cheddar cheese (about 1/3 cup), 1 dairy (75 calories)
- One 1-ounce slice whole-wheat bread, toasted, 1 grain (80 calories)
- ½ cup fresh strawberries, 1 fruit (25 calories)

Morning Snack (130 calories):

- 1 medium peach, 1 fruit (30 calories)
- 1 small low-fat granola bar, 1 grain (100 calories)

Lunch (330 calories):

- 3 cups mixed raw leafy greens and vegetables, 3 vegetables (60 calories)

- ¾ ounce shredded low-fat cheddar cheese (about 3 tablespoons), ½ dairy (40 calories)
- 1½ ounces skinless grilled chicken breast, ½ meat (75 calories)
- 2 tablespoons reduced-fat ranch dressing, 1 added fat (80 calories)
- One 4-inch whole-wheat pita pocket, 1 grain (75 calories)

Afternoon Snack (240 calories):

- 1 medium apple, 1 fruit (50 calories)
- 1-ounce unsalted mini pretzels (about ½ cup), 1 grain (110 calories)
- ½ cup nonfat vanilla yogurt, 1 dairy (80 calories)

Dinner (530 calories):

- 1 cup Fruity Chicken Stir-Fry (see recipe), 1 fruit, 1 vegetable, ½ meat (330 calories)
- 1 cup cooked brown rice, 2 grain (200 calories)
- Evening Snack/Dessert (75 calories)
- Half a ¾-inch slice Gingerbread (see recipe), ½ sweets (75 calories)

Nutrition analysis for the day:

1,585 calories, 6 grain, 4 fruit, 4 vegetable, 2½ dairy, 2 meat, 0 nuts/seed/legumes, 1 added fat, ½ sweets

1,600 CALORIES: DAY 18
Target:

6 grain, 4 fruit, 4 vegetable, 2 dairy, 1½ meat, ¼ nuts/seeds/legumes, 1 added fat, ½ sweets

Breakfast (280 calories):

- 1-ounce toasted oat cereal, 1 grain (100 calories)
- ½ cup sliced banana, 1 fruit (70 calories)
- 1 cup low-fat milk, 1 dairy (110 calories)

Morning Snack (105 calories):

- 1 cup red grapes, 2 fruit (105 calories)

Lunch (465 calories):

- 3 ounces sliced roasted beef tenderloin, 1 meat (150 calories)
- Two 1-ounce slices whole-wheat bread, 2 grain (160 calories)
- 1 cup shredded lettuce, 1 vegetable (20 calories)
- 4 slices tomato, 1 vegetable (20 calories)
- 1 teaspoon deli mustard (5 calories)
- One 1-ounce snack bag pretzels, 1 grain (110 calories)

Afternoon Snack (250 calories):

- 1-ounce whole-wheat snack crackers, 1 grain (130 calories)
- ¾ ounce (1 small slice) low-fat cheddar cheese, ½ dairy (40 calories)
- ¼ cup dried apricots, 1 fruit (80 calories)
- Cranberry sparkling water with a squeeze of lime (0 calories)

Dinner (395 calories):

- 1 Chicken Caesar Wrap (see recipe), 2 vegetable, ½ meat, 2 grain, ½ dairy, 1 added fat (395 calories)

Evening Snack/Dessert (60 calories):

- 1 snack-size peppermint patty, ½ sweets (60 calories)

Nutrition analysis for the day:

1,555 calories, 7 grain, 4 fruit, 4 vegetables, 2 dairy, 1½ meat, 0 nuts/seeds/legumes, 1 added fat, ½ sweets

1600 CALORIES: DAY 19
Target:

6 grain, 4 fruit, 4 vegetable, 2 dairy, 1½ meat, ¼ nuts/seeds/legumes, 1 added fat, ½ sweets

Breakfast (340 calories):

- 1 Low-Fat Blueberry Muffin (see recipe), 2 grain (200 calories)
- ½ cup raspberries, 1 fruit (30 calories)
- 1 cup low-fat milk, 1 dairy (110 calories)
- Morning Snack (160 calories)
- 1 cup sliced mango, 2 fruit (110 calories)
- ¾ ounce (1 small slice) low-fat cheddar cheese, ½ dairy (50 calories)

Lunch (325 calories):

- 1 Cobb Salad (see recipe), 4 vegetable, ½ dairy, ½ meat, 1 added fat (225 calories)
- 1 small chocolate chip granola bar, 1 grain (100 calories)

Afternoon Snack (160 calories):

- 4 celery sticks (5 inches each), 1 vegetable (5 calories)
- 1 tablespoon peanut butter, ½ nuts/seeds/legumes (100 calories)
- 2 tablespoons raisins, ½ fruit (55 calories)

Dinner (445 calories):

- Shrimp Scampi, 3 ounces shrimp with sauce (see recipe), 1 meat (145 calories)
- 1½ cups whole-wheat linguine, 3 grain (300 calories)

Evening Snack/Dessert (105 calories):

- 1 medium apple, 1 fruit (50 calories)
- 2 tablespoons low-fat caramel sauce, ½ sweets (55 calories)

Nutrition analysis for the day:

1,535 calories, 6 grain, 4½ fruit, 5 vegetable, 2 dairy, 1½ meat, ½ nuts/seeds/legumes, 1 added fat, ½ sweets

1,600 CALORIES: DAY 20
Target:

6 grain, 4 fruit, 4 vegetable, 2 dairy, 1½ meat, ¼ nuts/seeds/legumes, 1 added fat, ½ sweets

Breakfast (190 calories):

- 1 small low-fat granola bar, 1 grain (100 calories)
- ¾ cup 100% apple juice, 1 fruit (90 calories)

Morning Snack (110 calories):

- 3 cups air-popped popcorn, 1 grain (110 calories)
- Sparkling water with a squeeze of orange (0 calories)

Lunch (440 calories):

- Hummus sandwich with fresh tomatoes:
- One 7-inch whole-wheat pita pocket, 2 grain (170 calories)
- 2 tablespoons hummus, ¼ nuts/seeds/legumes (70 calories)
- 1-ounce slice low-fat swiss cheese, 2/3 dairy (55 calories)
- 3 thick slices tomato, 1 vegetable (15 calories)
- Bean sprouts, ½ cup, ½ vegetable (15 calories)
- 2 cups Simple Spinach Salad (see recipe), 2 vegetable, ¼ dairy, 1 added fat (115 calories)

Afternoon Snack (370 calories):

- 1-ounce unsalted mini pretzels (about ½ cup), 1 grain (110 calories)
- 1 cup nonfat vanilla yogurt, 1 dairy (160 calories)
- ¼ cup dried cherries, 1 fruit (100 calories)

Dinner (390 calories):

- 4½ ounces Poached Salmon (see recipe), 1½ meat (215 calories)
- ½ cup Roasted Brussels Sprouts (see recipe), 1 vegetable (50 calories)
- 2/3 cup Quinoa, Corn, and Black Bean Salad (see recipe), 1 grain, ¼ vegetable, ¼ nuts/seeds/legumes (125 calories)

Evening Snack/Dessert (90 calories):

- 1 cup fresh strawberries, 2 fruit (50 calories)
- 2 teaspoons chocolate syrup, ½ sweets (40 calories)

Nutrition analysis for the day:

1,590 calories, 6 grain, 4 fruit, 4¾ vegetable, 1¾ dairy, 1½ meat, ½ nuts/seeds/legumes, 1 added fat, ½ sweets

1,600 CALORIES: DAY 21
Target:

6 grain, 4 fruit, 4 vegetable, 2 dairy, 1½ meat, ¼ nuts/seeds/legumes, 1 added fat, ½ sweets

Breakfast (370 calories):

- 1½ ounces shredded wheat squares, 1½ grain (150 calories)
- 1 tablespoon flaxseeds, ½ nuts/seeds/legumes (40 calories)
- 1 cup low-fat milk, 1 dairy (110 calories)

- ½ cup sliced banana, 1 fruit (70 calories)

Morning Snack (210 calories):

- 1-ounce unsalted pretzels, 1 grain (110 calories)
- 1 cup grapes, 2 fruit (100 calories)

Lunch (375 calories):

- Toasted cheese sandwich:
- One 7-inch whole-wheat pita pocket, 2 grain (220 calories)
- 1½ ounces low-fat cheddar cheese (about 2 slices), 1 dairy (75 calories)
- 1 cup sliced carrots, 2 vegetable (50 calories)
- 2 tablespoons fat-free ranch dressing (30 calories)

Afternoon Snack (160 calories):

- 1 medium orange, 1 fruit (60 calories)
- 1-ounce unsalted whole-wheat mini pretzels (about ½ cup), 1 grain (100 calories)

Dinner (305 calories):

- 5 ounces baked cod, * 12/3 meat (150 calories)
- 1 cup (10–12 small spears) Roasted Asparagus (see recipe), 2 vegetable (80 calories)
- 1 cup mixed raw leafy greens, 1 vegetable (15 calories)
- 1 tablespoon Lemon Caper Vinaigrette (see recipe), 1 added fat (60 calories)
- Place fish on a baking sheet sprayed with cooking spray. Bake at 425°F for 15 minutes or until fish flakes with a fork.

Evening Snack/Dessert (190 calories):

- 2 graham cracker rectangles, 1 grain (120 calories)
- 10 mini marshmallows and 2 dark chocolate kisses, ½ sweets (70 calories)

Nutrition analysis for the day:

1,610 calories, 6½ grain, 4 fruit, 5 vegetable, 2 dairy, 12/3 meat, ½ nuts/seeds/legumes, 1 added fat, ½ sweets